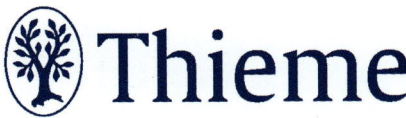

The Clinical Guide for Plastic and Reconstructive Surgery

A Practical Handbook

Veena K. Singh, MCh, DNB (Plastic Surgery)

Additional Professor & HOD
Department of Burns & Plastic Surgery;
Deputy Medical Superintendent, Superspecialty Hospital;
Nodal Officer, Rashtriya Bal Swasthya Karyakram (RBSK);
All India Institute of Medical Sciences, Phulwari Sharif
Patna, Bihar, India

Thieme
Delhi • Stuttgart • New York • Rio de Janeiro

Publishing Director: Ritu Sharma
Senior Development Editor: Dr Nidhi Srivastava
Director-Editorial Services: Rachna Sinha
Project Manager: Sumbul Jafri
National Sales Manager: Bishwajit Kumar Mishra
Managing Director & CEO: Ajit Kohli

Thieme Medical and Scientific Publishers
Private Limited.
A - 12, Second Floor, Sector - 2, Noida - 201 301,
Uttar Pradesh, India, +911204556600
Email: customerservice@thieme.in
www.thieme.in

Cover design: © Thieme
Cover image source: © Thieme

Page make-up by RECTO Graphics, India

Printed in India

5 4 3 2 1

DOI: 10.1055/b000000997

ISBN: 978-81-966914-9-3
Also available as an ebook:
eISBN (PDF): 978-81-966914-0-0
eISBN (epub): 978-81-966914-3-1

Important note: Medicine is an ever-changing science undergoing continual development. Research and clinical experience are continually expanding our knowledge, in particular, our knowledge of proper treatment and drug therapy. Insofar as this book mentions any dosage or application, readers may rest assured that the authors, editors, and publishers have made every effort to ensure that such references are in accordance with **the state of knowledge at the time of production of the book**.

Nevertheless, this does not involve, imply, or express any guarantee or responsibility on the part of the publishers in respect to any dosage instructions and forms of applications stated in the book. **Every user is requested to examine carefully** the manufacturers' leaflets accompanying each drug and to check, if necessary, in consultation with a physician or specialist, whether the dosage schedules mentioned therein or the contraindications stated by the manufacturers differ from the statements made in the present book. Such examination is particularly important with drugs that are either rarely used or have been newly released in the market. Every dosage schedule or every form of application used is entirely at the user's own risk and responsibility. The authors and publishers request every user to report to the publishers any discrepancies or inaccuracies noticed. If errors in this work are found after publication, errata will be posted at www.thieme.com on the product description page.

Some of the product names, patents, and registered designs referred to in this book are in fact registered trademarks or proprietary names even though specific reference to this fact is not always made in the text. Therefore, the appearance of a name without designation as proprietary is not to be construed as a representation by the publisher that it is in the public domain.

Thieme addresses people of all gender identities equally. We encourage our authors to use gender-neutral or gender-equal expressions wherever the context allows.

Contents

Contents

Foreword

I have seen the dominance of Western literature during the early part of my plastic surgery career but between the previous decade and now, there has been a sea change in the scenario. Currently, there are very effective textbooks, many reference books, and plastic surgery journals published in India. Designing, writing, and publication of this book *The Clinical Guide for Plastic and Reconstructive Surgery: A Practical Handbook* is a step forward in this direction.

Till now our young generation has been using books on clinical methods written for general surgery. The plastic surgery trainees and the teachers alike are looking for reading materials written by Indian authors. Dr. Veena Singh has aptly identified this vacuum in this area and has edited and written the book. The authors have presented 5 long cases and 18 short cases, which are the most commonly discussed clinical cases. Each chapter has been designed as if one is presenting the case in the examination, with relevant history, examination, diagnosis, and management. The icing on the cake is the question and answers at the end of each chapter. This book proves the point that we in India have a unique method of teaching, training, and evaluation.

I have no doubt that this book will become an essential part of teaching and learning in plastic surgery. This will be received by the plastic surgery fraternity with the enthusiasm that it rightly deserves.

Dr. Karoon Agrawal
Senior Consultant, Plastic Surgery
National Heart Institute, New Delhi
Former Director Professor and Head
VMMC & SJH, New Delhi and JIPMER, Puducherry
Editor-in-Chief, *Textbook of Plastic, Reconstructive, and Aesthetic Surgery*

The Clinical Guide for Plastic and Reconstructive Surgery: A Practical Handbook fills a gap in the plastic surgery literature and provides an invaluable resource for those studying and preparing for plastic surgery examinations. Dr. Veena Singh, aided by her residency batchmates, Dr. Rimpi Jain and Dr. Saurabh Gupta, has produced a unique book that will be eagerly sought after by students and established plastic surgeons alike. As she says in the preface, this is a clinical guide, not a textbook, but it is laid out in such a way as to allow the reader to structure his or her approach to a given problem. The book highlights both long and short cases and guides the reader on how to approach each challenge, what to seek in the history, how to conduct the physical examination, and what investigations might be relevant. As I said, there is no such book in our literature that I am aware of, and Dr. Singh is to be heartily congratulated for conceiving this concept.

Peter C. Neligan, MB, FRCS(I), FRCSC, FACS
Professor Emeritus
University of Washington
Seattle, Washington, USA

I congratulate Dr. Veena Singh for understanding the mental anguish of residents when they encounter a six- or seven-volume textbook, which can in no way be revised just before an examination. A clinical guide like this, which can serve both as a quick reference before a case presentation or a revision material to reorganize one's thoughts before a written test or a viva voce, will be of immense benefit to the residents. Residents often know a lot, but during an examination, in their anxiety, they fail to channel their thoughts and communicate effectively. This clinical guide will help them to do so. I am eagerly looking forward to the second volume of this book.

Dr. Surajit Bhattacharya
Past President, APSI
Past Editor, *IJPS*

This book contains chapters covering the entire spectrum of clinical cases that are commonly presented during the MCh/DNB Plastic and Reconstructive Surgery Examination. Each and every case is meticulously planned with very good clinical photographs, illustrations, and explanations about the clinical features and etiologies behind the presenting symptoms. The management of the cases is explained elaborately based on sound scientific principles. This book will be the best guide, not only for postgraduates but also for practicing plastic surgeons.

Dr. Nitin Mokal
President, APSI (2023)

This book covers almost all the long as well as short cases which are routinely allotted in the exams. The authors have taken great pains to guide the students regarding case preparation, presentation and complete range of questions, examiners can ask related to a particular case. Dr. Veena has great passion for teaching and has been instrumental in starting APSI- Post Graduate Medical Education Program during my tenure as President APSI in 2022. This initiative of hers is very popular amongst the residents and gives them exposure to potential examiners from all over the country.

Dr. Ravi K. Mahajan
Past President APSI

Preface

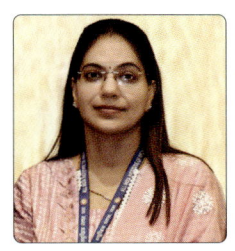

It gives me immense pleasure to present a concise but comprehensive clinical handbook for plastic surgery residents undergoing speciality training or appearing for exit examinations as well as for practicing plastic surgeons passionate in teaching profession.

In the plastic surgery curriculum, practical examination consists of long cases, short cases, radiology, operative viva, surgical instruments, and pathological specimens. However, a book on the clinical presentation of plastic surgery cases for students of MCh/DNB Plastic Surgery as well as consultant is currently not available. The concept behind this book *The Clinical Guide for Plastic and Reconstructive Surgery: A Practical Handbook* is to provide plastic surgery residents authentic information that is compiled at one place which can be used as ready reference and for channelizing their thought process. The inspiration for writing this book has been derived from the existing books in general surgery discipline such as *Clinical Surgery* by Dr. S. Das and *Bedside Clinics in Surgery* by Dr. M. L. Saha.

In my personal experience during the residency in plastic surgery, the trainee resident keeps struggling regarding the special type of history which needs to be taken or examination to be done for every case; thus, they refer to their seniors and colleagues before case presentation or viva voice. If the seniors or colleagues have noted the details of clinical presentation of each case during their training, only then information can be gathered; however, at the same time, lots of references from different textbooks are required, which makes it more complicated for a resident to gather information while simultaneously struggling with hectic schedule of managing patients in the ward. Learning from my own practical experience, I felt the need to compile all the information regarding the plastic surgery cases and organize the thinking process of residents from the very beginning of residency. This book will help them in clarifying all their doubts and fill the gap in the knowledge of a resident or a consultant.

The book consists of long and short clinical cases encountered during the entire teaching and training of Plastic Surgery Residency program. It includes a structured history, general and local examination, investigations, how to proceed, stepwise planning, and various surgical procedures to deal with a case. I am also planning to write a second volume of this book which will include the details about the various types of Table Viva including the radiology, pathological specimens or models, instruments, and grand viva. It will also include detailed surgical anatomy, the surgical steps, and comprehensive information related to the various surgical procedures followed in plastic surgery.

However, this book is mainly a clinical guide and not a textbook. Thus, residents must refer to the available standard textbooks in plastic surgery for a better understanding of the basic as well as advanced concepts. The suggested resource materials are mentioned towards the end of every chapter.

This is an initial and a sincere attempt by all the contributors to share authentic information by verifying the facts and to bring out the standard answers. Still, if any errors are found, the readers may email me at drsveena@aiimspatna.org and the same may be corrected in further editions. I will be happy to address any queries, comments, suggestions, or criticisms for the benefit of the readers.

Veena K. Singh, MCh, DNB (Plastic Surgery)
Additional Professor & HOD
Department of Burns & Plastic Surgery;
Deputy Medical Superintendent, Superspecialty Hospital;
Nodal Officer, Rashtriya Bal Swasthya Karyakram (RBSK);
All India Institute of Medical Sciences, Phulwari SharifPatna, Bihar, India

Acknowledgments

When I conceived the thought of writing a clinical handbook on plastic surgery during the year 2020, I could never have imagined the huge amount of work, research, and enlightenment that had to be put into this book to make it a reality. Text, words, and verbal terms may fail when I ought to depict my profoundest feelings of gratitude for the people who have rendered invaluable help and without whom, the voyage of this book would not have been accomplished. I sincerely convey my deepest sense of recognition and appreciation.

- To the Almighty God to whom I owe my very existence for providing me with this opportunity and granting me the capability to proceed smoothly and successfully.
- To all my learned and luminous teachers who have always been inspirational in my journey of becoming a teacher.
- To all my patients for being the richest source of study material and students, on whose needs this book is based upon.
- To All India Institute of Medical Sciences (AIIMS), Patna for the wonderful opportunity to be a part and parcel of this prestigious institute which has instilled faith and hope and provided me the resources for completion of this publication.
- To my plastic surgery residency batchmates—Dr. Rimpi Jain and Dr. Saurabh K. Gupta—for their enthusiasm in working on the same frequency and timely academic contribution.
- To my friend and an unconditional supporter, Dr. Meenakshi Tiwari, Associate Professor, Department of Biochemistry, AIIMS, Patna for providing insights and sharing her wisdom and knowledge that elevated my confidence. It was her idea only that no one else but the three batchmates (Dr. Veena, Dr. Rimpi, and Dr. Saurabh) can give shape to the book.
- To my department faculty members, Dr. Ansarul Haq, Dr. Sarsij Sharma, and Dr. Vishwadeep, for their immense help and warm cooperation in accomplishing my book and all other details pertaining to it.
- To my final year postgraduate student Dr. Anupama for her untiring efforts in picking up the correct instructions while collecting the clinical photographs of patients.
- To my postgraduates—Dr. Varun, Dr. Shreosi, Dr. Jatin, Dr. Niraj, and Dr. Sreepriya—for their timely support whenever required.
- Special thanks to Ms. Mary Francis and Mr. Saket Saurav for the excellent secretarial support they provided time and again.
- To my colleagues—Dr. Pritanjali and Dr. Sanjeev—and my own wanderlust family friends—Dr. Shruti, Dr. Prashant, Dr. Yogesh, Dr. Lokendra, Dr. Mukta, Dr. Divendu, and Mrs. Reena—for all the inspiration during the journey of this book, or even my life.
- To my beloved father Prof. Vinay Kishore Singh for his blessings and instilling pride in me, my brother and sister, parents in-law, my better (than me) half Dr. Santosh and kids Satyam, Samyak, and Varenya for their endless love, valuable prayers, unlimited sacrifices, and continual support and encouragement throughout the progress in completion of this book.

- To my dearest mother, late Mrs. Ramawati Singh, for sowing the seeds of an organized mind and perfectionism in me which has forever helped me evolve as a better plastic surgeon.
- Last but not the least, to the entire staff at Thieme publisher for their continuous painstaking efforts in the final shape of this book.

Veena K. Singh, MCh, DNB (Plastic Surgery)
Additional Professor & HOD
Department of Burns & Plastic Surgery;
Deputy Medical Superintendent, Superspecialty Hospital;
Nodal Officer, Rashtriya Bal Swasthya Karyakram (RBSK);
All India Institute of Medical Sciences, Phulwari Sharif
Patna, Bihar, India

Contributors

Saurabh K. Gupta, MCh, FICS (Plastic Surgery)
Associate Director
Department of Burns & Plastic Surgery
Jaypee Hospital
Noida, Uttar Pradesh, India

Ansarul Haq, MCh (Plastic Surgery)
Associate Professor
Department of Burns & Plastic Surgery
All India Institute of Medical Sciences
Patna, Bihar, India

Rimpi Jain, MCh (Plastic Surgery)
Senior Consultant
Department of Burns, Plastic and Cosmetic Surgery
Kalinga Super specialty Hospital
Bhubaneswar, Odisha, India

Anupama Kumari, MS
Third Year Senior Resident
Department of Burns & Plastic Surgery
All India Institute of Medical Sciences
Patna, Bihar, India

Veena K. Singh, MCh, DNB (Plastic Surgery)
Additional Professor & HOD
Department of Burns & Plastic Surgery;
Deputy Medical Superintendent, Superspecialty Hospital;
Nodal Officer, Rashtriya Bal Swasthya Karyakram (RBSK);
All India Institute of Medical Sciences, Phulwari Sharif
Patna, Bihar, India

1 Lower Leg Defect with Exposed Bone

Veena K. Singh

Learning Objectives

At the end of this chapter, the students will be able to:
1. Understand the anatomy of lower leg.
2. Describe the clinical presentation of a case of lower leg wound.
3. Demonstrate the motor and sensory examination of lower extremity.
4. Understand the approach to a lower limb injury.
5. Perform the appropriate flap reconstruction for coverage of leg wound.

Introduction

The management of lower limb wound starts with a thorough examination of the wound and leg both. The primary goal of reconstruction is the restoration of functionality. It includes not only a stable skeletal base but also robust surrounding soft tissues like muscles, neurovascular structures, and skin envelope. A very good understanding of the tissue loss and its replacement with like tissues along with prevention of chronic pain and wound infection are important key aspects for a successful outcome.

Chief Complaints of the Patient

- Wound over the lower leg.
- Inability to bear weight on the affected limb.
- Pain/Discharge from the wound.
- Restricted movements of the joints.

History of Present Illness

1. Duration of injury/leg defect/exposed bone/wound.
2. Mode of injury including velocity of the vehicle in case of road traffic accident (RTA).
3. Immediately, what happened after the accident:
   - Bleeding.
   - Dangling of limb.
   - Loss of consciousness/ear/nose bleed/vomiting.
   - Unable to move limb.
   - Condition of wound:
     - Bone/Fracture—visible/not visible.
     - Skin flaps avulsed/not visible.
   - Whether immediate splintage at injury site.
   - Associated trauma:
     - Vertebral fracture
     - Maxillofacial fracture
4. Primary aid was given/not given—Where and What?
   - Debridement of wound.
   - Application of plaster of Paris (PoP) slab/cast.
   - Blood transfusion received, if any.
   - Application of external fixator.
   - Condition of wound after external fixator.
   - Seen by plastic surgeon team/not (if yes—what advice/intervention).
   - Type and frequency of dressing.
   - Management of associated injury, if any.

5. Referral to plastic surgery after how many days.
   - What was the condition of wound as told by treating doctor?
   - What was the advice given?
   - Any intervention done at that time?
6. Associated pain/fever/inability to move the foot.
7. Bladder/Bowel function.
8. Sleep/Appetite.

Past History

History of diabetes, hypertension, tuberculosis, any other medical illness, and history of any surgery done in the past.

Personal History

Married/unmarried, number of children, socioeconomic status, diet, history of smoking/alcohol intake, tobacco chewing. Alcohol intake history would include whether a regular/occasional drinker, and amount on daily basis if a habitual drinker. Smoking history must include the no. of cigarettes/bidis pack per day and number in each pack. The detailed history will give an idea about the ischemic effects of nicotine if a pedicled flap is planned for coverage of the defect. Alcohol intake will provide information about the general status of the patient.

Family History

Parents—whether elderly and dependent, siblings.

History of Allergy

To any specific food or medicine.

Treatment History

Any intervention for fracture stabilization, history of blood transfusion, history of injection Penicillin.

General Physical Examination

- Conscious level.
- General temperature (one should have a thermometer).
- Build.
- Nutrition.
- Pallor/cyanosis/jaundice/clubbing/edema.
- Pulse/BP (must)/respiration.
- Neck veins/glands.
- General condition of skin.

Systemic Examination

- Abdomen.
- Central nervous system (CNS)
- Cardiovascular system (CVS).
- Respiratory system.

Refer to chapter 3 on Carcinoma oral cavity.

Local Examination

Take proper informed consent and examine the patient in adequate light.

Exposure

- Both limbs from the anterior superior iliac spine (ASIS) to the toes.
- Private areas need to be covered.

Important: If patient is ambulatory, observe the gait (if foot drop is present, then the cause must be looked for and also the level of nerve injury).

Inspection

1. Attitude and apparent shortening, if any.
2. Atrophy/Wasting—over thigh, leg, foot; always compare with the normal limb.
3. External fixator—extent and type of fixator needs to be described.
4. Pin tracts—granulation tissue/pus discharge, if any.
5. Wound (**Fig. 1.1**):
   - Site in terms of distance from anatomical landmarks.

- Proximally: Lower end of patella, medial/lateral femoral condyle.
- Distally: Lateral/medial malleoli.
- Medially: Anterior tibial border.
- Laterally: Posterior midline.
- Size: In longitudinal and transverse dimensions (approximately in cm).
- Margins: Whether epithelialization present or not.
- Granulation tissue: Fine/coarse, pink/beefy red, bleeds easily on touch or not so as to differentiate between healthy and unhealthy granulation tissue.
- Slough: Any visible dead and necrotic tissue.
- Discharge: Whether Yes/No. If yes, then amount, color, odor, consistency, from which part of wound.

6. Exposed Bone:
- Site: For example, patella/femoral condyles, upper/middle/lower third of tibia, ankle, malleoli, dorsum/sole of foot.
- Size.
- Fracture site and fragments: Visible/not visible.
- Alignment of the fracture fragments.
- Whether periosteum is intact.
- Appearance of the exposed bone:
  - Living bone: Ivory white, shiny.
  - Dead bone: Lusterless, yellowish, blackish.
- Whether anterior cortex/both cortex visible.

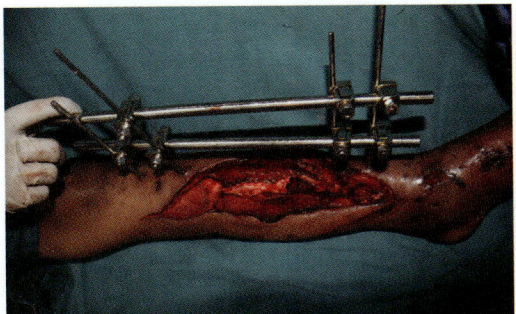

Fig. 1.1 Lower leg defect with exposed bone with external fixator in situ

- Any exposed hardware.
7. Surrounding skin:
- Presence of multiple scars, hypopigmentation.
- Corn/Callosities.
8. Joint above and below: Condition of the skin, any swelling.
9. Foot: Condition of the skin: Whether dry, flaky.
- Look for signs of ischemia: Shiny/stretched, hair present or not.
- Pedal edema: Pitting or nonpitting.

Palpation

1. Temperature: As compared with the other limb or normal part of the same limb.
2. Tenderness: At the wound site and at edges.
3. Findings of the inspection of the are then corroborated.
4. Palpate for the peripheral pulses (in a trauma case, be careful of a single-vessel limb).
- Dorsalis pedis artery (DPA) in the space between the first and the second metatarsals.
- Posterior tibial artery (PTA): Between the posterior border of medial malleolus and tendoachilles.
- Popliteal artery: Palpated in the popliteal fossa.
5. Sensations: In territory of all cutaneous nerves and grade it according to the Medical Research Council (MRC) scale.
- Over thigh and leg.
- Over foot—dorsum, first web space, sole, lateral and medial borders.
- Wound edges.

Movements

The active and passive range of movements at all joints of the lower limb must be checked and mentioned during the clinical examination.

1. Hip joint: Flexion, extension, abduction, and adduction.
2. Knee: Flexion and extension.

3. Ankle:
- Dorsiflexion and Plantarflexion.
  - Subtalar joint (talocalcaneal) joint.
- Eversion/abduction and Inversion/adduction.
  - Talocalcaneonavicular joint.

Measurements (After Squaring of Pelvis) (Fig. 1.2a, b)

1. Total limb length:
   - Keep the measuring tape from greater trochanter up to lateral malleolus.
   - To be measured on both affected and normal sides.
   - This gives the **apparent shortening** of the affected limb if it exists.
2. Leg:
   - The length is measured from medial joint line to tip of medial malleolus.
   - To be measured on both affected and normal sides.
   - This gives the **true shortening** of the affected side leg if it exists. This is because it excludes the shortening of the whole limb due to thigh defects.

3. Limb girth:
- From a fixed bony point (e.g., 10 cm from tibia tuberosity for leg).
- To be measured on both affected and normal sides to confirm the atrophy of muscles on the affected side.

X-Ray

Before making the provisional diagnosis, see the X-ray plates of the patient and describe under the following points (**Fig. 1.3a, b**):
- Which bones are visible.
- Which joints are visible.
- Location of fracture.
- Whether fracture fragments are displaced.
- Any osteomyelitis of bone.
- Presence of periosteal reaction.
- External fixator pins (type of screws).

Provisional Diagnosis

Must include the following points:
- Duration of injury (e.g., 3-month-old).
- Cause of injury (e.g., post-RTA).
- Side (Right/Left).
- Gustilo classification.

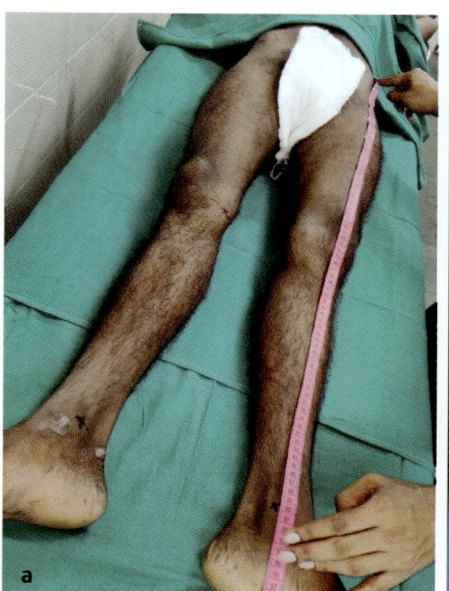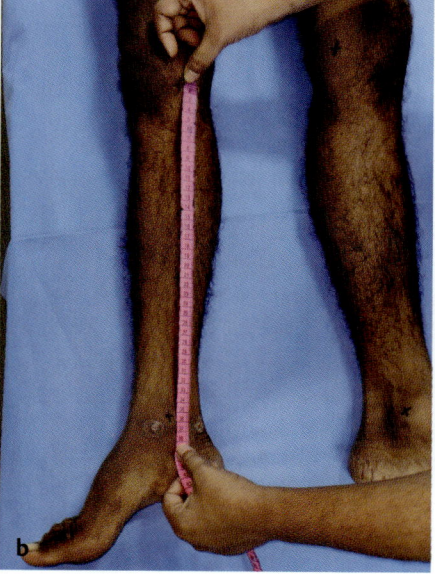

Fig. 1.2 **(a, b)** Measurement of apparent and true shortening in a leg.

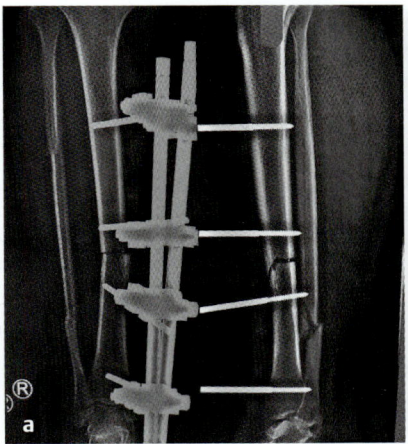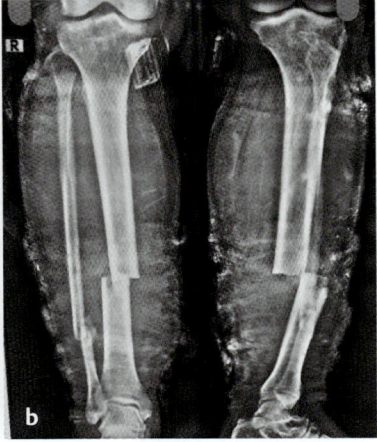

Fig. 1.3 (a, b) X-ray of fracture in both bones of leg.

- Site (thigh/leg/foot): Upper/middle/lower third.
- Exposed bone.
- Exposed fracture site (tibia/fibula).
- Granulation tissue (healthy/unhealthy).
- Discharge.
- Type of external fixator in situ.
- Whether foot drop/not.

For example, the provisional diagnosis can be: A case of 2 months old compound # both bone with exposed tibia lower third Gustilo type III-b with external fixator in situ with foot drop in a 40-year-old male patient.

Questions

Q1. How will you proceed?

The plan will be to get the baseline investigations done for preanesthesia checkup (PAC) fitness followed by surgery of the wound which will be debridement and flap cover of the exposed bone.

Whatever your first plan is, it should be supported by rationality.

1. Stages of surgery required.
   - Single stage if no bone gap exists—Only flap is required.
   - Two-stage surgery if bony gap exists.
     - First stage: Flap cover.
     - Second stage: Bone replacement.
   - Both stages can be combined: In cases of rail road fixators and Ilizarov's fixator.
2. Always make a local flap as one of the plans. Options could be:
   - Fasciocutaneous flaps.
   - Muscle flap.
   - Cross-leg.
   - De-epithelialized inverted flaps.
3. Plan for bone defect:
   - How much is the defect (exact size).
   - Options ⟨ Single stage / Two-stage
   - In case of staged surgery, how much is the gap between the two stages—6 to 12 weeks between soft tissue cover and bony reconstruction.
   - Options for bone defects:
     - Nonvascularized bone graft for defect up to <4 cm.
     - Ilizarov for 4- to 8-cm bone gap.
     - Vascularized bone graft (for defects up to 24 cm).
     - From same leg or contralateral leg.
4. Doppler examination must be done during examination of cases:
   - Where pulses are not palpable.
   - Perforators for marking a local flap.
   - Recipient vessels when planning a free flap.

5. In cases of pedicled fasciocutaneous flap:
   • Markings for triangularization of the defect (**Fig. 1.4**).
   • Whether medial/lateral.
   • Whether superiorly/inferiorly based.
6. Think about whether propeller/perforator flap/islanded flap is an option.

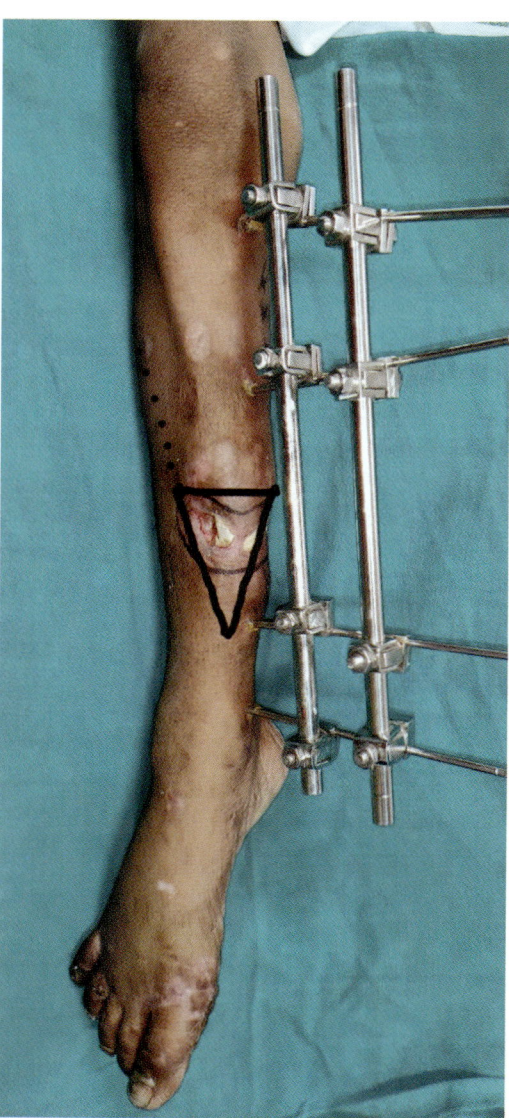

Fig. 1.4 Triangularization of defect for transposition fasciocutaneous flap.

7. If free muscle flap is the first plan:
   • Whether muscle + split-skin thickness skin graft (SSG) or musculocutaneous.
   • Advantages/disadvantages of both.
   • If plan is for muscle flap—test for its presence and power.
8. Think about all options for defects over proximal/middle/distal third.

Q2. How will you classify the open wounds of leg?

Gustilo classification:
   • I—Open Fracture with wound <1 cm.
   • II—Open Fracture with wound >1 cm without extensive soft tissue damage.
   • III—Open Fracture with soft tissue damage.
   • IIIa—III with adequate soft tissue damage.
   • IIIb—III with soft tissue loss with periosteal stripping and bone exposure.
   • IIIc—III with arterial injury; requires repair.

Q3. How will you manage a case of lower extremity trauma?

   • Lower extremity trauma is usually a part of polytrauma encountered in RTA. Advanced Trauma Life Support (ATLS) protocol needs to be followed.

   Start with Primary Survey
   ↓
   A—**A**irway is secured with stabilization of cervical spine
   ↓
   B—**B**reathing is maintained
   ↓
   C—**C**irculation is checked and maintained
   ↓
   D—**D**isability assessment

   • Central nervous system examination (Glasgow coma scale [GCS] is used to assess it).

- Head-to-toe examination is also done by completely exposing the patient but preventing hypothermia.

	Glasgow coma scale	Score
Eye opening	Spontaneously	4
	To speech	3
	To pain	2
	None	1
Verbal response	Oriented	5
	Confused	4
	Inappropriate	3
	Incomprehensible	2
	None	1
	None—Intubated	1T
Motor response	Obeys commands	6
	Localizes to pain	5
	Withdraws to pain	4
	Flexion to pain (decorticate)	3
	Extension to pain (decerebrate)	2
	None	1
	Maximum score	15
	Minimum score	3
		3T if intubated

- After primary survey, a secondary survey is done with history-taking, appropriate radiologic and laboratory investigations.
  - Focused assessment with sonography in trauma (FAST).
  - Computed tomography (CT).
  - Angiography.
  - X-rays of extremities.
  - Arterial blood gases (ABG).
  - Full biochemical profile.

Q4. What are the immediate quick examinations in acute limb injuries?

The examination is done under the following headings:

1. Vascular:
   - Examine the pulse, color, temperature, and turgor of the foot.
   - Doppler may be performed when pulses are not palpable.
   - CT angiography is done for the confirmation.
2. Bone:
   - Fracture fragments.
   - Any visible fracture line or loss of bone segment is there.
   - Associated periosteal stripping.
   - X-rays are mandatory to evaluate the bones.
3. Soft tissue:
   - Loss of skin, subcutaneous tissues, muscles, periosteum.
   - Any avulsed or crushed tissue.
   - Check for soft tissue viability.
   - Serial debridement confirms the difference between viable and nonviable tissues.
4. Neurologic assessment:
   - Should be done in the sensory zones of peroneal and tibial nerve.
   - Look for the action of muscles.

Q5. How do you decide that the limb is salvageable or not?

Limb viability is evaluated by assessing the vascular, bone, soft tissue, and nerve injuries.

- Mangled extremity severity score (MESS) is used to guide whether to go for salvage or amputation.
- Based on the following four criteria:
  - Skeletal or soft tissue injury.
  - Vascularity of limb.
  - Presence of shock.
  - Age of the patient.

Variables	Score
Skeletal/soft-tissue injury	
Low energy (stab; simple fracture; pistol gunshot wound)	1
Medium energy (open or multiple fractures, dislocation)	2
High energy (high speed MVA or rifle gunshot wound)	3
Very high energy (high speed trauma + gross contamination)	4
Limb ischemia	
Pulse reduced or absent but perfusion normal	1^2
Pulseless; paresthesias, diminished capillary refill	2^2
Cool, paralyzed, insensate, numb	3^2
Shock	
Systolic BP always >90 mmHg	0
Hypotensive transiently	1
Persistent hypotension	2
Age (years)	
<30	0
30–50	1
>50	2

- A score of ≥7 is an indication of amputation.
- Maximum possible score is 16.
- Score gets doubled if ischemia time is >6 hours.

Q6. What are the risk factors that predict the requirement of an amputation?

- Gustilo IIIC injury.
- Sciatic/tibial nerve injury.
- Ischemia time >6 hours.
- Crush injury.
- Significant contamination of the wound.
- Severely comminuted fractures with segmental loss of bone.
- Old age along with severe comorbidities.

Q7. What is the approach to lower extremity trauma management?
Flowchart 1.1.

Q8. What is the reconstructive approach in a lower limb injury?
Flowchart 1.2.
Indications for amputation:
- Completely severed limb.
- Segmental tibia loss >6 hours.
- Ischemia time >6 hours.
- Severance of posterior tibia.

Q9. What are the characteristics of bones in lower leg?
- Tibia provides 85% of weight-bearing capacity.
- Fibula mainly serves as an anchoring bone for the muscle and fascial attachments. It contributes in the formation and stability of the ankle joint.
- Both are attached proximally at tibiofibular joint, in the midportion at interosseous membrane (IOM) and distally at tibiofibular syndesmosis.

Q10. What are the techniques of fracture fixation in leg?
- Traction fixation:
  - More in thigh.
  - Temporary measure in sick patients.
- Cast immobilization: In closed injuries (plaster cast introduced by Ollier).
- Intramedullary (IM) nailing:
  - Reamed nails—rigid fixation.
  - Nonreamed nails (Nailing for minimally comminuted # with no bone loss).
- Internal fixation: With plates and screws.
- External fixation

Q11. What are the compartments of the leg?
There are four compartments in the leg **(Fig. 1.5):**
- Anterior.
- Lateral.
- Posterior.
- Deep posterior.
1. Anterior compartment:
   - Comprises of four muscles: Tibialis anterior, extensor hallucis longus (EHL),

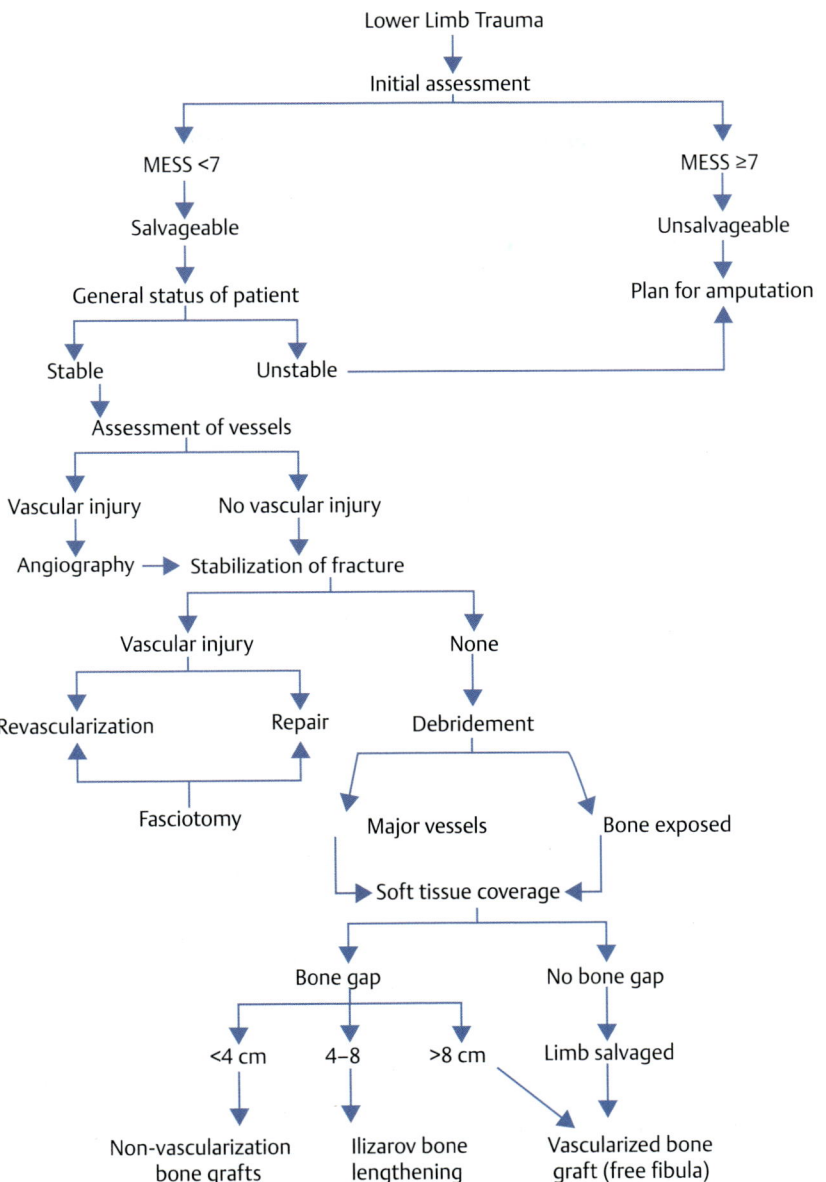

Flowchart 1.1   Lower extremity trauma management and reconstruction plan.

extensor digitorum longus (EDL), and per-oneus tertius (PT).
- All muscles are dorsiflexors of the foot. The primary dorsiflexors is tibialis anterior which is also the inventor of the foot.
- EHL extends the great toe.
- EDL extends the remaining four toes and also dorsiflexes the foot.
- PT is a dorsiflexor and evertor of foot.

- The blood supply of all four muscles is anterior tibial artery and innervated by deep peroneal nerve.
2. Lateral compartment:
   - Two muscles: Peroneus longus (PL) and peroneus brevis (PB).
   - Both are plantar flexors and evertors of the foot.
   - Nerve supply by peroneal nerve.

Lower Extremity Trauma

Salvageable — Unsalvageable

Debridement and bony stabilization — Amputation

Clean wound + No bony defect — Dirty wound + Negative pressure wound therapy (NPWT)

Soft tissue coverage — Wound clean

Flowchart 1.2 Reconstructive approach in a lower limb injury.

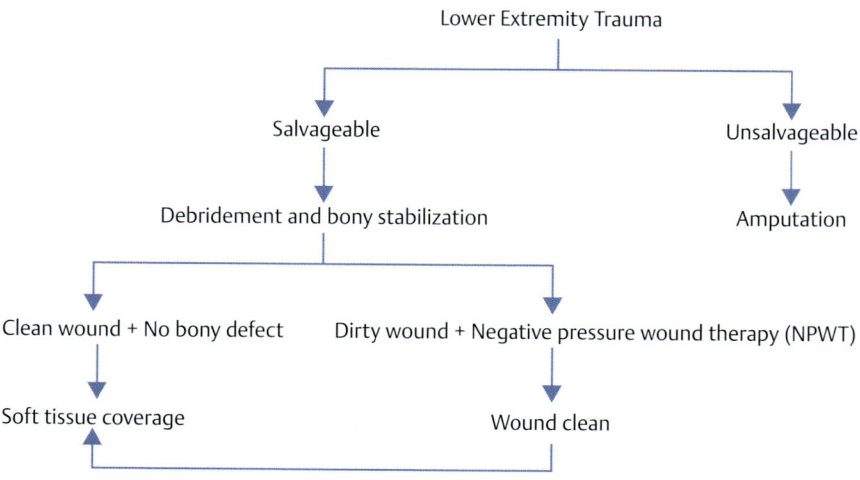

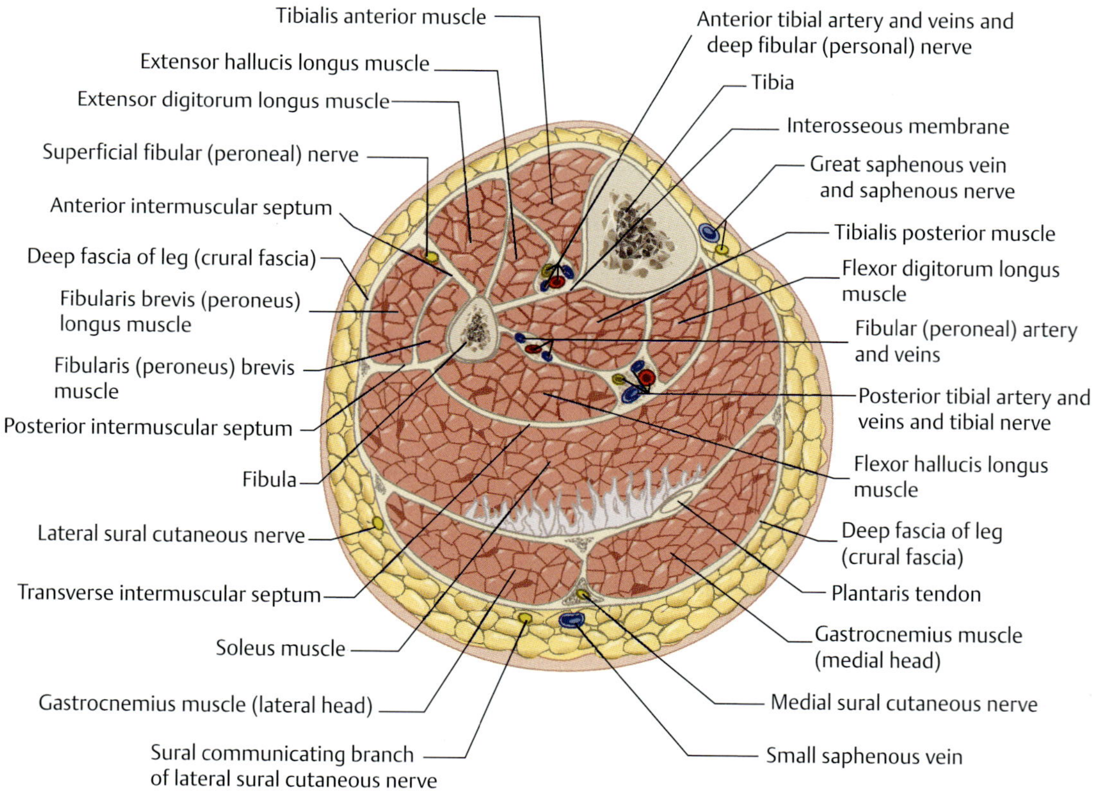

Tibialis anterior muscle
Extensor hallucis longus muscle
Extensor digitorum longus muscle
Superficial fibular (peroneal) nerve
Anterior intermuscular septum
Deep fascia of leg (crural fascia)
Fibularis brevis (peroneus) longus muscle
Fibularis (peroneus) brevis muscle
Posterior intermuscular septum
Fibula
Lateral sural cutaneous nerve
Transverse intermuscular septum
Soleus muscle
Gastrocnemius muscle (lateral head)
Sural communicating branch of lateral sural cutaneous nerve

Anterior tibial artery and veins and deep fibular (personal) nerve
Tibia
Interosseous membrane
Great saphenous vein and saphenous nerve
Tibialis posterior muscle
Flexor digitorum longus muscle
Fibular (peroneal) artery and veins
Posterior tibial artery and veins and tibial nerve
Flexor hallucis longus muscle
Deep fascia of leg (crural fascia)
Plantaris tendon
Gastrocnemius muscle (medial head)
Medial sural cutaneous nerve
Small saphenous vein

Fig. 1.5 Cross-section of leg showing compartments.

- PL receives blood supply by both anterior tibial and peroneal arteries.
- PB is supplied by peroneal artery.

3. Posterior compartment:
   - Muscles: Gastrocnemius, soleus, plantaris, popliteus.
   - Nerve supply by tibial nerve.
     - Gastrocnemius: Blood supply by sural branches of popliteal artery.
     - Plantar flexes the foot and flexes the knee.
     - Soleus: Blood supply from posterior tibial, peroneal, and sural arteries.
     - Plantar flexor of foot.
     - Plantaris: Blood supply from sural branches of popliteal artery.
     - Plantar flexor of foot.
     - Popliteus: Flexes the knee and rotates the tibia.
     - Blood supply from genicular artery (branch of popliteal artery).

4. **Deep posterior compartment:**
   - Three muscles:
     - Flexor hallucis longus (FHL).
     - Flexor digitorum longus (FDL).
     - Tibialis posterior (Tib. Post).
   - Nerve supply by tibial nerve.
   - FHL: Flexor of great toe.
     - Blood supply from peroneal artery.
   - FDL: Flexor of the other four toes and also helps in plantar flexion of foot.
     - Blood supply from PTA.
   - Tib. Post: Plantar flexor and invertor of foot.
     - Blood supply from peroneal artery.

Q12. What is the motor supply in lower limb?

Just proximal to the popliteal fossa, sciatic nerve divides into tibial and common peroneal nerves.
- Within the popliteal fossa, the tibial nerve runs lateral to popliteal artery and then enters into the deep posterior compartment of the leg.
- All the muscles of the deep and superficial posterior compartment of the leg are supplied by tibial nerve except the gastrocnemius.

- At the level of the deep and superficial posterior compartment of the leg are supplied by tibial nerve except the gastrocnemius.
- At the level of distal ankle, deep to the flexor retinaculum, the tibial nerve divides into three branches: calcaneal, medial, and lateral plantar nerves. These nerves provide motor supply to all the muscles of the foot except extensor digitorum brevis (EDB) muscle.
- The common peroneal nerve passes around the head of the fibula and divides into superficial and deep branches.
- The deep peroneal nerve supplies the muscles of anterior compartment and exits the extensor retinaculum to supply EDB.
- The superficial peroneal nerve supplies the muscles of the lateral compartment and then pierces the deep fascia to lie in a subcutaneous plane and provides sensation to the lateral aspect of lower leg and dorsum of foot.

Q13. What is the sensory supply of leg and foot (Fig. 1.6a–c)?

- Superficial peroneal nerve (root value: L4, L5, and S1):
  - It descends down in the lateral compartment to supply the anterolateral skin in the upper one-third of the leg.
  - At 10 to 12 cm above the ankle joint, it becomes subcutaneous and descends superficial to the extensor retinaculum and supplies the dorsum of the foot and all toes except for the lateral side of the fifth toe, which is supplied by the sural nerve, and the first web space, which is supplied by the deep peroneal nerve.
- Deep peroneal nerve (root value: L4, L5, and S1): Descends down the anterior compartment and passes deep to extensor retinaculum to supply the ankle and midfoot joints and first web space.
- Sural nerve (root value: L5 and S1):
  - It is formed by joining of medial sural and lateral sural branches of tibial and common peroneal nerves, respectively.

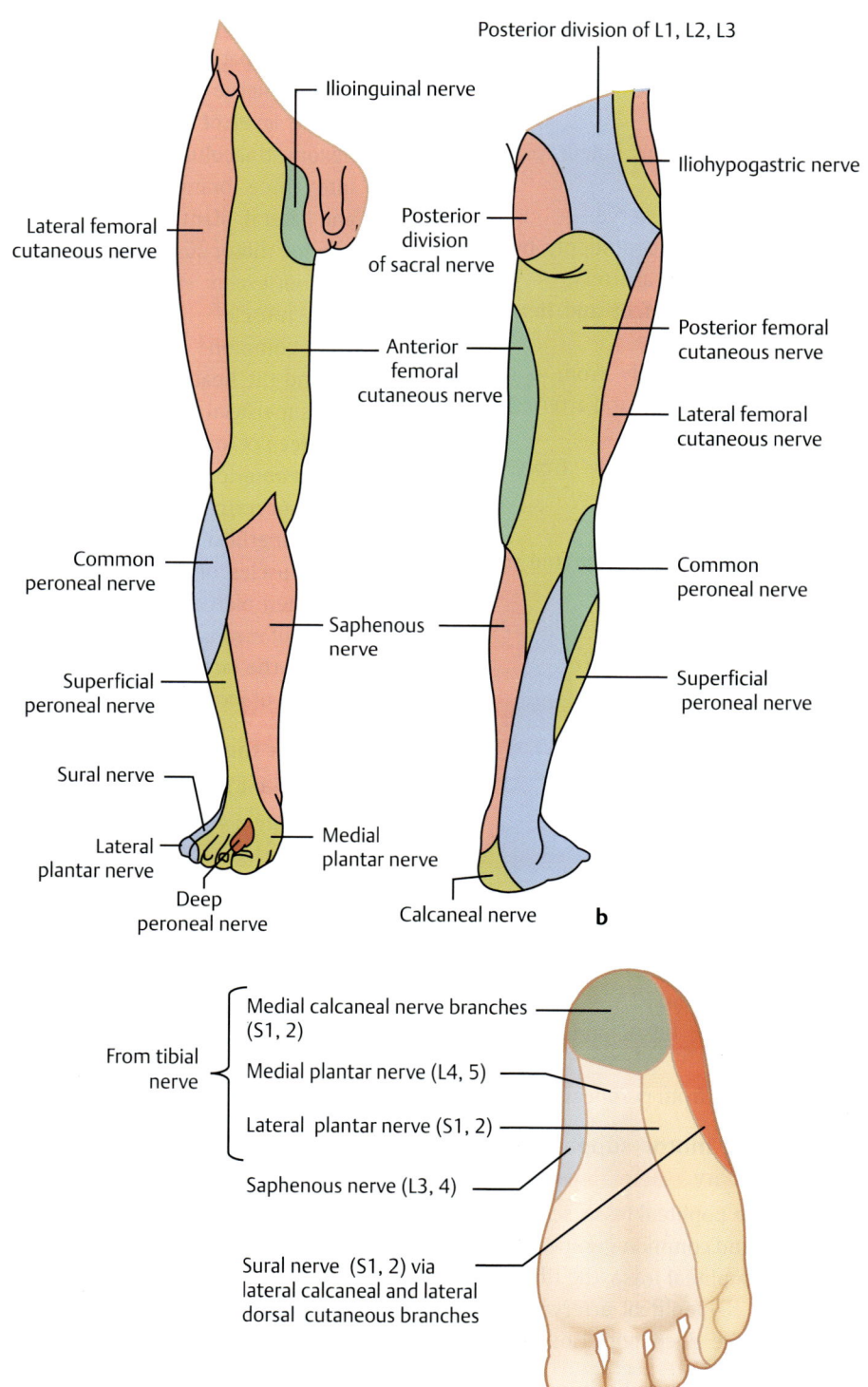

Fig. 1.6   **(a–c)** Sensory mapping of leg and foot.

- It descends into the leg in the posterior compartment along with lesser saphenous vein and provides sensory supply to the posterior and lateral third of the leg.
- It then passes between the tendoachilles and lateral malleolus and supplies the dorsolateral aspect of foot and the fifth toe.

- Saphenous nerve (root value: L5 and S1): It is a cutaneous branch of femoral nerve and supplies the skin over the medial half of leg and dorsomedial aspect of the foot.
- Medial and lateral plantar nerves:
  - Posterior tibial nerve divides into three branches:
    - Calcaneal branch (S1 and S2): It supplies the medial aspect of the heel.
    - Lateral plantar nerve (S1 and S2): It supplies the lateral two-thirds of the sole and lateral half of the fourth toe and the fifth toe.
    - Medial planter nerve (L4 and L5).

It supplies the medial one-third of the sole and the first, second, third toes and medial half of the fourth toe.

Q14. What is the vascular anatomy of leg?

The vascular supply of lower leg is from popliteal artery.

- Femoral artery after exiting from adductor canal continues as popliteal artery.
- It gives off multiple genicular branches around the knee to form a network.
- The superior genicular artery anastomoses with the descending branches from lateral femoral circumflex artery and the superficial femoral artery.
- After exiting from the popliteal fossa, popliteal artery divides into anterior tibial artery (ATA) and tibioperoneal trunk.
  - The ATA descends down between the two heads of tibialis posterior and runs on the anterior surface of the IOM. It crashes the anterior compartment of the leg and passes over the anterior

surface of the ankle between the lateral and medial malleoli and continues in the foot as DPA.

The tibioperoneal trunk divides into the peroneal and posterior tibial arteries. Both the vessels travel into the deep posterior compartment of the leg.

- Peroneal artery runs near the posterior surface of the fibula.
- The PTA travels down the leg, initially at a deeper plane and gradually becomes more superficial as it crosses the ankle posterior to medial malleolus where it is only covered by skin and subcutaneous fat.
- It then divides into the medial and lateral plantar arteries which are its terminal branches.
- Vascular supply of foot includes three vessels: Dorsalis pedis (branch of ATA), branches of PTA, and peroneal artery branches.
  - DPA:
    - It crosses deep to the extensor retinaculum between the tendons of EHL and EDL and EDB.
    - As it passes between the first and second metatarsals, it gives a main terminal branch which dips into the first metatarsal space and enters into the foot to anastomose with lateral plantar artery so as to complete the plantar arch.
    - Another major branch from DPA is first dorsal metatarsal artery that supplies the skin over the dorsum of the first and second toes.
    - Few septocutaneous perforators are given by DPA in the area of midfoot and forefoot. These perforators supply the medial two-third skin on the dorsum of foot which can be harvested as a dorsalis pedis fasciocutaneous flap.

- PTA—medial and lateral plantar arteries:
  - The terminal branches of PTA are medial and lateral plantar arteries which lie between the first and second layer of the muscles.
  - The division of PTA into two terminal branches occur under the adductor hallucis muscles.
  - Medial plantar artery runs along the medial side of the foot and is the smaller branch. It gives branches to the plantar digital arteries to the first, second, and third toes.
  - Lateral plantar artery is larger in caliber and the dominant blood supply of the foot. It anastomoses with the major terminal branch of DPA to form plantar arch. This arch provides metatarsal arterial branches to toes which join with the branches of medial plantar artery.
- Branches from peroneal arteries:
  - The branches from peroneal arteries anastomose with lateral malleolar and calcaneal branches of PTA at the level of ankle and heel.
  - Peroneal arterial magna.
  - In 5% of the population, the blood supply of the entire foot may come from peroneal artery.

Q15. How will you mark the perforators?

There are two perforator lines on either side of the leg:

- Medial perforator line (**Fig. 1.7a**):
  - The perforators along this line arise from PTA through the medial intermuscular septum between the anterior and posterior compartment.
  - Either mark a line from medial knee joint line to the tip of medial malleolus.
  - Or, mark a line at 3 cm from medial border of tibia.
  - Five to six perforators are present at a distance of 4.5 cm, 6 cm, 9 to 12 cm, 17 to 19 cm, 22 to 24 cm from the tip of medial malleolus on this line.
- Lateral perforator line (**Fig. 1.7b**):
  - These perforators arise from peroneal artery through the lateral intermuscular septum between the lateral and posterior compartment.
  - Mark a line from the head of fibula to the tip of lateral malleolus.
  - Five perforators are present on this line at 4 to 8 cm, 10 to 13 cm, 15 to 20 cm from the 5 to 6 cm from the tip of lateral malleolus and the proximal most is 5 to 6 cm from the fibular head.

Q16. Enumerate the types of flaps for leg defect.

A. Muscle Flaps

1. Gastrocnemius (**Fig. 1.8**).
   - **Indication:**
     - Arc of rotation of medial gastrocnemius is inferior thigh, knee, and upper third of tibia.

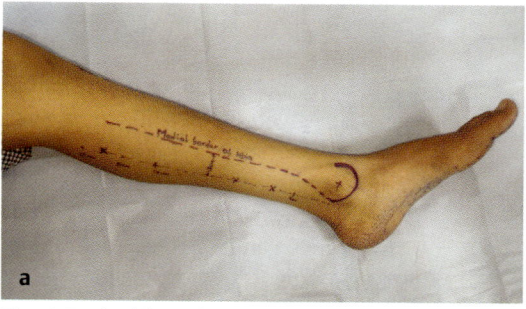
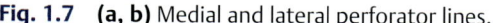
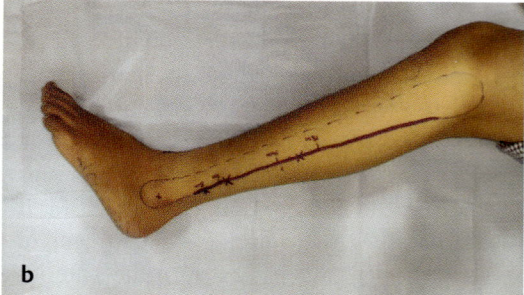

Fig. 1.7 (a, b) Medial and lateral perforator lines.

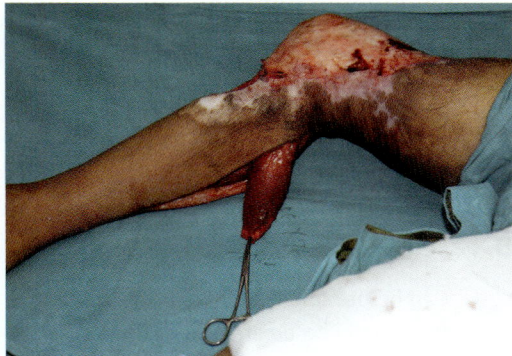

Fig. 1.8 Gastrocnemius flap for cover of exposed bone in the upper third of leg.

- – Arc of rotation of lateral head of gastrocnemius is up to suprapatellar region, knee, and upper third of tibia.
- • Anatomy:
  - – Attachments:
    - ▪ Medial head takes its origin from the medial condyle of femur.
    - ▪ Lateral head originates from lateral condyle of the femur.
    - ▪ Both form the Achilles tendon and insert into calcaneum.
  - – Vascular supply:
    - ▪ It is a Mathes-Nahai Type I muscle.
    - ▪ Medial and lateral sural arteries are supplied by branches of popliteal artery.
  - – Nerve supply:
    - ▪ Motor branches of tibial nerve.
    - ▪ Sensory supply to skin over medial gastrocnemius is via saphenous nerve and over lateral gastrocnemius is via sural nerve.
  - – Actions:
    - ▪ Both the heads bring plantar flexion of the foot.
  - – Markings:
    - ▪ A Lazy-S incision is marked over the posterior midline from popliteal crease up to the junction of middle and distal third of the leg.
    - ▪ It gives exposure to both the heads.
    - ▪ Care is taken to safeguard the sural and saphenous nerves and short saphenous vein.

- ▪ The key structure to differentiate between the gastrocnemius and soleus is plantaris which runs in between the two.
- ▪ Distally, the tendinous insertion is sharply cut from the Achilles tendon with 2 cm of gastrocnemius tendon for robust anchoring with the wound edges.
- ▪ Proximally, muscle is separated from soleus with blunt dissection using fingers.
- ▪ In case lateral head is being used, care has to be taken regarding the compression of common peroneal nerve while passing the muscle through the subcutaneous tunnel, over the head of fibula.
- ▪ Cutaneous paddle overlying the muscles can also be included in case of requirement but creates an unsightly scar at the donor site.

2. Soleus (**Fig. 1.9a–c**).
   - • Indication:
     - – For coverage of defects over the middle third of leg.
   - – Anatomy:
     - ▪ Attachments:
       - ○ The muscle has two bellies—A medial and a lateral separated by intermuscular septum.
       - ○ Medial belly takes its origin from the medial border of tibia in its middle third.
       - ○ Lateral belly takes its origin from the posterior surface of head and body of fibula.
       - ○ Both bellies along with medial and lateral gastrocnemius and plantaris form the Achilles tendon and insert into the calcaneum.
     - ▪ Vascular supply:
       - ○ It is a Mathes-Nahai Type II muscle. Its dominant pedicle is from the popliteal, posterior tibial, and peroneal arteries.
       - ○ Minor pedicles supplying the soleus arise from the posterior tibial and peroneal arteries.

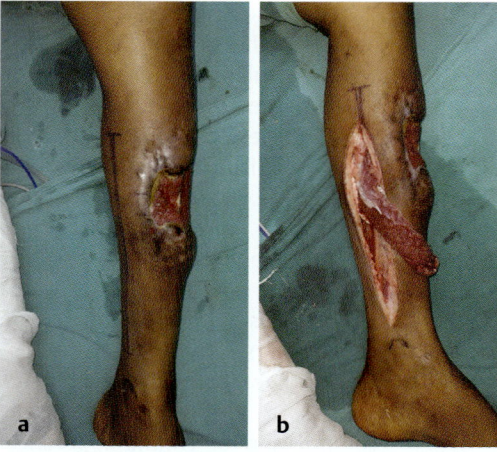

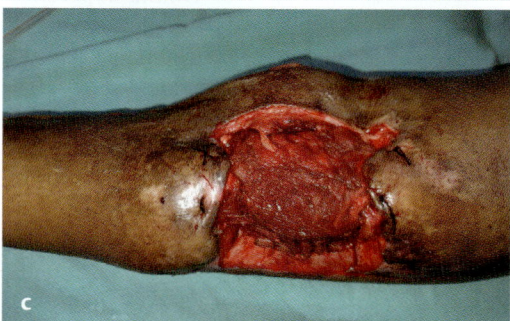

Fig. 1.9 **(a–c)** Hemisoleus muscle flap for defect in middle third.

- ■ **Nerve supply:** Motor branches from posterior tibial and peroneal nerves.
- ■ **Actions:** Both the heads bring plantar flexion of the foot.
- **Markings:**
  - A line is drawn 2 cm medial to the medial border of tibia or along the lateral border of fibula for exposure of medial and lateral bellies of soleus, respectively.
  - To reach soleus, one has to enter the posterior compartment and blunt dissection is done to separate from overlying gastrocnemius in the proximal part and sharp dissection in the distal part.
  - For proximally based flaps, distal pedicles are divided and the muscle is divided at midline raphe to elevate a hemisoleus flap.

- Hemisoleus flap is preferred to increase the arc of rotation and preservation of the muscle function.
- Reversed hemisoleus flaps are also used to cover the defects over distal third of the leg.

B. Fasciocutaneous Flaps of Leg

- Can be proximally based or distally based. Proximally based are more robust.
- Can be located on medial or lateral aspect of leg along the medial or lateral perforators. It can also be designed on the posterior aspect of the leg.
- Can be used as transposition flap (**Fig. 1.10a–d**) or cross-leg flap (**Fig. 1.11a, b**).
- If elevated on a single perforator, it is known as "perforator-based flap" (**Fig. 1.12a–c**).
- 5.The flap can also be rotated on a perforator like a propeller blade of an aircraft. Such a flap is known as "propeller flap." It can be rotated up to 180 degrees depending upon the location of the defect.

1. Propeller flap (**Fig. 1.13**):
   - It is an islanded fasciocutaneous flap which can rotate at an angle of more than 90 degrees.
   - It has two blades of unequal length and pivot point for rotation lies at the perforator.
   - The perforator chosen by a handheld Doppler device should lie as close to the defect as possible.
   - Length of proximal blade = distance between the perforator and distal part of the defect + 1 cm (for easy rotation and tension-free suturing of the flap).

Part of the propeller blade.
- Proximal to the perforator part of the flap which covers the donor defect distal to the perforator.
- Distal part of the blade which covers some of the donor defect proximal to the perforator.

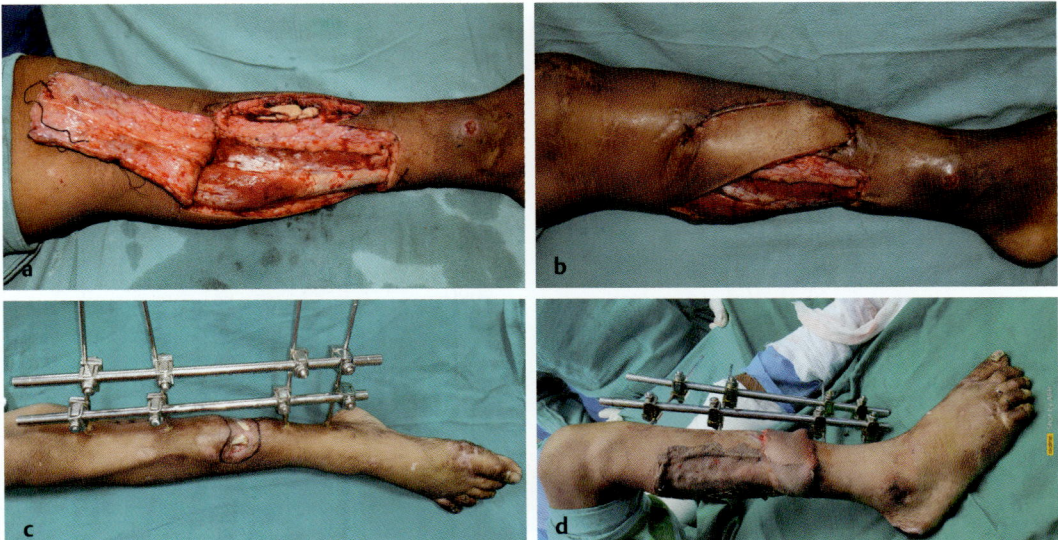

Fig. 1.10   (a–d) Pedicled fasciocutaneous flaps.

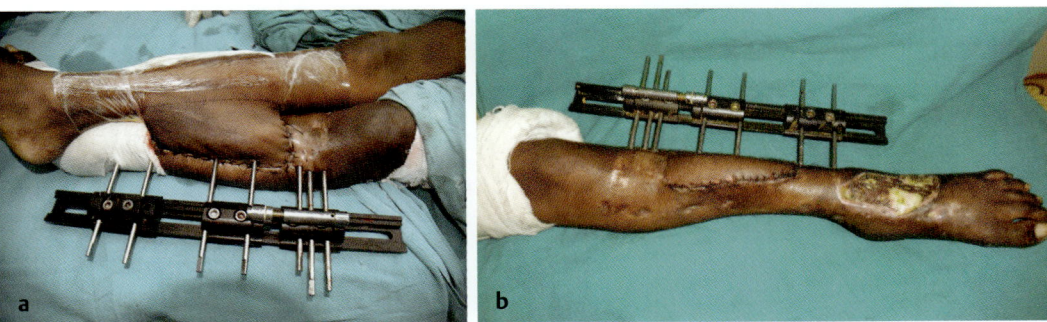

Fig. 1.11   (a, b) Cross-leg flap.

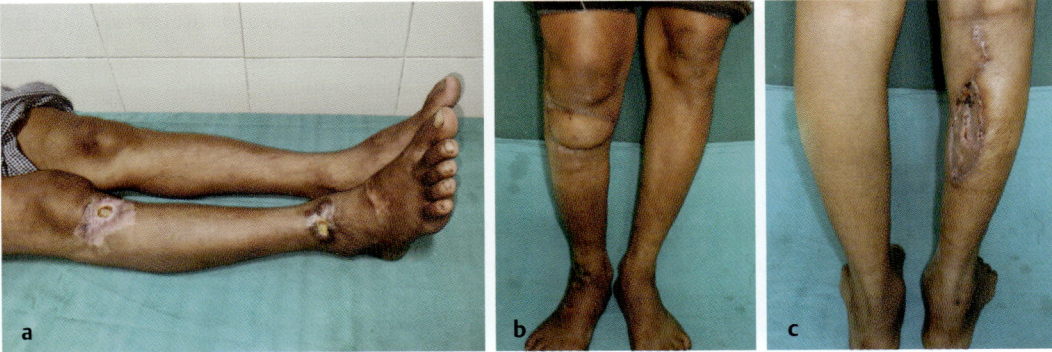

Fig. 1.12   (a–c) Perforator flap.

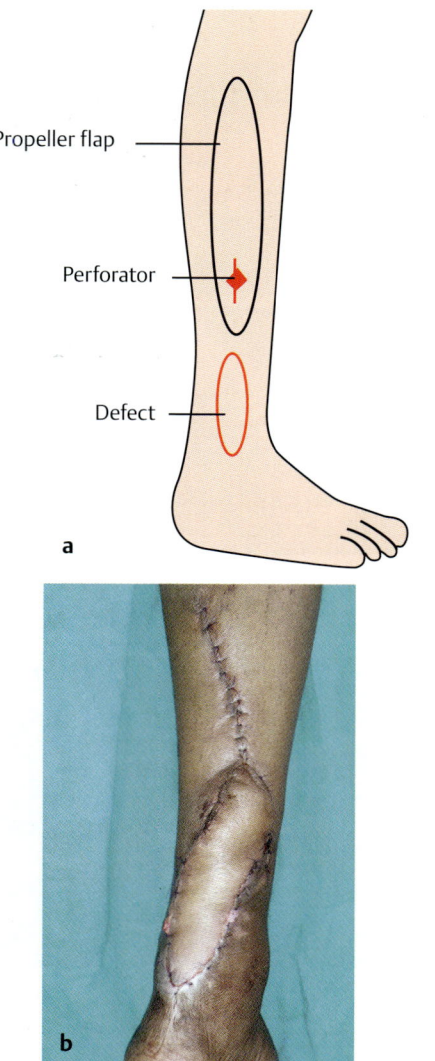

Fig. 1.13   **(a, b)** Propeller flap for coverage of exposed tendoachilles.

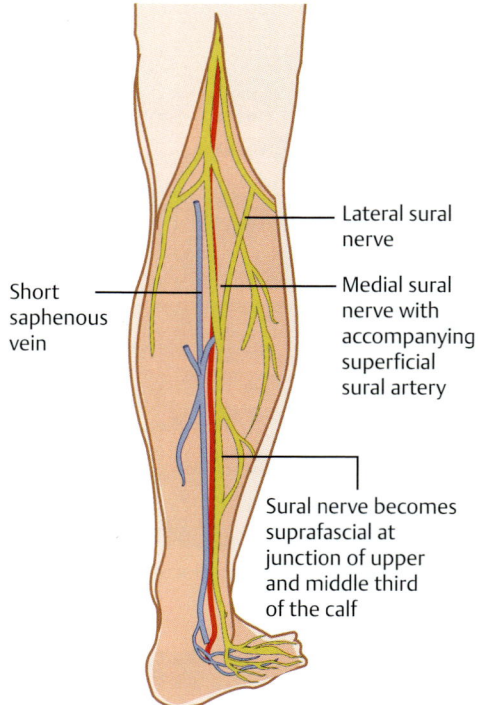

Fig. 1.14   Sural artery flap (antegrade) .

2. Sural flap
- Anatomical boundaries: Distal to the popliteal fossa up to the midportion of the posterior leg. It lies between the two heads of gastrocnemius.
- Vascular basis.
  - Based on median sural artery which is the terminal branch of popliteal artery (**Fig. 1.14**).
  - Venous drainage is via the short saphenous vein.

- Indications:
  - It is used as proximally based flap over knee, popliteal fossa, and upper third of leg.
  - As distally based flap, it receives its supply in a reverse flow through anastomosis between the peroneal artery perforator and accompanying vascular network of medial sural nerve. This flap is used to cover defects over lower leg, ankle, and heel region.
    - The flap is elevated deep to deep fascia along with the sural nerve and short saphenous vein.

Q17. Describe the types of flaps of foot.
Regions of foot and ankle are divided into five anatomic areas.
- Ankle and dorsum.
- Plantar forefoot.
- Plantar midfoot.
- Plantar hind foot.
- Area of tendoachilles.

1. Ankle and dorsum: EDB muscle flap, supramalleolar flaps, and free flaps are the reconstructive options for larger wounds.
   - Lateral supramalleolar flap (Fig. 1.15):
     – For defects over lateral malleolus and ankle.
     – Vascular basis is the perforator from the peroneal artery located 5 cm proximal to the tip of lateral malleolus. It is a fasciocutaneous flap with territory over the skin between the fibula and tibia.
     – It is a distally based flap.
2. Plantar forefoot:
   - Forefoot is the part of foot which lies anterior to midmetatarsal level.

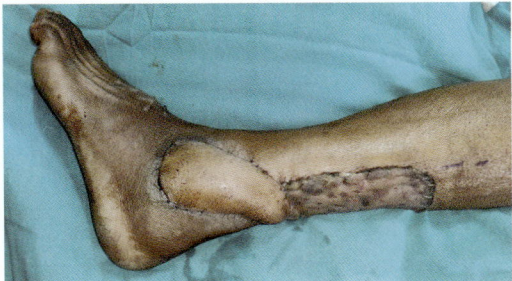

Fig. 1.15 Lateral supramalleolar flap for exposed lateral malleolus.

- Local fasciocutaneous flaps can be used to cover defects in this region as advancement, rotational, or transpositional flap.
- Other options can be fillet toe flap, neurovascular island flap, and free flap.

3. Plantar midfoot:
   - Area between midmetatarsal distally and proximal tarsal bones proximally is midfoot.
   - Same options of flap reconstructions as in forefoot.
4. Plantar hind foot:
   – Includes the area of hind foot.
   – Intrinsic muscle flaps such as abductor hallucis brevis muscle flap, flexor digitorum brevis muscle flap, and abductor digiti minimi muscle flap may be used to reconstruct small defects or larger defects.
   – Medial plantar artery flap, heel pad flaps, retrograde sural artery flap, and free flaps (**Fig. 1.16a, b**, **Fig. 1.17a–c**, and **Fig. 1.18a–d**) are the options.

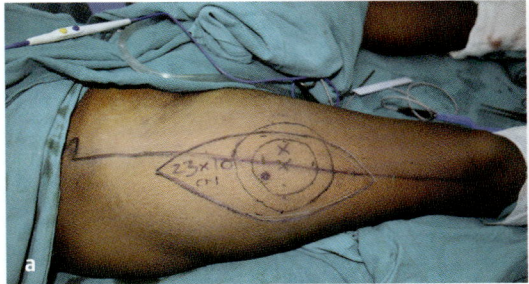
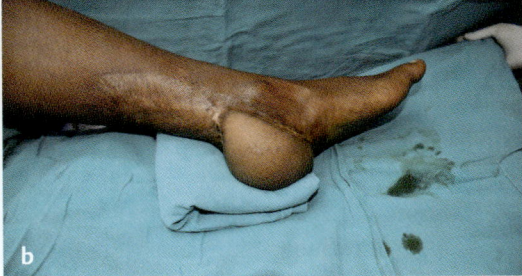

Fig. 1.16 **(a, b)** Free anterolateral thigh (ALT) flap for hind foot defect.

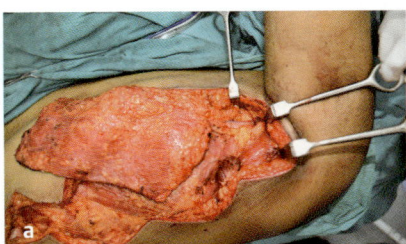
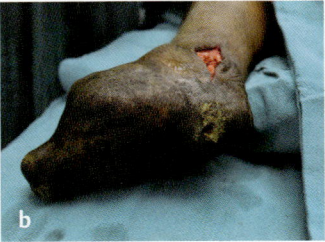
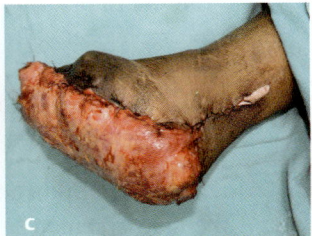

Fig. 1.17 **(a–c)** Free latissimus dorsi (LD) muscle-only flap for defect of sole.

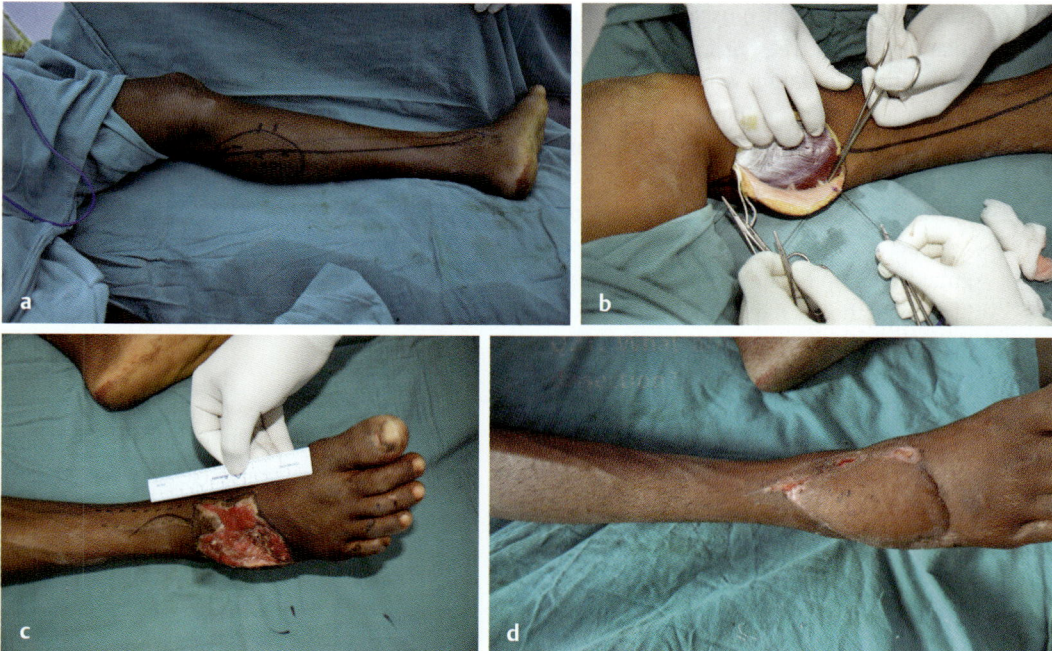

Fig. 1.18 **(a–d)** Free medial sural artery flap for defect over dorsum.

- Medial plantar artery flap (**Fig. 1.19a, b**):
  - It is a fasciocutaneous flap from the instep area of the foot and based on the medial plantar artery.
  - The medial plantar neurovascular pedicle lies in the intermuscular septum between adductor hallucis brevis and flexor digitorum brevis muscles.
  - It can also be used as a sensate flap.
- Retrograde sural artery flap (**Fig. 1.20a–c**):
  - Vascular basis is the arterial plexus around the sural nerve which receives the retrograde flow from a perforator of peroneal artery located 5 cm proximal to the tip of lateral malleolus.
  - The transitory of the flap lies over the raphe between the two heads of gastrocnemius.
  - This flap is used to cover the defect over ankle, tendoachilles, and heel region.

Q18. How to deal with chronic osteomyelitis?
Tibia is the most common site of posttraumatic chronic osteomyelitis.

- The key process in the development of persistent infection is the formation of a "biofilm" which is an aggregation of microbe colonies.
- Most common organism is *Staphylococcus aureus* and may be *Pseudomonas*.
- The four types of osteomyelitis are:
  - Medullary (intramedullary).
  - Superficial (bone surface).
  - Localized (full-thickness cortex with nodular extension).
  - Diffuse (circumferential bone).
- Investigations:
  - Biochemical: Erythrocyte sedimentation rate (ESR), C-reactive protein (CRP).
  - Radiological: X-ray, magnetic resonance imaging (MRI), Technetium-99 bone scan, and the gold standard is bone culture.
- Five criteria for diagnosis of chronic osteomyelitis:
  - Presence of exposed bone with drainage >6 weeks.

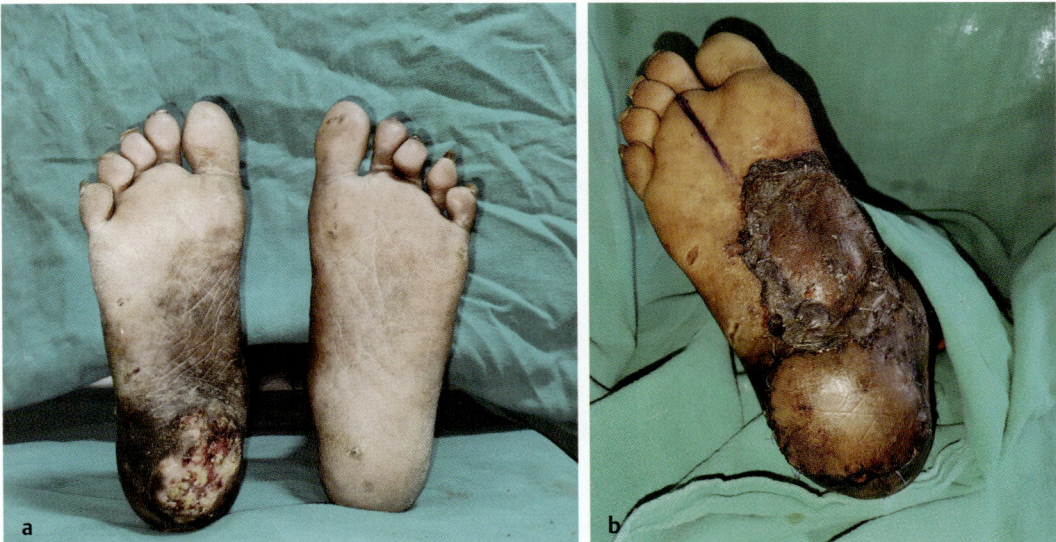

Fig. 1.19   (a, b) Medial plantar artery flap for hind foot defect.

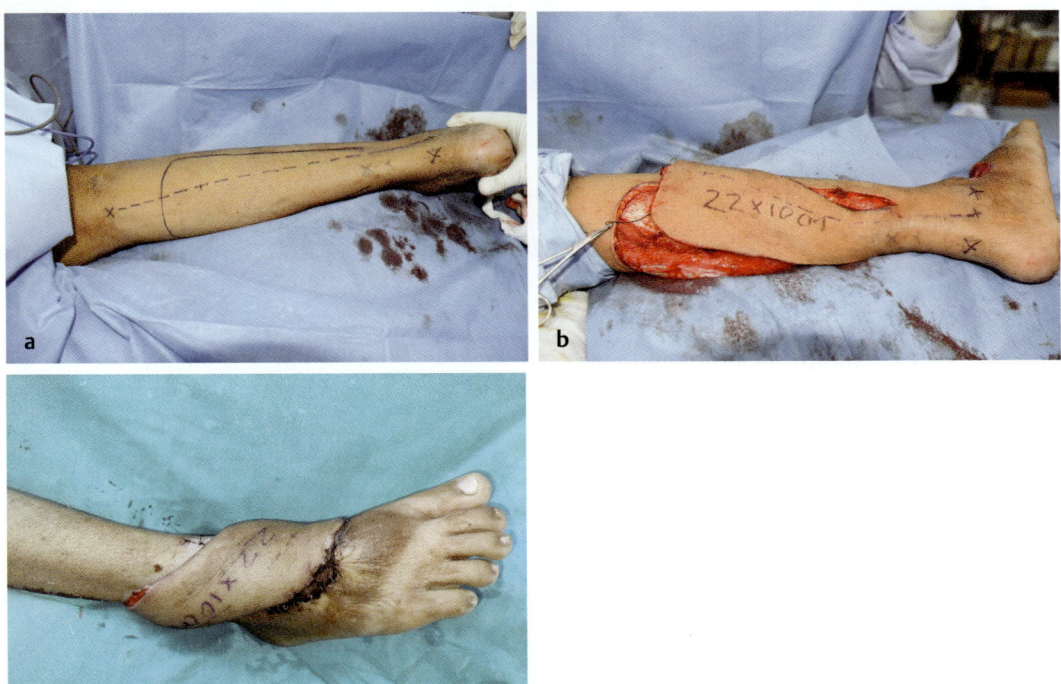

Fig. 1.20   (a–c) Retrograde sural artery flap for heel defects.

- Positive culture from wound debridement.
- Positive bone histologic response (biopsy—gold standard).
- Consistent X-ray findings.
- Bone scan consistent with chronic infection (within 1–2 wk).
- Treatment principles:
  - Debridement.
  - Vascularized soft tissue coverage.
  - Antibiotics
  - Muscle flaps are preferred.
  - Bone defects can be managed according to the bone gap.

Q19. What are the types of fixators in plastic surgery? What are the safe zones for fixator application?

Types (**Fig. 1.21a–c**):
- Type 1—Unilateral uniplanar.
- Type 2—Unilateral biplanar.
- Type 3—Bilateral uniplanar.

Multiplanar: According to planes:
- Planar—Hoffman.
- Circular—Ilizarov.

Other external fixators:
- Ilizarov external fixator.
- Universal mini external fixator.
- Modular external fixator.

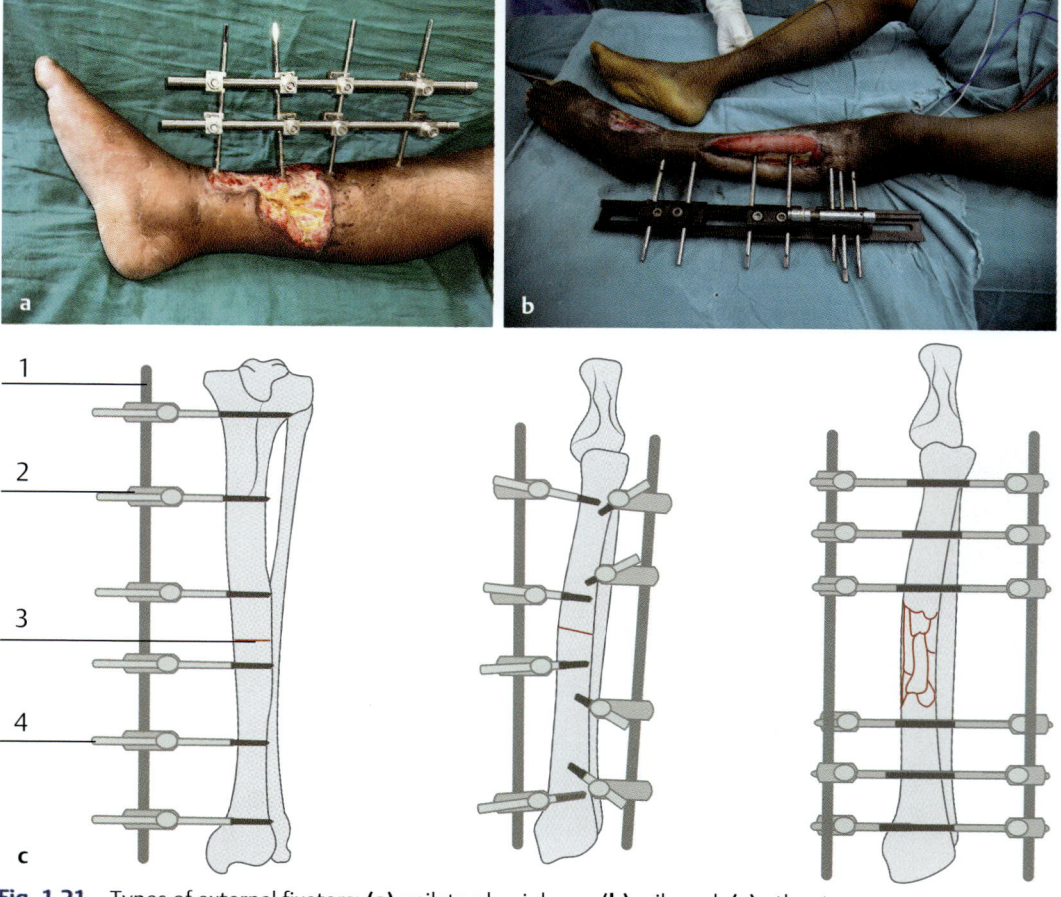

Fig. 1.21   Types of external fixators: **(a)** unilateral uniplanar, **(b)** rail-road, **(c)** other types.

The components of an external fixator are:
- The Schanz screw: 4.5- to 5-mm-long threaded pins.
- Clamp: Universal clamps.
  - Open-ended clamps.
  - Tube to tube clamp.

Safe zones in tibia:
- Proximal part of the proximal tibia.
- Proximal third: Distal to the tibial tuberosity.
- Mid shaft.
- Distal third: Distal to the shaft of tibia.

Advantages of external fixators:
- Can be applied without additional soft tissue injury.
- It causes minimum devascularization of the bone.
- Provides access to wound care.
- Provides an option for bone lengthening (if Ilizarov can be applied simultaneously).

Q20. What is Ilizarov technique?

It is an external fixator in a ring shape (**Fig. 1.22**). It can also be used for distraction and hence limb lengthening.
- It is most stable among all external fixators. There are minimum of three circular rings with three to four connecting rods between each ring to provide stable anchorage to the whole apparatus.
- The rings are anchored to the bone via Schanz screws.

There are two approaches:
- If bone gap is present, gap is obliterated and then bone lengthened.
- Distract one or both segments to fill the bone gap.

Q21. How will you differentiate a corn from a callosity?
- Corns:
  - Consists of a conical wedge of highly compressed keratotic epithelial cells.
  - Limited area, impinges on nerve endings leading to pain.
- Callosities:
  - It is distributed over a larger area.
  - It is a highly thickened and cornified skin.

Related topics to be read:
- Angiosome concept.
- Concept and types of delay.
- Fascial plexus supply to skin.

Suggested Readings

1. Sur YJ, et al. Management of lower extremity trauma. In: Chang J, Neligan PC, eds. Plastic surgery: lower extremity, trunk and burns. Vol. 4. 4th ed. Canada: Elsevier; 2018:53–82
2. Mackenzie DJ. Reconstructive surgery: lower extremity coverage. In: Mathes SJ, Hentz VR, eds. Plastic surgery: trunk and lower extremity. Vol. 6. 2nd ed. Saunders Elsevier; 2006: 1355–1382

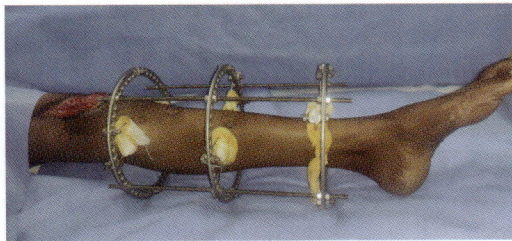

Fig. 1.22 Ilizarov ring fixator.

Post-Burn Contracture (PBC) Neck

Rimpi Jain

Learning Objectives

At the end of this chapter, the students will be able to:
1. Describe the clinical presentation of PBC neck.
2. Demonstrate the examination of patients with PBC neck.
3. Understand the pathophysiology of burn contracture.
4. Understand the planning and management of neck deformity.
5. Demonstrate the markings for surgery and relevant flaps in PBC neck.

Introduction

Neck is a vital part of the body required for keeping the head straight which is required for maintaining erect posture. Its functional impairment leads to various problems like difficulty in walking, sleeping, eating, distortion of cervical spine. As these contractures cause major functional and cosmetic problems with resultant economic and psychosocial implications, operative correction is recommended. A detailed assessment is needed for planning the release and skin cover, and postoperative rehabilitation is highly recommended in these cases.

History

Particulars of the patient (same as for general case like name, age, sex, gender, occupation, residence, etc.).

Chief Complaints

- Inability to straighten the neck completely.
- Inability to look upward.
- Restricted side-to-side movements of neck.
- Thickened scar over neck.
- Itching over scar.

History of Present Illness

- Patient was apparently well before he/she sustained burn months/years back.
- Whether accidental/suicidal/homicidal (includes acid burn attacks).
- Write about the cause of burn—whether flame burn, scald burn, chemical burn.
- Write in details about the temperature (hot/very hot/extremely hot) and duration of contact.
- Ask about history of facial burn, inhalation injury, difficulty in breathing.
- Ask about the history of blisters.
- After sustaining burns, whether immediate cooling with water done or not and for how long.
- Enquire about the treatment received after burns:
  - About medication.
  - Whether open or closed dressing done.
  - Whether dressing done by patient at home or by doctor/paramedics.
- Ask about the history of progression of contracture, and time taken in developing contracture.
- History of any surgical intervention.
- Any physiotherapy or splintage provided or not.

- Ask about the condition of the wound at the time of discharge.

Negative History

- Any difficulty in mouth opening and closing.
- Difficulty in eating and drinking.
- Drooling of saliva, if any.
- Difficulty in speech.
- Ask about the range of vision and presence of restriction, if any.
- History of itching over scar—how severe, frequency, any self-medication for the relief.
- Any discharge from the scar or history of recurrent wound breakdown and healing.
- History of pain.

Past History

History of diabetes mellitus, hypertension, tuberculosis, or any other medical illness.

Any surgery done in the past for the current problems.

Personal History

History of addiction including alcoholism, smoking, marital status, number of kids, employment status. In case of females, ask for the date of last menstrual period (LMP).

Family History

Number of family members dependent on the patient.

Treatment History

History of allergy to food or medications.

General Physical Examination

General physical examination as for other cases. (Refer chapter 1.)

- In general examination, observe whether patient is malnourished, anemic, or hypoproteinemic.
- Apart from general examination, look for bilateral thighs for graft donor sites.
- Examine oral hygiene—may be poor in these patients.
- Look for healed scars or wound over other areas in the body.

Systemic Examination

- Abdomen
- Central nervous system (CNS)
- Cardiovascular system (CVS)
- Respiratory system

Refer to chapter 3 on Carcinoma Oral Cavity.

Local Examination of Neck and Face

Inspection

1. **Neck:**
   - Look for attitude of neck. Neck will be in flexion in case of PBC.
   - Look for extent of scar and contracture in terms of definite landmarks like:
     - Mental tubercle.
     - Mandibular angle.
     - Mastoid process.
     - Suprasternal notch.
     - Midpoint of clavicle.
     - Tip of shoulder.
2. **Scar:**
   - Whether raised or not, approximate thickness in millimeters.
   - Color of scar.
   - Margin of scar.

- Surface of scar.
- Pigmentation—hyper- or hypopigmentation.
- Always better to tell in terms of Vancouver Scar scale.
- Any pits or sinuses in scar.

Vancouver Burn Scar Assessment Scale

Pigmentation

0—Normal: Color that closely resembles the color of the rest of the body.

1—Hypopigmentation.

2—Hyperpigmentation.

Vascularity

0—Normal: Color that closely resembles the color of the rest of the body.

1—Pink.

2—Red.

3—Purple.

Pliability

0—Normal.

1—Supple: Flexible with minimal resistance.

2—Yielding: Giving way to pressure.

3—Firm: Inflexible, not easily moved, resistant to manual pressure.

4—Banding: Rope like tissue that blanches with extension of the scar.

5—Contracture: Permanent shortening of the scar producing deformity or distortion.

Height

0—Normal: Flat.

1—<2 mm.

2—<5 mm.

3—>5 mm.

3. Cervicomental angle obliterated or not.
   - Normal—cervicomental angle is between 105 and 120 degrees (**Fig. 2.1**).
   - It is decreased in neck contractures (**Fig. 2.2**).

4. Mouth opening present or not and how much, in terms of interincisal distance or patient's own fingerbreadths.
   - Look for Mallampati grading.
     Mallampati Grading
     Class 1—faucial pillars, soft palate, and uvula can be visualized.

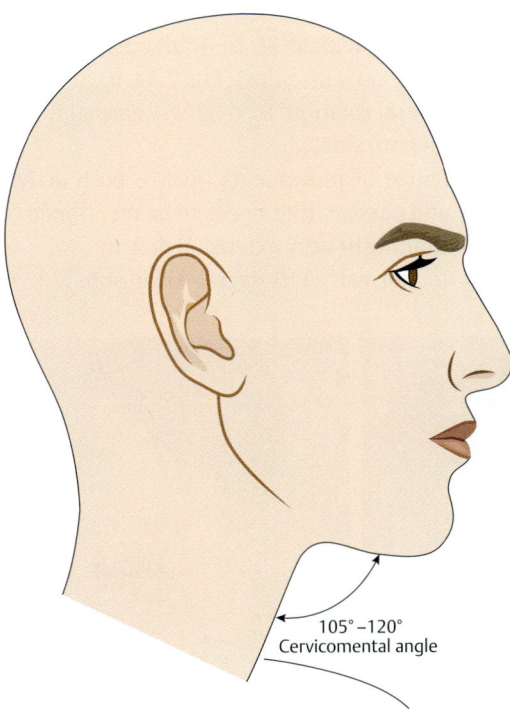

105°–120°
Cervicomental angle

Fig. 2.1 Illustration showing normal range of cervicomental angle.

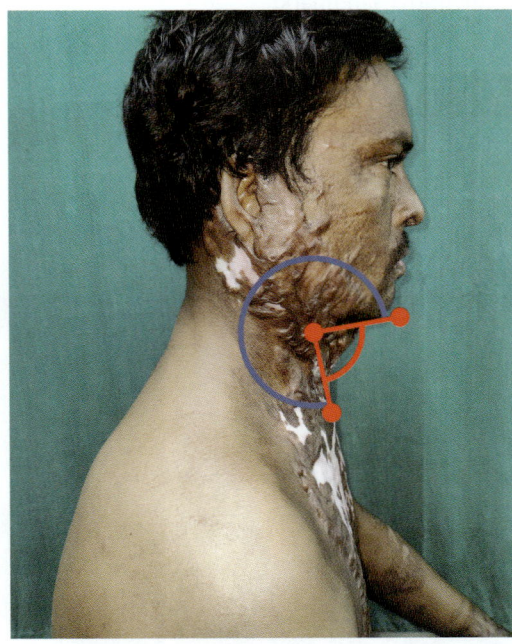

Fig. 2.2 Photograph of a patient showing decreased cervicomental angle in post-burn contracture (PBC) neck.

Class 2—faucial pillars and soft palate can be visualized but uvula is masked by the base of the tongue.

Class 3—only soft palate is visualized.

5. **Eye:** Palpebral aperture in straight gaze both horizontal and vertical.
   - Status of puncta—everted or not.
   - Condition of eyebrows, eyelashes, Xerosis, corneal opacity.
   - Look for conditions of nose and ear also if burnt.
6. **Lips:** Ectropion of lip.
   - Exposure of lower gingiva present or not.
   - Deviation of angle of mouth.

6. Consistency—pliable or nonpliable.
7. Blanching present or not—with index finger, apply pressure over the scar for few seconds and then release it immediately and look whether the color of the scar returns immediately or after sometime. If it returns slowly, then it is said that blanching is present.
8. Able to pinch the scar or not—try to pinch the scar in between thumb and index finger and lift the scar from the overlying tissue.
9. Scar details may be observed in terms of Vancouver burn scar scale.
10. Check the sensations over scar to assess the depth of burn.

Palpation

1. Local temperature over the scar.
2. Local tenderness over the scar.
3. Corroboration of all inspectory findings.
4. Thickness of the scar—to be measured with a calipers or scale (in millimeters).
5. Extent of the scar—size measurement in both longitudinal and transverse dimension from a definitive landmark.
   - Mental tubercle.
   - Mandibular angle.
   - Mastoid process.
   - Suprasternal notch.
   - Midpoint of clavicle.
   - Tip of shoulder.

Movements

- Flexion: 80 to 90 degrees (normal range).
- Extension: approximately 70 degrees (normal range) (**Fig. 2.3a–c**).
- Total range of cervical motion from full flexion to full extension is approximately 130 degrees.
- Lateral flexion: 20 to 45 degrees (normal range on both sides) (**Fig. 2.4a, b**).
- Lateral rotation: 90 degrees (normal range on both sides).
- Range of movements (ROM): both active and passive ROM needs to be mentioned.
- Grading of neck extension deficit:
  - Normal: >110-degree extension.

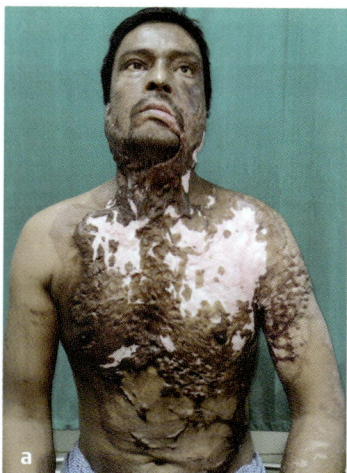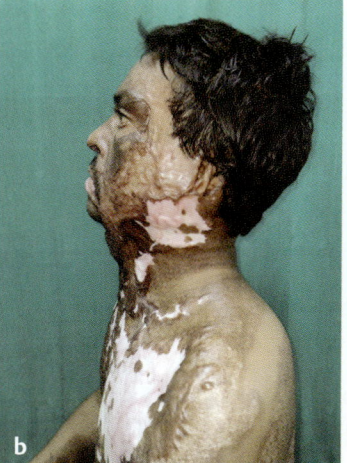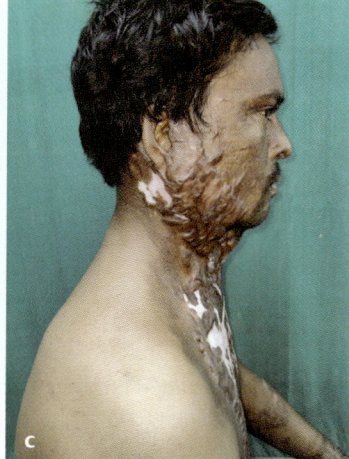

Fig. 2.3 **(a–c)** Examination of neck extension. **(a)** Anterior view; **(b)** left lateral view; **(c)** right lateral view.

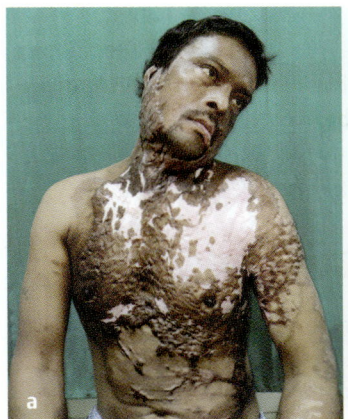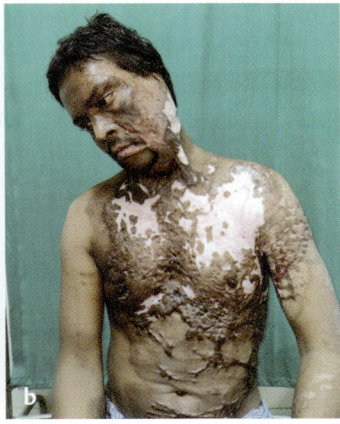

Fig. 2.4 **(a, b)** Examination of lateral flexion.

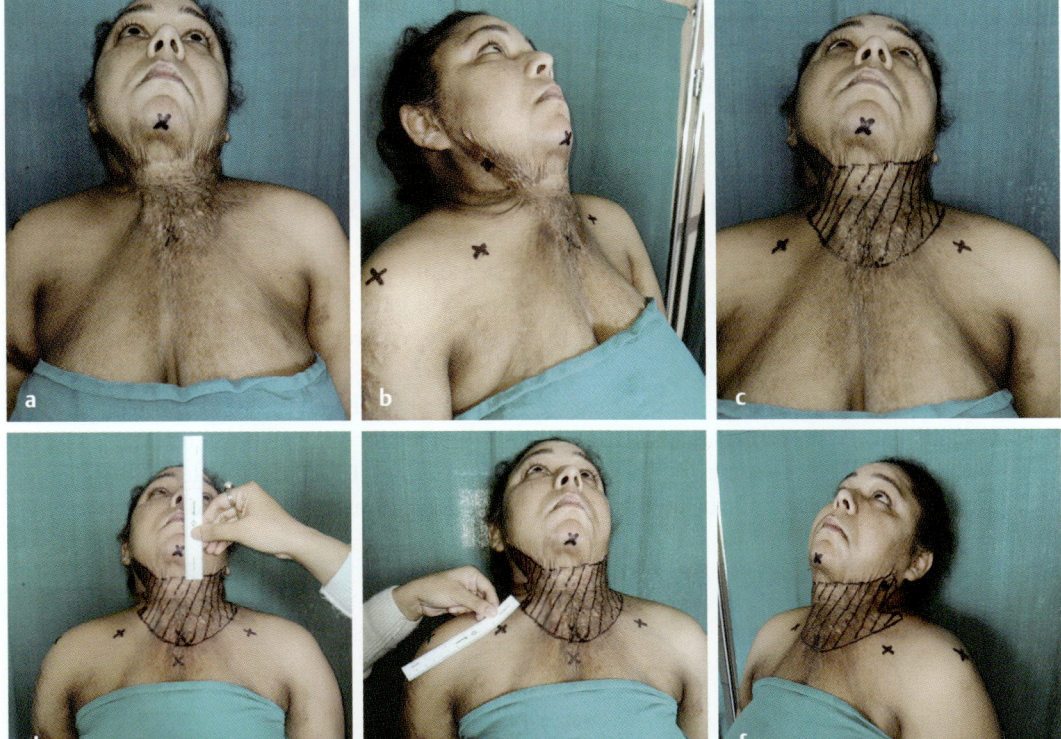

Fig. 2.5 **(a–f)** Measurement of apparent defect.

- E1: 95 to 110 degrees; beyond horizontal plane and parallel to the ground.
- E2: 85 to 95 degrees; extension and vison limited to the horizontal plane.
- E3: <85 degrees; mentosternal synechiae where a patient has a visual range only below the horizontal plane.

Measurement of Defect

Apparent and True Defect

Apparent Defect (Fig. 2.5a–f)

- Measure the extent of scar both in longitudinal and transverse planes with appropriate landmarks as mentioned above.

- This represents the defect occupied by the scar and therefore, it is "apparent."
- The landmarks are fixed ones:
  - For vertical measurements:
    Midline: Above—symphysis mentum.
    Below—sternal notch.
    Lateral: Above—midpoint of mandible body.
    Below—midpoint of clavicle.
    Posterior: Above—mastoid process.
    Below—acromion process.
  - For transverse measurements:
    Above: Anterior—symphysis mentum.
    Posterior—angle of mandible.
    Below: Anterior—sternal notch.
    Posterior—acromion process.

True Defect (Fig. 2.6a–c)

- Measure the same distance from same landmarks on the normal side if the burn is unilateral and mark the points.
- Join all the points in sequence to get the "true" defect which represents the exact size of flap or graft required.
- If burn is on bilateral sides, then measure that distance with same landmarks in a normal individual of same age, sex, and build to get the extent of true defect.

- Prepare a template of true defect.
- Mark the true defect only after assessing whether you are going to excise/release the contracture (also keep in mind the quality of the skin available for resurfacing).

Provisional Diagnosis

- Give a complete diagnosis mentioning:
  - Side.
  - Contracture.
  - Grading of contracture.

For example: This is a case of 9 months old PBC neck with moderate grade with ectropion lip with involvement of nose, ear, and eye in a 30-year-old female.

Questions

Q1. How will you proceed?
I will prepare the patient for surgery that is release of contracture and cover with split-thickness skin graft (STSG). First, baseline investigations are required to assess fitness of the patient for surgery.

Baseline Investigations:

- Blood for hemoglobin (Hb), total leukocyte count (TLC), differential leukocyte count (DLC), erythrocyte sedimentation rate

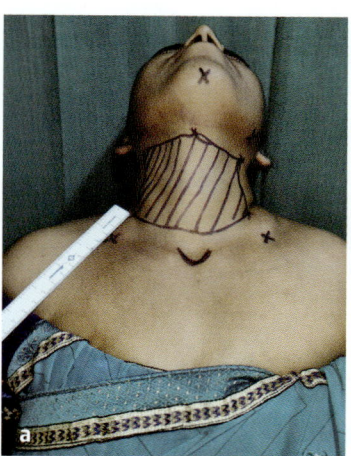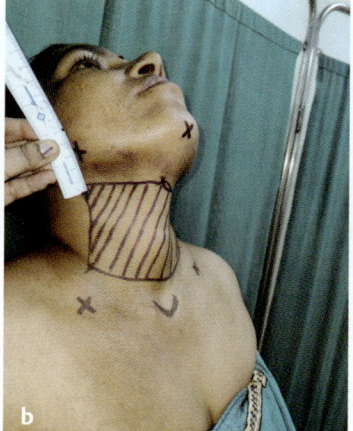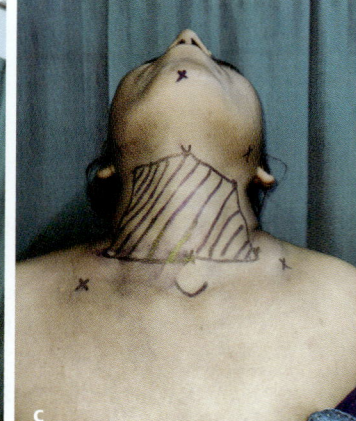

Fig. 2.6 **(a–c)** Measurement of true defect in a normal female of same age group with appropriate landmarks.

(ESR), prothrombin time/international normalized ratio (PT/INR).

- Blood for sugar, urea, creatinine, electrolytes.
- Chest X-ray—posteroanterior (PA) view.
- Electrocardiography (ECG) in 12 leads.
- Arrange for blood if Hb <10 g/dL.
- Arrange for fiberoptic intubation.

Q2. What are the options if there is difficult intubation?

The options are:
- If facility for fiberoptic intubation is there, it should be used because due to restricted extension of neck, the vocal cords cannot be seen by laryngoscope and intubation becomes difficult. If there is thick scar on neck, still there will be difficulty in intubation in spite of good neck extension, as, again, there will be difficulty in visualizing the vocal cords.
- Release the contracture under local anesthesia (Ketamine) and then go for intubation.

Q3. What is the role of X-ray neck in long-standing post-burn neck contracture?

A lateral view of X-ray neck helps in locating the position of trachea.

Q4. What is the difference between contraction and contracture?

Wound contraction is a healing process which starts after injury due to the involvement of fibroblasts, myofibroblasts, and collagen deposition while contracture is the end result of wound contraction which leads to deformity.

Q5. What is the pathophysiology of burn wound contracture?

- The healing of a burn wound is accomplished either by restitution (complete regeneration) or substitution.
- Restitution is possible only if the skin is burnt as deep as the stratum papillare and all the specialized cells of the organ are preserved.

- The epithelial cells, in these cases, are derived from the epithelial appendages such as pilosebaceous units and sweat glands in the central portion and wound edges at the periphery.

↓

- These appendages extend into the deeper dermis and may even penetrate into the subcutaneous fat and survive in partial-thickness injuries.

↓

- The sequence of cellular events that comprise epithelialization include cellular detachment, migration, proliferation, and differentiation.
- If the skin is affected deeper in the zone of stratum reticulare, the defect is covered by substitutive unspecialized connective tissue.

↓

- The final result is demonstrated by a lesser or more extensive formation of the cicatrix, with full-thickness loss of skin, wound contraction, and epithelialization from the margins leading to contracture.
- Wound Contraction:
  - Contraction is an active biological process by which an area of skin loss in an open wound is decreased due to concentric reduction in the size of the wound.
  - The reduction in the size of wound causes lesser degree of connective tissue deposition and the amount of epithelialization needed is decreased.
  - Wound contraction involves an interaction of fibroblasts, myofibroblasts, and collagen deposition and is a satisfactory mechanism when the tissue loss is small, in a noncritical area and surrounded by loose skin.
- Scar contracture, on the other hand, is the end result of the process of contraction.

Q6. Why blanching occurs?

Blanching is a normal process when the skin color returns slowly to normal after becoming white/pale due to digital pressure. Presence of blanching indicates immature scar with increased vascularity. It is misleading in hypopigmented areas of the scar due to dermal vessels lying immediately beneath the epidermis, and the color returns promptly after releasing the digital pressure.

Q7. How do you grade neck contracture?

- Mild:
  - Scar appears only during neck extension.
  - Loss of cervicomental angle.
  - Neck extension ranges from 95 to 110 degrees.
- Moderate:
  - Scar appears in resting position, which hinders any more neck extension.
  - Neck extension ranges from 85 to 95 degrees.
- Severe:
  - Neck is already in the flexed position and the scar is limiting any neck.
  - Movement and the neck extension <85 degrees.

Another classification of neck contracture can be seen in **Table 2.1** (**Fig. 2.7a-d**).

Q8. Why itching occurs in a burn scar and how can it be treated?

- After burn injury there is inflammation in the body which causes release of histamine, due to which there is itching in the body. Some itching may occur as a part of the normal process of wound healing also.
- There is a grading of the itching ranging from 0 to 10, where 0 is "no itch" and 10 is "worst itch imaginable."
- To describe how itching affects life, there is a 5-D Itch Scale. This is a set of questions that the patient can be asked:
  - Duration (number of hours per day).
  - Degree (intensity).
  - Direction (whether it is getting better or worse).
  - Disability (impact on activities).
  - Distribution (location on your body).
- **Treatment:**
  - Moisturizers can be used to prevent itching. They help to maintain skin moisture and hydration and so they are applied frequently.
  - Diphenhydramine cream blocks histamine and is sometimes helpful.
  - Antihistaminic drugs: pheniramine maleate, promethazine, etc.
  - Gabapentin.
  - Massage with steroid-containing cream.

Q9. What is the pathophysiology of a hypertrophic scar?

- A hypertrophic scar is a thick raised scar that occurs due to an abnormal response to wound healing.
- Hypertrophic scar following a burn is caused by the excessive deposition of

Table 2.1 Classification of neck contracture

Type I	Mild anterior contracture. Patient able to flex the neck and bring the neck and jaws to the anatomical position Extension Inability to place an object located on the ceiling (**Fig. 2.7a**)
Type II	Moderate anterior contracture. Patients are able to flex the neck and bring the neck and jaws to the anatomical position while erect. Extension away from the anatomical position result in a significant pull at the (uninvolved) lower lip (**Fig. 2.7b**)
Type III	Severe anterior contracture. Neck in the flexed position and the chin restrained to the anterior trunk. Unable to reach anatomical position of the neck and jaws. Extension: the superior limbus of the unaffected eye is covered and the inferior limbus of the unaffected eye is clearly seen, also it usually pulls on the (uninvolved) lower lip (**Fig. 2.7c**)
Type IV	Posteriorly located contracture. Contracting band at the back of the neck prevents full neck flexion and may hold the neck in some degree of extension (**Fig. 2.7d**)

collagen resulting in an exaggerated wound healing response.

- It usually occurs in deeper burns.
- With deeper wounds (into the dermis layer and lower), body responds by making collagen to repair the wound. Collagen is thicker than the rest of the skin.
- This thicker, less flexible tissue becomes a scar.

Q10. What is the treatment of hypertrophic scars?

- Compression garments.
- Silicone gel sheets.
- Intralesional injections of triamcinolone every 4 weeks.

Q11. How pressure garments work?

- It diminishes the number of myofibroblasts, erythema, thickness, and firmness of hypertrophic scar and accelerates its maturation.
- These are due to hypoxia of scar tissue by occlusion of microvasculature, increased collagenase-mediated collagen breakdown due to pressure-induced decrease in capillary blood flow, reduction in tissue edema.

Q12. What is the mechanism of silicone gel sheet?

- Increase the temperature of scar thereby enhancing the activity of collagenase.
- Increase pressure leading to hypoxia.
- Lower oxygen tension.

Q13. How the wound contracture can be prevented?

Following are the methods by which wound contracture can be prevented.

- Wearing a splint: Neck splint should be applied in the position of extension to prevent the flexion contracture of the neck.
- Range of motion exercises: Exercises of the neck should be done in lateral and backward position.
- Surgery: Close the wound as early as possible using split-skin grafts in deep dermal and full-thickness burns.

Q14. How to decide the timing of surgery in PBC neck?

- If less than 6 months, excise the scar as scar is immature. If we go for incision of the scar at this time, there will be more bleeding and more inflammation which further causes the formation of hypertrophic scar.
- More than 6 months: After 6 months to 1 year scar usually gets matured so incision of the contracture is usually preferred.

Q15. What are the principles of neck contracture release?

- Contracture should be released completely up to normal tissue.
- Avoid damage to any important underlying structure—artery, vein, nerves.
- Incision should begin across the point of maximum tension, (i.e., where the contracture is most tight).
- Fish tailing of the incision on either side should be done to avoid linear scar contracture.
- Ideal material for covering should be thin, supple, large well-vascularized healthy tissue.
- Intermediate-thickness graft is appropriate as compared to split thickness.

Q16. How to ensure that contracture has been released adequately?

- To ensure that contracture over neck has been adequately released, there should not be any visible soft tissue contracture band. And after release, the patient's chin should be parallel to the ceiling and eyes be facing the back wall.

Q17. How will you resurface the defect after release?

There are several methods:

- STSG: If the burn is superficial, then STSG is preferred.
- Intermediate-thickness skin graft: If the burn is deep, then intermediate-thickness skin graft is preferred as it contracts less and provides better contour.

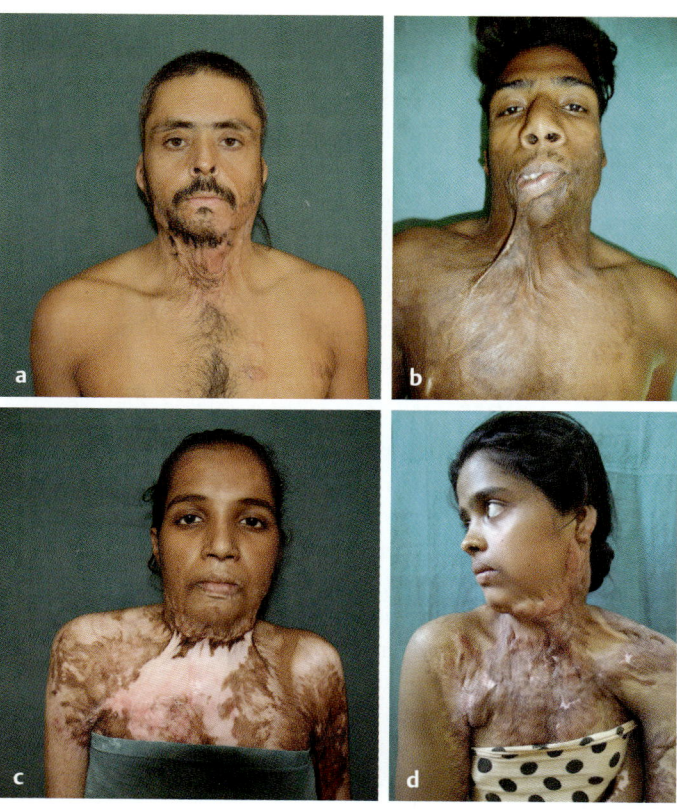

Fig. 2.7 (a–d) Grading of neck contracture.

- Flaps: Pedicled.
- Free flaps: Groin and free radial artery flap (FRAFF).

Q18. What are the indications of flap cover in post-burn contracture neck?

- If after release of contracture, vessels are exposed then flap cover is required.
- If after release of contracture, bone gets exposed then flap cover is required.
- If there is infection, then also flap cover is required.

Q19. What are the advantages and disadvantages of flap?

Advantages:

- Chances of recontracture are less in flap cover.
- Color matching is good in case of flap cover as compared to graft.
- Itching is less in flap cover.

Disadvantages:

- The normal cervico-mental angle is not restored.
- Donor site deformity may develop.

Q20. What are the disadvantages of putting thick graft?

- There are problems in healing of donor site.
- Chances of hypertrophic scar formation may be there over donor as well as recipient site.

Q21. How will you do dressing in a case of neck release + SSG?

The SSG must be secured with tie-over dressing over which sterile pads are placed to bring a convex profile of the entire dressing. It is then immobilized with dynaplast as shown in **Fig. 2.8a.**

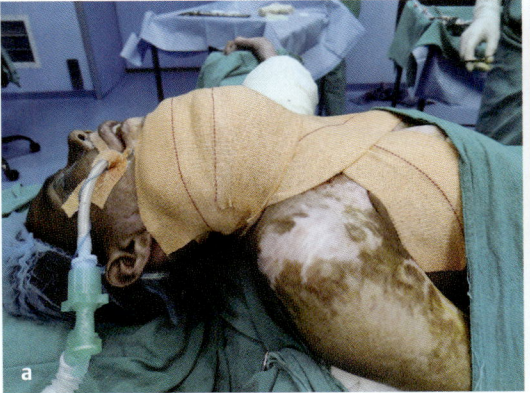
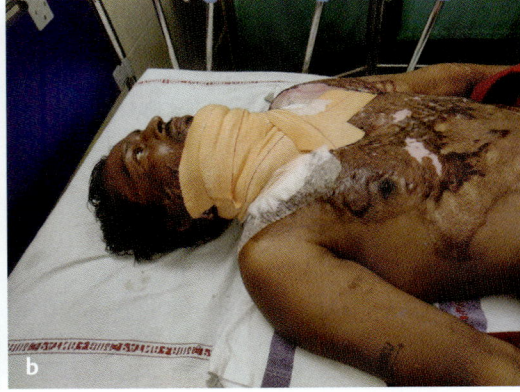

Fig. 2.8 **(a)** Photograph showing dressing in a case of post-burn contracture (PBC) neck (look at the convex profile of the dressing). **(b)** Postoperative position of patient.

Q22. What are the important postoperative instructions?

- Advise nasogastric tube feeding: No movement at the neck due to swallowing.
- Round the clock prophylactic antiemetics should be added to the medications for first few days as postoperative nausea/vomiting is common in these patients.
- Keep the neck in extension by putting a pillow underneath the shoulder (**Fig. 2.8b**).
- There should be strict instructions in the ward regarding "NO PILLOW UNDER THE HEAD."
- Monitor for severe pain at donor site or any soakage.
- In case of doubt about intraoperative hemostasis, first check dressing can be done after 48 hours.
  - If sure about adequate hemostasis during the surgery, then normally first dressing is done on postoperative day (POD) 7 to 10.
  - If during check dressing, any hematoma is seen, then a nick with no. 11 sterile blade is given over the skin graft and clots are flushed out with copious irrigation.
- Cervical collar application after 10 days once the graft uptake is established.

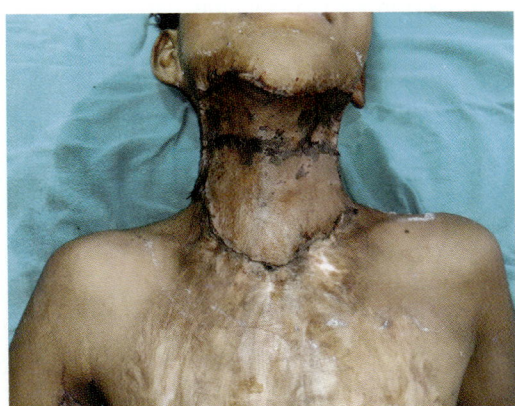

Fig. 2.9 Healed split-thickness skin graft (STSG) at 4 weeks.

Q23. What are the instructions to be given at discharge?

- Neck should be kept in extension while sleeping by putting a pillow beneath the shoulder.
- Collar should be applied. Soft cervical collar is preferred as the patients are more compliant toward it as compared to hard cervical collar.
- No pillow under the head.
- Avoid sunlight to prevent hyperpigmentation of graft.
- Gentle massage with moisturizer or coconut oil over the graft (**Fig. 2.9**).

Q24. What is bony deformity of mandible in post-burn contracture neck?

Apertognathia (open bite deformity): In cases of long-term post-burn contracture neck there is restriction of mandibular growth which results in open bite deformity.

Treatment is done in two stages:

- First stage: Releasing the neck contracture and covering with graft or flap.
- Second stage: It is done after 6 to 8 weeks. Intraoral segmental osteotomy of mandible along with advancement is done.

Q25. Which flaps are used for covering the neck defect?

- Occipitocervico-shoulder flap.
- Supraclavicular flap.
- Bilobed flap.
- Epaulette flap or charretera flap (acromiocervical).
- Expanded skin flaps.

Key aspects of occipitocervico-shoulder flap:

Three variants of occipitocervical shoulder flaps are (**Fig. 2.10**):

- Occipitocervico-pectoral flap based on the pectoral region.
- Occipitocervico-shoulder flap based on the clavicular region.
- Occipitocervico-dorsal flap based on the back region.
  - Their arterial supply is by the descending cutaneous branch of the transverse cervical artery.
  - If the vascular territory does not reach the distal part of the flap, then thinning of the distal part can be done.
  - These flaps provide a large skin paddle and a great arc of rotation.

Key aspects of supraclavicular flap:

- Flap is based on the patient's shoulder.
- Fusiform designs are preferred as we can close the donor site primarily.
- Maximum dimension of the flap is 11 cm in width and 21 cm in length.
- If the flap width is less than 10 cm then donor site can be closed primarily.
- If the donor site width is >10 cm split-skin graft or local flaps are required to close the donor site.
- This flap has a wide arc of rotation which ensures a 180-degree anteroposterior mobilization.

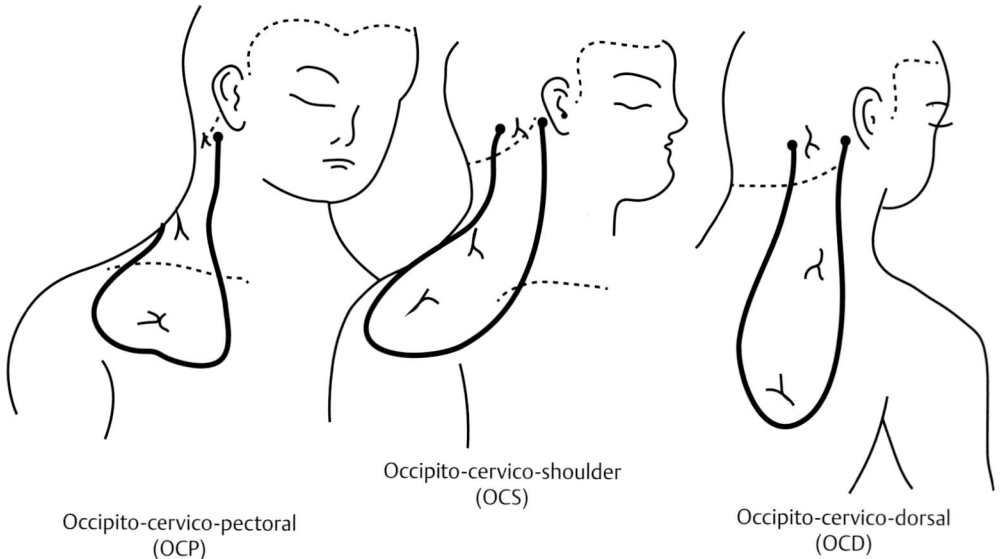

Occipito-cervico-pectoral
(OCP)

Occipito-cervico-shoulder
(OCS)

Occipito-cervico-dorsal
(OCD)

Fig. 2.10 Occipitocervical-pectoral, occipitocervical-shoulder, and occipitocervical-dorsal flaps.

- **Vascular basis of the flap:**
  - Preop Doppler is required to identify the supraclavicular artery.
  - Supraclavicular artery arises from transverse cervical artery which is a branch of the first part of subclavian artery.
  - Pedicle of supraclavicular artery flap lies in the posterior triangle of the neck which is bounded anteriorly by the posterior border of sternocleidomastoid, posteriorly by anterior border of trapezius, and inferiorly by the clavicle (**Fig. 2.11**).
  - Flap can reach distant sites due to a 20-cm-long subcutaneous pedicle.

Q26. What are the free flaps used in PBC neck?

Free flaps used for skin resurfacing in PBC neck are:

- Radial artery.
- Groin flap.
- Anterolateral thigh flap.

Key aspects of free radial artery forearm flap:

- It is a Type C fasciocutaneous flap.
- Allen test should be performed to confirm the presence and patency of an intact ulnar artery and complete superficial or deep arch or both.
- **Vascular basis of the flap:**
  - Brachial artery divides into its two terminal branches, the radial and ulnar arteries approximately 2.2 cm inferior to the transverse crease of the elbow.
  - Radial artery courses between the extensor and flexor groups of muscles in the lateral intermuscular septum.
  - Proximally it lies between the supinator muscle and the fibrous origin of flexor digitorum sublimis muscle. In the medial one-third of the forearm, it lies anterior to the pronator teres muscle. Distally, it courses anterior to the flexor pollicis longus muscle.
  - Throughout the proximal two-thirds of its course, it lies posterior to the fleshy belly of the brachioradialis muscle.
- **Points to remember:**
  - Average flap dimensions are 10 to 12 cm in width and 20 to 30 cm in length (two-thirds of forearm).
  - If lengthy pedicle is required, the flap is positioned distally.
  - Proximal positioning is useful if the recipient pedicle is of suitable length.
  - Flap is designed so that its lateral one-third is located lateral to the course of the radial artery (**Fig. 2.12**).
- **Advantages:**
  - There is an infrequent occurrence of atherosclerosis in the radial artery.
  - Donor flap can be dissected under regional anesthesia with tourniquet control.
  - There is limited immobilization and operative pain.
  - Vascular pedicle is lengthy and of large external diameter (2.5–3.5 mm).

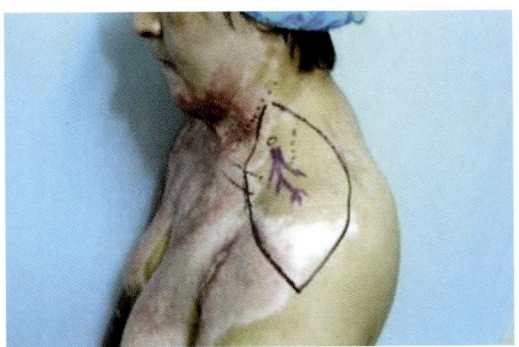

Fig. 2.11 Marking of supraclavicular artery flap.

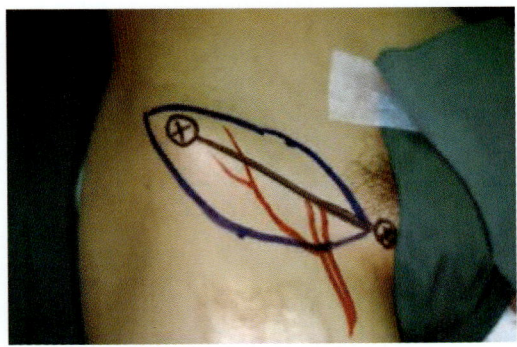

Fig. 2.12 Marking of free groin flap.

- Two teams can operate simultaneously.
- Forearm skin is thin, pliable, and relatively hairless.
- **Disadvantages:**
  - There is conspicuous donor deformity of the forearm.
  - A dominant forearm artery is sacrificed.
  - The graft taken at the distal forearm is less than in the central or proximal forearm because of the superficially located tendons.

Key aspects of free groin flap:
- First free flap to be described in PBC neck.
- Dimensions of flap are 10 cm wide and 25 cm long. The length can be increased with distal delay (distal 10–12 cm random).
- **Vascular basis of the flap:**
  - Superficial circumflex iliac artery (SCIA) is a direct cutaneous artery.
  - Arises from femoral artery. The SCIA arises 2.5 cm inferior to the inguinal ligament.
  - The pedicle length before branching into a superficial and deep branch is 1.5 cm.
- **Markings (Fig.2.12):**
  - Femoral artery is palpated. Medially femoral vein is outlined. A line is drawn from anterior superior iliac spine (ASIS) to the pubic tubercle indicating the inguinal ligament.
  - The origin of SCIA 2.5 cm inferior to the inguinal ligament on the femoral artery is identified.

- Margins of the flap are outlined.
  - Medially, over the femoral vessels.
  - Laterally, 8 to 10 cm from the ASIS.
  - Superiorly, 2 to 3 cm parallel to the inguinal ligament.
  - Inferiorly, 7 to 8 cm parallel to the inguinal ligament.
- **Advantages:**
  - There is concealment of the donor deformity.
  - Can close the donor site primarily.
  - This is a cutaneous flap of large dimension (length can be extended with delay); width extension requires closure of the donor site with STSG.
  - This is a non-hair-bearing flap.
- **Disadvantages:**
  - There is a short arterial pedicle.
  - The arterial anatomy is variable.
  - The artery has a small external diameter (0.8–1.8 mm).
  - An interpositional vein or artery graft is frequently required.
  - Anesthesia in the lateral cutaneous nerve distribution is common.
  - There is a poor color match at the recipient site.

Suggested reading

1. Textbook of Plastic, Reconstructive, and Aesthetic Surgery Volume 5: Burns. Thieme; 2020.

3 Carcinoma Oral Cavity

Veena K. Singh

Learning Objectives

At the end of this chapter, the students will be able to:
1. Describe the clinical presentation of patients with carcinoma oral cavity.
2. Demonstrate the examination of a patient with malignant growth/ulcer.
3. Recall the various management strategies according to site and stage of carcinoma oral cavity.
4. Demonstrate the steps in surgical reconstruction—excision, calculation of defect, and planning of flap.
5. Demonstrate the standard markings of various flap options.

Introduction

Ninety percent of all head and neck carcinomas are squamous cell in origin. Advances in reconstructive strategies using micro- and super-microvascular techniques have enabled the plastic surgeons to reconstruct any possible defect in a single stage. A sound clinical examination and critical assessment of the defect created after ablative procedures provides a strong foundation for functional and aesthetic outcomes.

Chief Complaints

- Ulcer over the tongue/anywhere inside the mouth (location and duration in terms of patient language).
- Growth/swelling over the cheek or inside the mouth.
- Swelling in the neck.
- Pain over ulcer/growth/swelling.
- Loose tooth.

History of Present Illness

- Onset: Whether sudden/insidious.
- How did the patient notice it?
- Progression: Increase in size (sudden/gradual). Any recent increase in size and also change in color, discharge, fungation, bleeding, smell, etc.
- In case of loose tooth, any consultation with a dentist or any history of extraction of tooth or denture use or ear ache (ill-fitting denture may lead to chronic inflammation and an ulcer).
- Pain: The lesion may be initially painless but as the size increases and ulcer develops, there may be associated intermittent/persistent, mild/moderate/severe, dull aching pain over the ulcer. Pain may also increase during eating and speaking if ulcer is around the areas of upper and lower lip. Requirement of medication must also be asked as it indicates the severity of pain.
- Bleeding: May be associated with the ulcer, spontaneous or on trivial trauma like scratching.
- History of consultation/intake of homeopathic medicines.
- Any history of biopsy from the lesion.
- History of excessive salivation.
- History of pain on chewing food or neck pain.

- History of difficulty in swallowing food.
- History of fever (due to infection in the ulcer or growth) or bad smell of the breath (due to tumor necrosis).
- History of alteration in speech: Patient with ulcer over the lips finds difficulty in speaking loudly as the air passes over the ulcer making it painful, and in cases of large ulcer, there may be escape of air.
- History of neck swelling if any.
- History of restricted mouth opening.
- History of sleep/appetite/weight loss/ recent loosening of clothes.
- History of bladder and bowel function.

Negative History

- History of chest pain/hemoptysis/ breathlessness.
- History of bony pain.
- History of convulsion/severe headache/ nausea.

Past History

Refer to chapter on "Basal Cell Carcinoma. (Chapter 15)"

Personal History

- Refer to chapter on "Lower Leg Defect." (Chapter 1)
- Socioeconomic status (bidi/cigarette).
- Tobacco: Whether smoker/gutkha/pan/ betelnut chewer, or tobacco user in any other form. How much tobacco consumption per day? Whether having habit of reverse smoking?
- Alcohol intake: What alcohol, how much, frequency of intake, for how many years.

Family History

Refer to chapter on "Lower Leg Defect." (Chapter 1)

Treatment History

- Any treatment for the present ulcer/swelling/growth or whether intake of homeopathic/ayurvedic medication.

History of Allergy

To food or medications.

General Physical Examinations

- Level of consciousness: Whether oriented to time, place, and person.
- Whether cooperative/irritable.
- Build: The bony stature of the patient (whether small/medium/tall build).
- Nutrition: Look whether cancer cachexia is present or not, if patient looks malnourished.
- Decubitus.
- Facies: Any obvious deformity or evidence of facial nerve palsy or facial distortion due to pain.
- Pallor: Carefully look for pallor as a patient with malignancy may be pale due to anorexia.
- Cyanosis: Look for it as patient might have respiratory distress due to chronic obstructive pulmonary disorder (COPD) (in chronic smokers) leading to cyanosis.
- Jaundice: May be present in cases of extensive liver metastasis or alcoholic liver disease.
- Clubbing: May be present if the patient is having concomitant COPD due to smoking.
- Pedal edema.
- Pulse rate/min, rhythm, volume, any irregularity.
- Blood pressure (BP): Must be measured as many of these patients may be hypertensive.
- Respiration: Rate/min rhythm, thoracoabdominal.
- Body temperature: Patient might have fever due to superadded infection.

- Neck veins: Look for external jugular and internal jugular veins, if they are engorged.
- Neck nodes: In details (refer to chapter on "BCC"). (Chapter 15)
- Any other deformity/scar elsewhere in the body.
- Any skin abnormality/similar lesions in the body.

Systemic Examination

- Abdomen: Feel of the abdomen is soft.
  - No organomegaly felt.

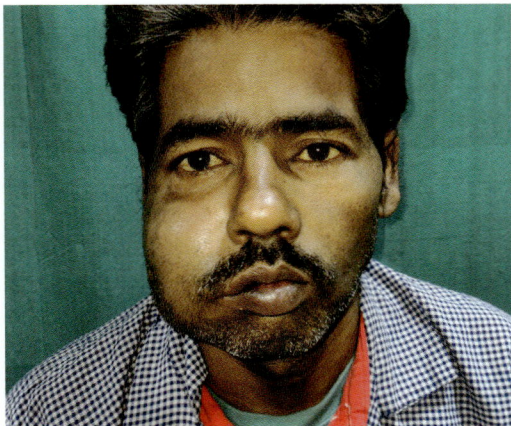

Fig. 3.1   Facial bulge in a case of CA buccal mucosa.

- CNS: Orientation and consciousness.
- CVS: Apex beat location.
  - S_1S_2: Audible.
  - No murmur or any other added sound.
- Respiratory system: Breath sounds.
  - Whether bronchial or vesicular type.
  - Whether bilateral.
  - Air entry is equal.

Local Examination

Inspection

1. Facial symmetry:
   - Affected side must be compared to the other side.
     - If any bulge seen (in CA buccal mucosa/gingivobuccal sulcus), it may be mentioned in detail (**Fig. 3.1**).
2. Lips: Whether black staining due to smoking present.
3. Intraoral examination:
   - Mouth opening: Interincisal distance (in cm) (**Fig. 3.2**).
     - How many finger-breadths wide (patient's fingers to be used).
   - Halitosis: Whether present or not.
   - Dental hygiene: Whether tobacco staining on teeth/presence of caries (**Fig. 3.3**).

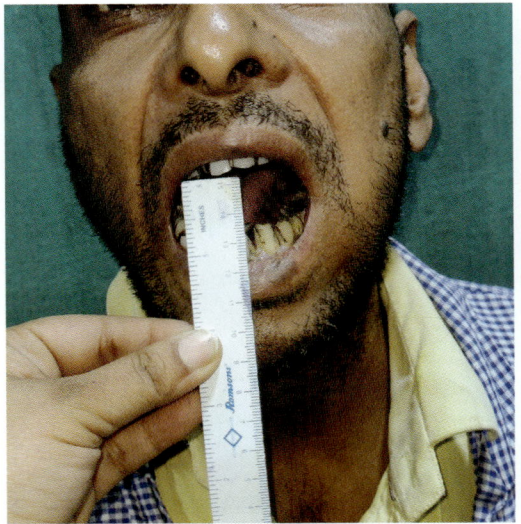

Fig. 3.2   Measurement of interincisal distance.

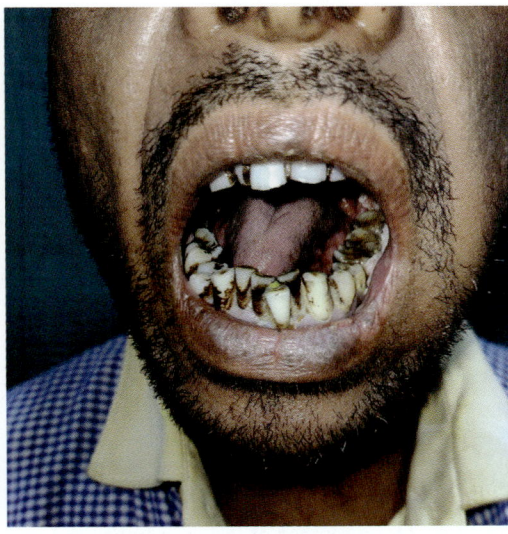

Fig. 3.3   Tobacco staining on teeth/presence of caries.

- Dentition: Whether edentulous/partially.
  - Write the dental formula for the patient.

$$\frac{\times 7\,6\,5\,4\,3\,2\,1 \mid \times 2\,3\,4\,5 \times\times\times}{8\,7\,6\,5\,4 \times\times\times \mid \times\times 3\,4\,5\,6\,7\,8}$$

  (The above is an example in a partially edentulous patient.)

- Ulcer:
  1. Extent: Inferior and superior extent should be in terms of lower and upper jaw teeth-
     - Anterior and posterior extent should be in terms of distance from midline and retromolar trigone, respectively.
  2. Size: Approximate size in cm; both in horizontal and vertical dimensions.
  3. Color: Reddish, yellowish, or blackish.
  4. Margins: Whether regular or irregular.
  5. Surface/Floor: Covered with granulation tissue/necrotic tissue/blood clot.
  6. Discharge: If any.
  7. Whether similar lesions present in the oral cavity.
  8. Condition of oral cavity mucosa.
     - Location of parotid duct (Stenson's duct) opening (normally, it opens opposite the maxillary second molar).

- Look at the tonsillar fossa and the posterior aspect of tongue.

Palpation

Always do a digital palpation with a gloved hand.

1. Temperature: Must be compared to the normal area.
2. Tenderness.
3. Whether bleeds on touch.
4. Other inspectory findings to be corroborated.
5. Exact size must be measured with a scale—in both vertical and horizontal dimensions (**Fig. 3.4**).
6. Fixity to skin: Check it by pinching the overlying skin and trying to lift it up from underlying lesion (**Fig. 3.5**).
7. Base of the ulcer: Whether induration present/not.
8. Look for the movement of tongue: Whether freely mobile or restricted.
9. Bimanual palpation: Is done using index fingers of both hands, one finger inside the mouth and other finger on the skin. It is done to assess the lesions in the floor of mouth (**Fig. 3.6**).
10. Fixity to the underlying bone (mandible/maxilla) is checked by holding the lesion

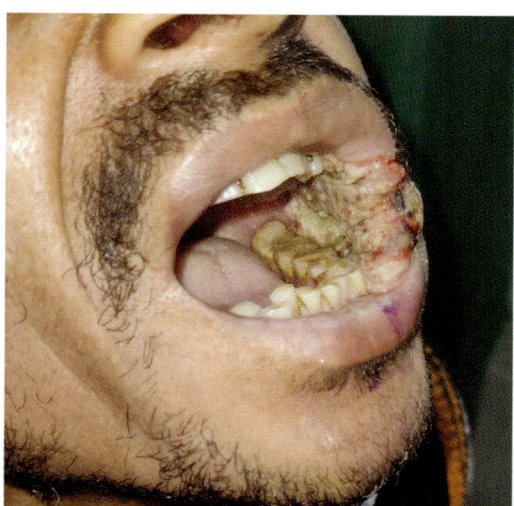

Fig. 3.4 Measurement of lesion in horizontal and vertical dimensions.

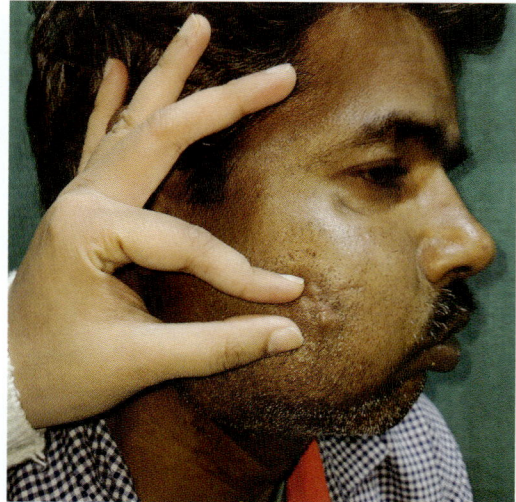

Fig. 3.5 Checking of fixity of overlying skin from the underlying lesion.

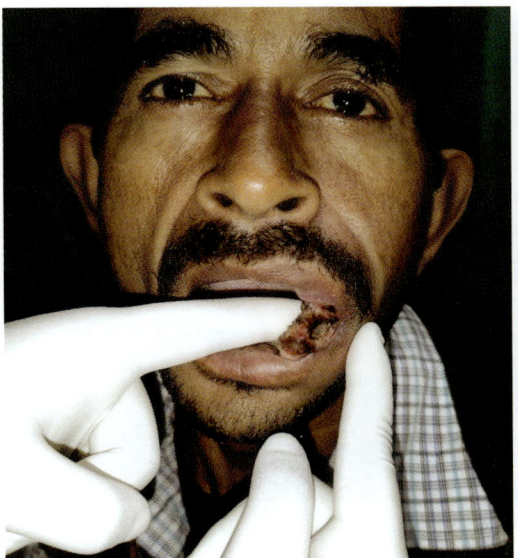

Fig. 3.6 Bimanual palpation of the lesion.

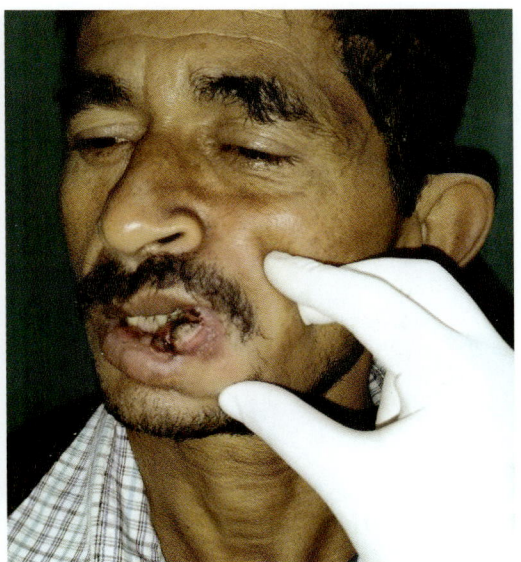

Fig. 3.7 Checking the fixity of lesion to the underlying bone.

between thumb, index, and middle fingers and try to move it over the bone (**Fig. 3.7**).

11. Lower lip sensation:
- Due to extension of lesion in the floor of mouth or gingivobuccal sulcus up to the mental nerve leading to anesthesia of the lower lip.
- It indicates bony involvement.

Measurements

Calculation of Soft Tissue Defect (Fig. 3.8)

- First mark the margins of the lesion, then mark the induration on all sides.
- Add the measurement (1 cm) for wide local excision to calculate the soft tissue defect and accordingly requirement of flap.
- Get the dimensions of the excision in both horizontal and vertical planes.

  For example:
  - Size of the lesion = 5 cm × 3 cm induration = 0.5 cm on all sides.
  - Size of the lesion after adding the induration:

- Horizontal dimension: 5 cm + 0.5 × 2 = 6 cm.
- Vertical dimension: 3 cm + 0.5 × 2 = 4 cm.
- 1-cm-wide margin is added for macroscopic clearance of the tumor.
- Size of the defect:
  - Horizontal: 6 cm + 1 cm × 2 (on both sides) = 8 cm.
  - Vertical 4 cm + 1 cm × 2 (on both sides) = 6 cm.
- So, final defect size = soft tissue requirement = 8 cm × 6 cm.
- The calculation is similar on both skin and mucosal side so defect should be calculated separately for both.
- If reconstruction of both skin (covering) and mucosa (lining) is required then add 1 cm extra to the total soft tissue requirement for folding of the flap, if reconstruction is planned by a single flap.

Calculation of Bone Defect

- Length of involvement of bone + 1 cm × 2 (1-cm-wide margin on both sides).

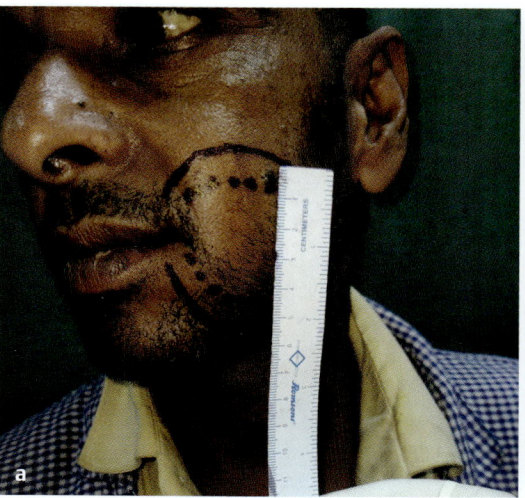
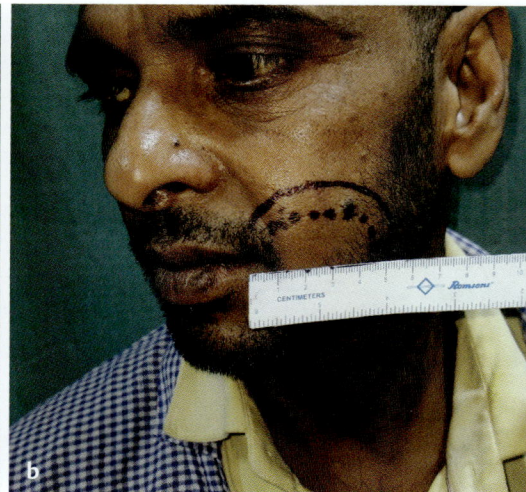

Fig. 3.8 (a, b) Markings for the calculation of the soft tissue defect.

- Add 1 cm to the total bone requirement for every osteotomy.
  For example:
  - Involvement of ramus and body of mandible = 3 cm + 4 cm = 7 cm.
  - Total bone defect = 7 cm + 1 cm × 2 = 9 cm.
  - One osteotomy for angle is required = 1 cm.
  - So, total bone requirement = 9 cm + 1 cm = 10 cm.

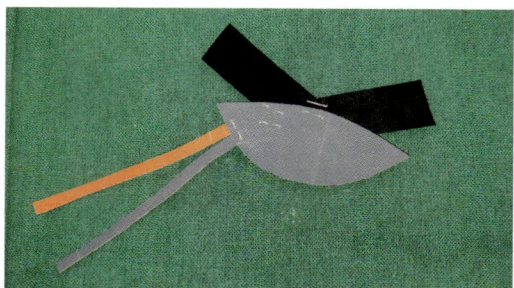

Fig. 3.9 Preparation of a flap template.

Pedicle Length

- Mark the facial artery and vein (preferred vessels for anastomosis) at middle of body of the mandible.

↓

- Imagine the orientation of the flap so that vascular pedicle lies as much close to facial vessels as possible.

↓

- Measure the length of the pedicle required in the flap but pedicle length is harvested to its maximum and safer length so the anastomosis can be done to the superior thyroid vessels also, in case it is required.

Preparation of the Flap Template

- For demonstrating the requirement of soft tissue + bone + pedicle length.
  - For soft tissue, a lint piece is used.
  - For bone, an unusable X-ray is used.
  - For pedicle, part of lint piece is only used.
- Combine all three as a real composite flap would look like (**Fig. 3.9**).
- For any CA oral cavity, always plan a flap with and without bone and accordingly two templates need to be prepared.

Note: In a case, always mark margins of excision (including induration), flap markings (with template prepared), course of facial artery and external jugular vein.

Provisional Diagnosis

It is a case of carcinoma gingivobuccal sulcus (GBS)/cheek/tongue/buccal mucosa/lower lip most likely to be squamous cell carcinoma (SCC) stage T3NoMo.

Questions

Q1. How will you proceed?

I would like to first confirm my diagnosis.

- **Confirmation of diagnosis:** If biopsy has not been done previously, then go for a punch biopsy to confirm the diagnosis.
- **Radiological investigations to see the extent of bony involvement, if any:**
  - Orthopantomogram (OPG) especially in tumors of floor of mouth/GBS to see anterior mandible.
    - Widened mental foramen indicates tumor involvement of nerve and bone.
    - OPG is not helpful in detecting the initial involvement of bone because at least 50% of calcified component of bone must be lost before any changes are seen in OPG.
  - Computed tomography (CT) face + neck (**Fig. 3.10**).
  - Magnetic resonance imaging (MRI) with gadolinium enhancement to see the invasion of posterior tongue by an invasive tumor.
- **Metastatic work-up:**
  - Chest X-ray (CXR)—Posteroanterior (PA) view to exclude second primary or distant metastasis in lung and other site-specific X-rays in case of bony pain.
  - USG abdomen + liver function tests.
  - In case of any doubt on CXR or USG, a CT with contrast or MRI is indicated.
  - A bronchoscopy may also be needed to see the invasion of posterior tongue by an invasive tumor.

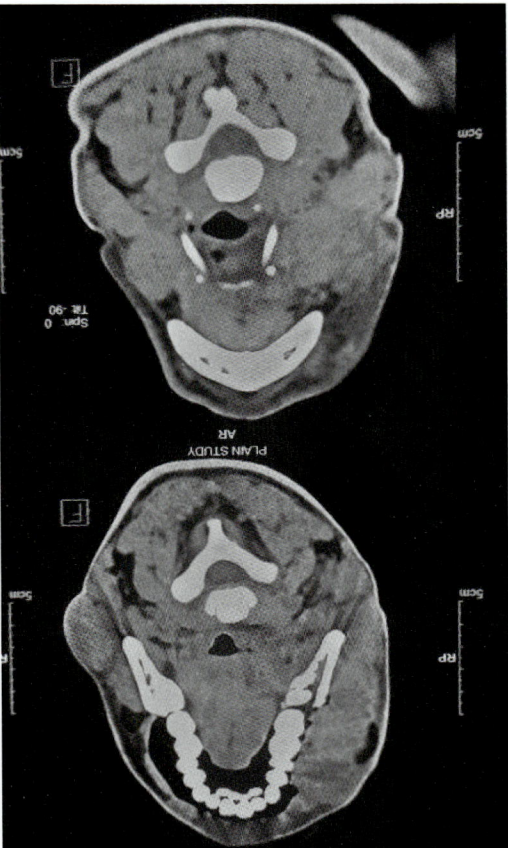

Fig. 3.10 Computed tomography (CT) scan of face in a patient with mandibular involvement.

- **Baseline and other investigations for preanesthetic fitness:**
  - Complete blood count, prothrombin time/international normalized ratio (PT/INR).
  - KFT, S. electrolytes, blood sugar.
  - Electrocardiogram (ECG) in 12 leads.
  - Echocardiography if any complaints related to heart and a cardiology opinion.
  - Dental evaluation.
- **Surgical plan:**
  - Wide local excision (WLE) ± segmental/hemi-mandibulectomy neck dissection (depends on the "N" stage) ± reconstruction.

– The choice of the flap depends upon the location of ulcer/growth, tumor staging, and involvement of bone.

- **If only soft tissue involvement:**

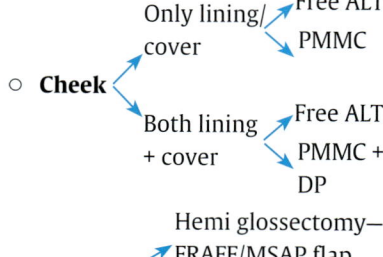

○ **Cheek**
- Only lining/cover → Free ALT / PMMC
- Both lining + cover → Free ALT / PMMC + DP

○ **Tongue**
- Hemi glossectomy— FRAFF/MSAP flap
- Total glossectomy— Free ALT

○ **Lower lip**: Free radial artery forearm flap/Anterolateral thigh (FRAFF/ALT).
○ **Palate**: FRAFF/MSAP (medial sural artery perforator) flap.
○ **Floor of mouth**/Gingivobuccal sulcus:
  i. FRAFF/MSAP flap.
  ii. If concomitant bony involvement, then free fibula osteocutaneous (FFOC) flap.

- **If mandible/maxilla involvement:**
  ○ Bony reconstruction with FFOC flap.
- **Neck nodes involvement:** Mentioned in detail later in the chapter.

Q2. How do you perform a tumor biopsy?

- Punch biopsy is the preferred technique.
- Specimen includes a piece of tissue containing the tumor and should not contain a larger amount of necrosis.
- The biopsy is always done under local anesthesia.
- The pathologist will then evaluate the depth (thickness) of the tumor along with the tumor-host interface.
- A biopsy is always preferred over fine-needle aspiration cytology (FNAC) because of the above-mentioned reasons.

Q3. What are the other techniques of biopsy?

- **Wedge biopsy:**
  - Generally taken in a nonhealing ulcer where a wedge of tissue is removed including the ulcer part and normal skin.
  - It can be performed as four-quadrant biopsy to exclude malignant changes at all margins of a nonhealing ulcer.
- **Incisional biopsy:**
  - Includes tissue from the periphery of the lesion.
  - Wedge biopsy is also one type of incisional biopsy.
- **Excisional biopsy:**
  - In small lesions or highly suspicious lesion, it can be done to minimize the waiting time for report to be available.
- **Shave biopsy:**
  - Tangential biopsy from a skin lesion.
  - A razor-blade-like instrument is used for the same.
- **Needle biopsy:**
  - Includes FNAC.
  - Core needle biopsy.
  - Vacuum-assisted biopsy.

Q4. When you will clinically suspect the tumor involvement of mandible?

- Clinical suspicion arises in two situations:
- When there is presence of a loose tooth in the vicinity of a cancerous lesion.
- On palpation of mandible, if bony irregularity is felt.

Q5. What are the signs of a locally advanced tumor?

Stage II to IVA are locally advanced tumors.

Q6. What are the signs of irresectability?

- Neurovascular invasion.
- Involvement of prevertebral fascia.
- Infiltration into trachea, esophagus, or mediastinum.
- Infiltration into skull base or orbit.
- Spreads to dura or brachial plexus.

Q7. How will you test the mobility of a lesion over the tongue?

Ask the patient to protrude the tongue so that the muscles become taut and then try to mobilize the lesion in both anteroposterior and side-to-side directions. If the lesion does not move, it is fixed to the underlying muscles of tongue.

Q8. What are poor prognostic indicators in carcinoma oral cavity?

These include:

- Multiple levels of positive lymph nodes.
- Extracapsular extension of the cancer in a lymph node.
- Deep invasion of the primary tumor.
- Neurovascular invasion.
- Tumor margins clearance <5 mm.

Q9. Why do patients of carcinoma tongue complaint of earache/otalgia?

This is a referred pain carried by auriculotemporal nerve due to infiltration of cancer cells into the lingual nerve.

Q10. Why there is drooling of saliva in carcinoma tongue?

Drooling of saliva is due to excessive salivation either due to irritation caused by lesion in the tongue or inability to swallow the saliva due to infiltration into the floor of the mouth.

Q11. What are modes of spread of head and neck malignancies?

- Squamous cell carcinoma is the most common type of cancer of the lip, oral, and oropharynx.
- Other types present are primary tumors of minor salivary glands, lymphoma, sarcoma, and melanoma.
- **Modes of spread:**
  - **Local extension:** SCC presents in one of three ways:
    - Superficial exophytic.
    - Infiltrating spread along the mucosal surface.
    - Ulcerating—invades early producing an "Iceberg" effect.
      - Ulcerating fungating tumors metastasize earlier.

- **Regional metastasis:**
  - Oral cavity cancers initially drain into submental and supraomohyoid nodes (Zone I) then to upper deep jugular chain (Zone II and III).
  - B/L nodal involvement is seen in patients with large tumors that cross midline and also in tumors originating from midline (e.g., floor of mouth).
  - The location of the tumor also dictates the spread in L.N.:
    - Invasive T1 and T2 of tongue will spread early to L.N. as compared to same stage lip cancers.
  - In oropharynx, primary drainage site is to jugulodigastric (Level II) L.N.
- **Distant metastasis:**
  - Cancer of lip, and oral cavity or oropharynx do not present as metastatic lesion below the clavicle. The chances of such a tumor to be a secondary primary one is more likely.
  - The most distant site is lung.
  - The treatment of two synchronous primary has a better prognosis as compared to treatment of primary tumor with a distant metastasis.

Q12. How does lymphatic spread take place?

The lymphatic spread to different chains of lymph nodes varies according to the anatomic site of the primary tumor.

Cervical lymph nodes:

- Tumor cells spread via lymphatic channels to reach the regional nodes which in turn begin to replace the lymph nodes.
- The nodes enlarge because of:
  - Reactive response to the cancer cells.
  - Reactive response to the bacteria in the oral cavity that invade the tumor ulcer to cause a local infection.
  - Tumor replacement of the lymph node parenchyma.
- L.N. need to enlarge at least 1 cm in size before they can be clinically detectable.
- 1-cm node is completely replaced by cancer harbors 109 tumor cells.

- When an L.N. is fixed, it represents the continued growth of the tumor within the lymph node which has broken through the capsule and grown into and become attached to the adjacent structures.

Q13. How will the lymphatic spread from tongue cancers take place?

- Tip into submental (1a) lymph nodes on either side.
- Anterior two-thirds: into submandibular (Ib), jugulodigastric (II), and jugulo-omo-hyoid (III).
  - Usually, level I, II, and III nodes are involved in carcinoma tongue which require supraomohyoid neck dissection.

Q14. How will the lymphatic spread from carcinoma lip take place?

- Lower lip: into level Ia, Ib, and II nodes.
- Upper lip: into preauricular Ib and II nodes.
- Commissure: to all nodes draining upper and lower lip.

Q15. What is TNM staging?

- **Primary Tumor (T):**
  - TX: Primary tumor cannot be assessed.
  - T0: No evidence of primary tumor.
  - Tis: Carcinoma in situ.
  - T1: Tumor 2 cm or less in greatest dimension.
  - T2: Tumor more than 2 cm but not more than 4 cm in greatest dimension.
  - T3: Tumor more than 4 cm in greatest dimension.
  - T4:
    - **For Lip CA:** Tumor invades the adjacent structure (e.g., through cortical bone, tongue, skin of neck).
    - **For oral cavity and oropharynx:** Tumor invades adjacent structures (e.g., through cortical bone, soft tissues of neck, deep [extrinsic] muscle of tongue).

- **Regional Lymph Nodes (N):**
  - NX: Regional lymph nodes cannot be assessed.
  - N0: No regional lymph node metastasis.
  - N1: Metastasis in a single ipsilateral lymph node, 3 cm or less in greatest dimension.
  - N2: Metastasis in a single ipsilateral lymph node, more than 3 cm but not more than 6 cm in greatest dimension; or in multiple ipsilateral lymph nodes, none more than 6 cm in greatest dimension.
    - N2a: Metastasis in a single ipsilateral lymph node more than 3 cm but not more than 6 cm in greatest dimension.
    - N2b: Metastasis in multiple ipsilateral lymph nodes, none more than 6 cm in greatest dimension.
    - N2c: Metastasis in bilateral or contralateral lymph nodes, none more than 6 cm in greatest dimension.
  - N3: Metastasis in lymph node > 6 cm in greatest dimension.
- **Distant Metastasis (M):**
  - MX: Presence of distant metastasis cannot be assessed.
  - M0: No distant metastasis.
  - M1: Distant metastasis.

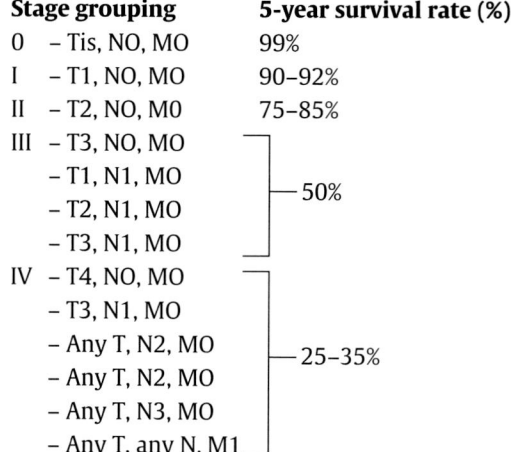

Stage grouping	5-year survival rate (%)
0 – Tis, N0, M0	99%
I – T1, N0, M0	90–92%
II – T2, N0, M0	75–85%
III – T3, N0, M0	
– T1, N1, M0	
– T2, N1, M0	50%
– T3, N1, M0	
IV – T4, N0, M0	
– T3, N1, M0	
– Any T, N2, M0	
– Any T, N2, M0	25–35%
– Any T, N3, M0	
– Any T, any N, M1	

Q16. What is the management approach to tumors of oral cavity?

- Multimodal approach is used:
  - Surgery alone.
  - Radiation therapy alone.
  - Surgery combined with postoperative radiation therapy.

- The third option is used by most of the head and neck surgeons when there are poor prognostic indicators.
  - Multiple levels of positive lymph nodes.
  - Extracapsular extension of the cancer in lymph node.
  - Deep invasion of the primary tumor.
  - Neural and vascular invasion.
  - Tumor margins less than 5 mm.

Q17. What is the treatment protocol according to clinical staging?

The treatment algorithm for cancer of the oral cavity is as shown in **Flowchart 3.1**:

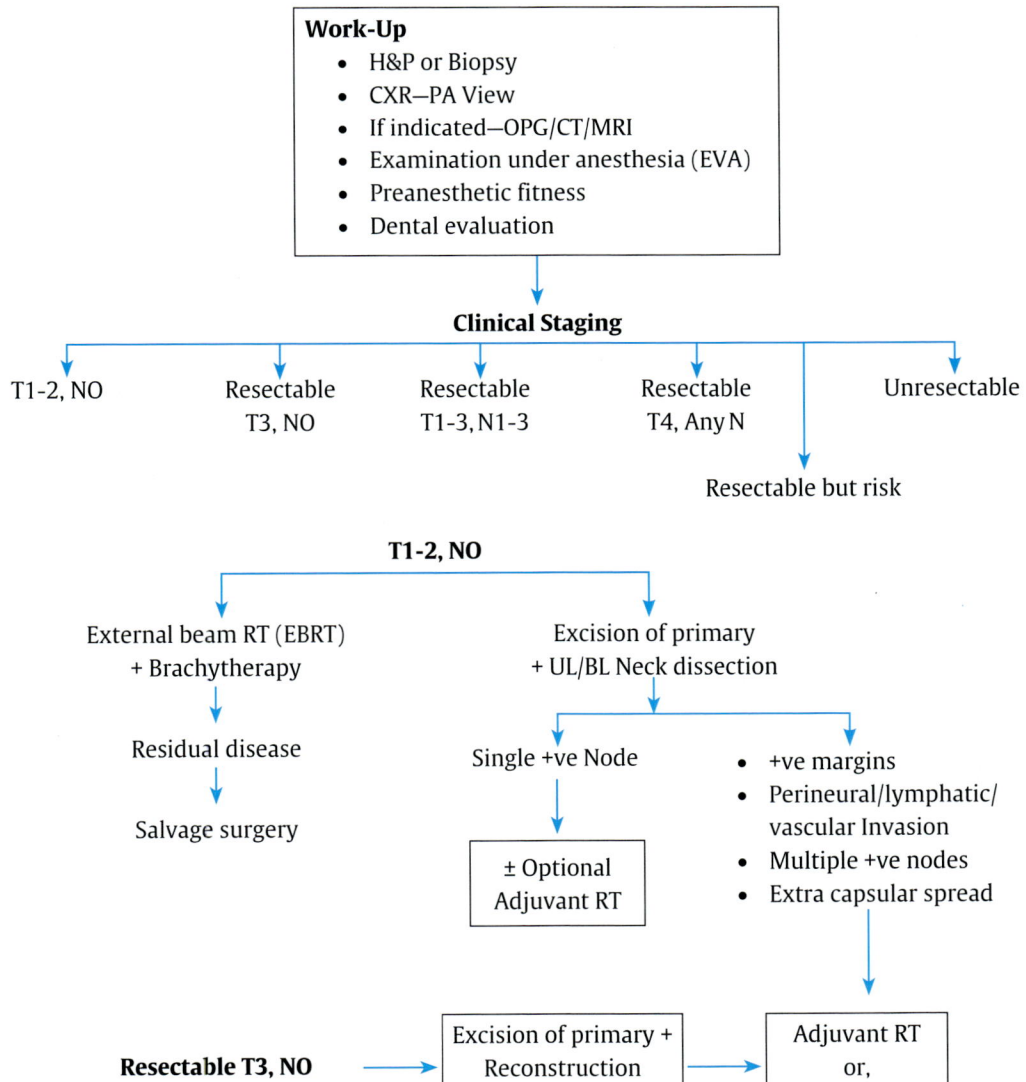

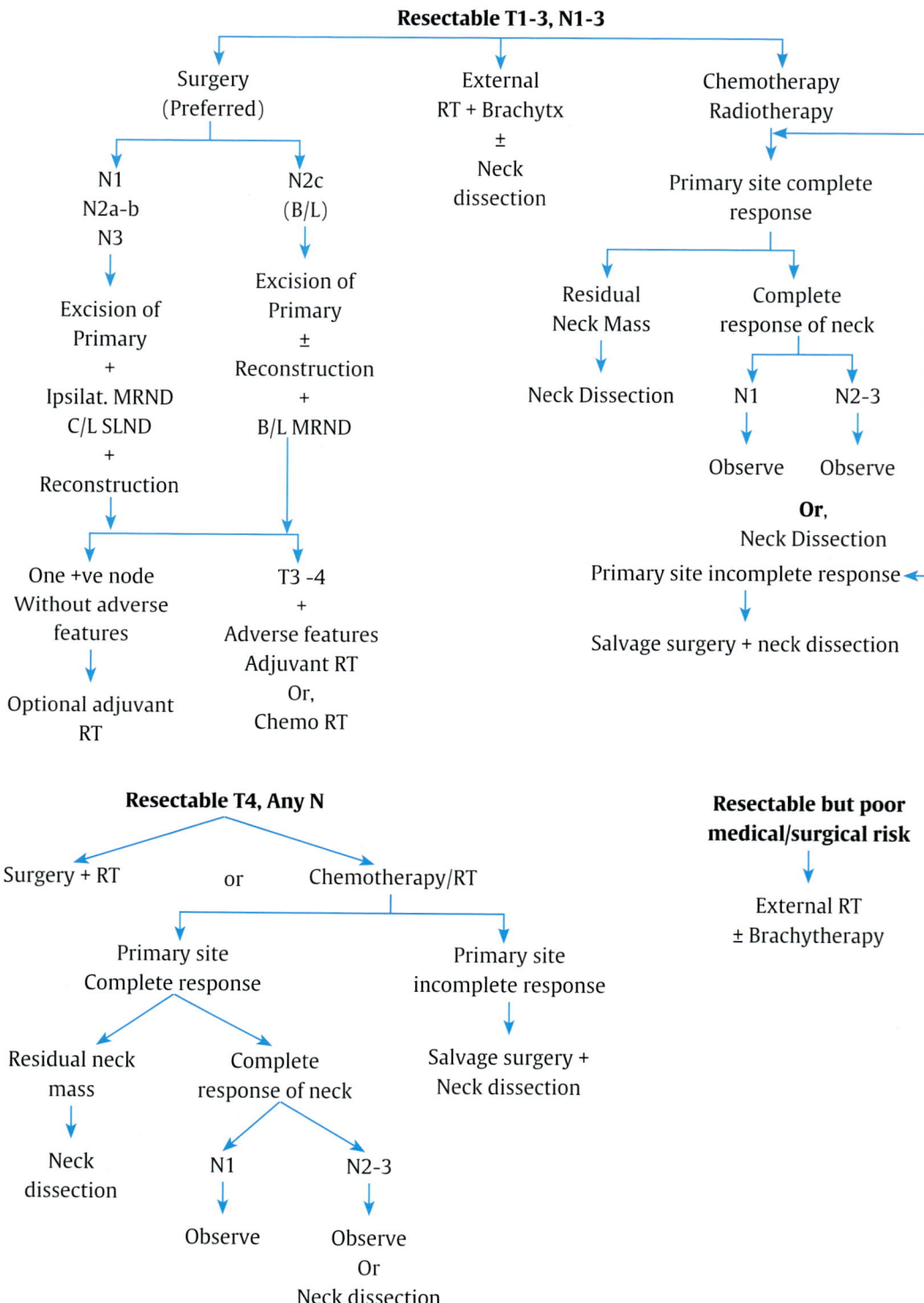

Flowchart 3.1 Treatment algorithm for cancer of oral cavity.

Follow-up:

- Physical exam: Every 1 to 3 months in Year 1.

  Every 2 to 4 months in Year 2.

  Every 4 to 6 months in Year 3 to 5.

  Every 6 to 12 months in >Year 5.

- Chest imaging annually or earlier if indicated.
- Thyroid-stimulating hormone (TSH) test every 6 to 12 months in case of neck radiotherapy.

Q18. What are the surgical approaches to site-specific tumors?

Resections can be done by the following surgical approaches:

- Transoral.
- Mandible sparing (pull-through).
- Mandibulectomy.
- Composite resection (including mandible and associated neck dissection).
- **Transoral resection:**
  - Is used for easily accessible and smaller lesions.
  - Such location may include:
    - Anterior and superficial lesions of floor of mouth.
    - Anterior two-thirds of tongue.
    - Buccal mucosa.
    - Palate.
  - Lesions are T1 or early T2 exophytic.
  - One variation is resection of upper half of the mandible as a marginal mandibulectomy (no reconstruction is usually required).
- **Mandible sparing (pull-through procedure):**
  - Ideal for moderate-size lesions on anterior and lateral floor of mouth.
  - Maintains the contour of mandible.
  - Defect is usually reconstructed with a free flap.

- **Mandibulectomy:**
  - For large tumor of posterior oral cavity or oropharynx when there is no bone involvement.
  - Known as mandibular swing as the mandible is divided lateral to midline (anterior to mental foramen) after doing predrilled holes for fixing the mandible later.
  - It is the most common approach for lesion over retromolar trigone, base of the tongue, tonsil, and lateral pharyngeal wall.
- **Composite resection with mandibulectomy:**
  - When mandible is also involved by the tumor, it is removed as a full-thickness, segmental mandibulectomy.
  - Reconstruction of both bone and soft tissue is important.

Q19. What are the principles of reconstruction?

The principles of cancer reconstruction are:

- Tissue used for reconstruction should not compromise the ablative surgery.
- The standard time is immediate reconstruction in the same sitting.
- Reconstructive procedures should not add to the morbidity of ablative surgery.
- Replace "like tissue with like tissue."
- The reconstruction must be tailored to the patients' need.

Q20. How will you manage the neck?

1. Surgical:

- **Types of neck dissection:**
  - **Classic radical neck dissection (RND):**
    - All level of lymph nodes are removed.
    - Sternocleidomastoid (SCM), internal jugular vein (IJV), spinal accessory nerve (SAN), and submandibular salivary gland are all sacrificed.

- **Modified radical neck dissection (MRND):**
  - Either of SCM, JIV, or SAN is preserved.
  - In cases where no palpable L.N. (N0) but still a high (>15%) chance of presence of microscopic disease based on the location of primary tumor.
- **Selective neck dissection:**
  - Only selected level of L.N. on the basis of understanding of the common pathways for spread of head and neck cancers to regional nodes.
- **Comprehensive neck dissection:**
  - Includes all L.N. that are included in a classic neck dissection.
- **Types of selective neck dissection:**
  - Supraomohyoid neck dissection (SOND):
    - Includes level I, II, III, and superior parts of level V.
    - Removes nodes associated with metastasis from oral cavity.
  - Lateral neck dissection:
    - Level II, III, and IV.
    - Removes nodes most commonly involved with cancers of pharynx, oropharynx, and larynx.
  - **Superficial T1, N0**—No prophylactic neck dissection.
    - Very rarely (<10%) risk of spreading to regional nodes.
  - **Invasive T1-2, N0**—Supraomohyoid neck dissection (SOND).
  - **T3-4, N0**—RND on same side.
    - In case a tumor crosses the midline, an SNOD is indicated on the other side.

2. Radiotherapy:

- "N" zero (N0) neck (No Surgery).
  - 50 Gy for 5 to 6 weeks.
  - Early tumors (T1)—66 Gy.
  - Larger tumors (T2 and T3)—70 Gy.

- The fractionation/frequency is once a day for 5 d/wk at 2 Gy/fraction.
- Hyperfractionation—smaller doses two to three times/d.
- Hypofractionation—one large dose every 2 to 3 days.
- Brachytherapy—artificially produced isotopes are placed in implants that are put directly into tumor-bearing tissue.

Q21. What are the skin incisions for neck dissection?

- **Hockey stick** (**Fig. 3.11a**):
  - Vertical limb starts at mastoid process superiorly.
  - Extends toward clavicle inferiorly across the posterior triangle.
  - Superior part of this vertical limb extends across the upper part of sternocleidomastoid (SCM).
  - Lower part lies behind the sternal head of the muscle paralleling its posterior border.
- Inverted hockey stick (**Fig. 3.11b**).
- Modified Schobinger's incision (**Fig. 3.11c**).
- Ariyan incision (posterior neck incision) (**Fig. 3.11d**).
- Lahey's lateral utility incision (**Fig. 3.11e**).
- Apron flap incision (**Fig. 3.11f**).
- Y-incision of Crile (**Fig. 3.11g**).
- Double Y-incision of Martin (**Fig. 3.11h**).
- Conley's incision (**Fig. 3.11i**).
- MacFree double transverse incision (**Fig. 3.11j**).
- "H" incision (**Fig. 3.11k**).

Q22. What are the 6S' of head and neck cancers?

6S' are:
- Smoking.
- Spirit.
- Spices.
- Sharp tooth.
- Sideropenic dysphagia.
- Syphilis.

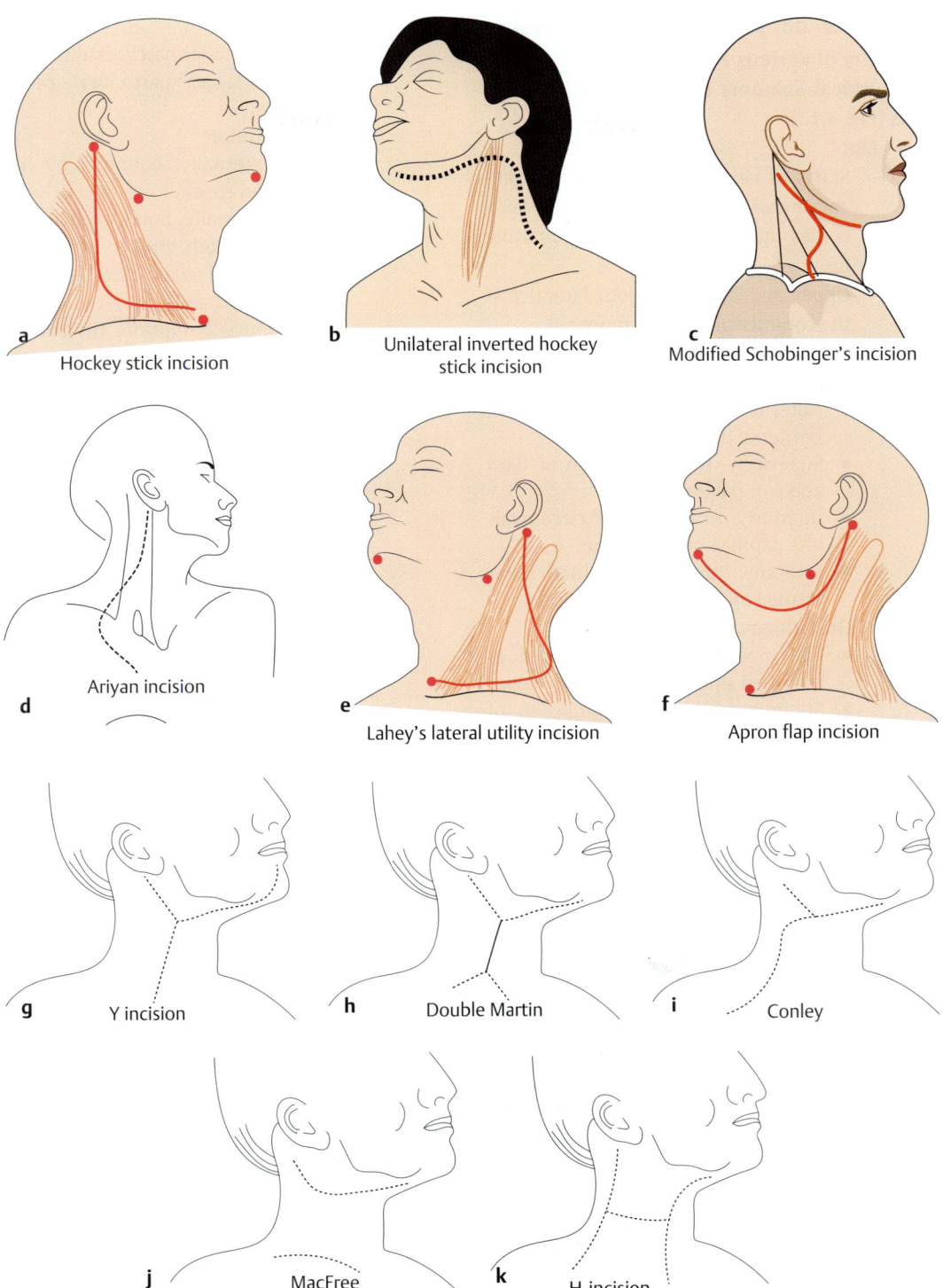

Fig. 3.11 Various incisions for neck dissection. **(a)** Hockey stick. **(b)** Inverted hockey stick. **(c)** Modified Schobinger's incision. **(d)** Ariyan incision (posterior neck incision). **(e)** Lahey's lateral utility incision. **(f)** Apron flap incision. **(g)** Y-incision of Crile. **(h)** Double Y-incision of Martin. **(i)** Conley's incision. **(j)** MacFree double transverse incision. **(k)** H-incision.

Q23. How do you describe the surgical anatomy of various areas?

The surgical anatomy of oral cavity is as follows (Fig. 3.12):

- **Lip:**
    - Starts at vermilion border of the skin and includes that part of the lip which comes into contact with the opposing lip.
    - Upper and lower lips join laterally at the commissures of the mouth.
- **Oral cavity:**
    - **Boundaries:**
        - Anteriorly, extends from vermilion border of lips.
        - Superiorly, to the junction of hard and soft palate.
        - Inferiorly, to the line of circumvallate papillae of the tongue.
        - Laterally, anterior tonsillar pillar formed by palatoglossus muscle.
    - **Oral mucosa:**
        - The oral mucosa is composed of stratified squamous epithelial cells.
        - Submucosal layer is composed of loose fatty connective tissue. It is absent in the areas of hard palate and gingiva.

- It consists of:
    - Outer smaller part: vestibule.
    - Inner larger part: oral cavity proper.
    - **Vestibular:**
        i. Externally, bounded by lips and cheek.
        ii. Internally, bounded by gums and teeth.
        iii. Parotid gland duct/Stenson's duct opens into the buccal mucosa opposite the second upper molar tooth.
        iv. On either side of the maxillary/mandibular arch, alveolar mucosa covers the alveolus bone and fuses with gingival mucosa.
        v. The alveolar mucosa behind the mandibular third molar extends upward along the inner surface of ramus of the mandible making up the area of retromolar trigone. It is continuous with the maxillary tuberosity.
    - **Oral cavity proper:**
        i. Contains lingual gingival and alveolar mucosa, floor of

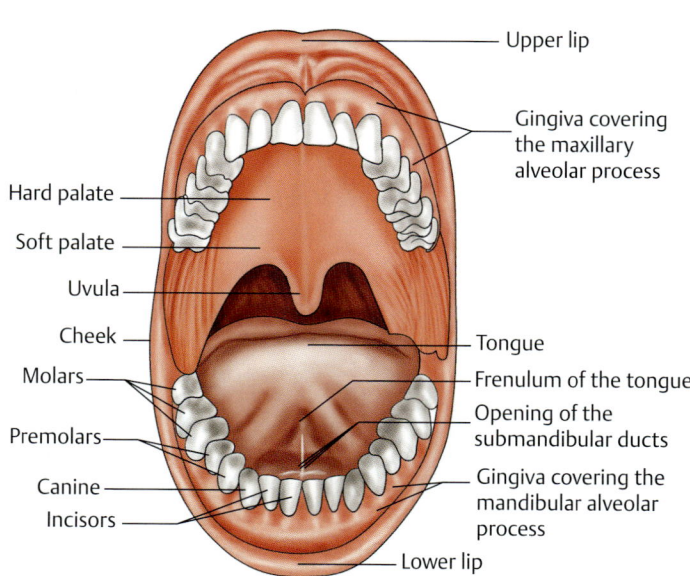

Fig. 3.12 Anatomy of lip and oral cavity.

mouth, oral tongue, and hard palate.

- ○ **Buccal mucosa:**
  - i. Epithelial lining of the inner surface of lips and oral surface of cheeks.
  - ii. Superiorly, line of attachment of mucosa.
  - iii. Inferiorly, alveolar ridge of upper and lower jaws.
  - iv. Posteriorly, attachment at the retromolar trigone (pterygomandibular raphe).
- ○ **Alveolar ridge:**
  - i. Consists of upper (maxillary) and lower (mandibular) osseous alveolar processes.
  - ii. The alveolus supports dentition with its overlying gingiva.
- ○ **Retromolar trigone:**
  - i. Area of the mouth posterior to the last mandibular tooth.
  - ii. Superiorly, apex at the tuberosity of the maxilla.
  - iii. Lateral limit is buccal mucosa.
  - iv. Medial limit is anterior tonsillar pillar.
- ○ **Floor of the mouth:**
  - i. Extends from the inner surface of lower alveolar ridge.
  - ii. Up to the ventral surface of the tongue.
  - iii. Posterior border is the base of the anterior tonsillar pillar.
  - iv. Surface area is divided into halves on either side of the frenulum of tongue.
  - v. Wharton duct (submandibular gland duct) opens at sublingual papilla near the base of lingual frenulum.
- ○ **Hard palate:**
  - i. Upper alveolar anteriorly.
  - ii. Soft palate posteriorly.
  - iii. Lateral alveolar ridges laterally.
- ○ **Oral tongue (Fig. 3.13):**
  - i. The anterior two-thirds of tongue is freely mobile.

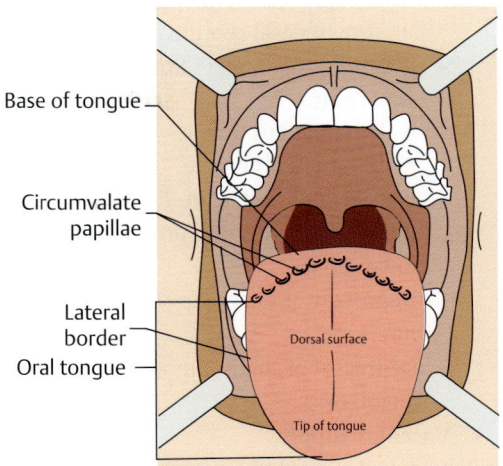

Fig. 3.13   Anatomy of oral tongue.

  - ii. It extends posteriorly to the circumvallate papilla.
  - iii. Inferiorly on each side, to the junction with the floor of the mouth.
  - iv. Tongue is divided longitudinally into two halves by the median sulcus and underlying lingual septum.
  - v. Sulcus terminalis, a V-shaped groove separates the oral tongue from the base of the tongue.
  - vi. Anterior two-thirds is composed of four areas:
    - a. Tip.
    - b. Lateral borders.
    - c. Dorsum.
    - d. Undersurface.
  - vii. Extrinsic muscles include genioglossus, hyoglossus, styloglossus, and palatoglossus.

Q24. What are the anatomical considerations in lip reconstruction?

- • **Muscles:**
  - – The orbicularis oris muscle of lip is composed of:
    - ▪ Horizontal fibers starting at modiolus and inserting into opposite philtral column.

- Oblique fibers run from the commissure to nasal septum and nasal floor.
  - Elevators of upper lip—Levator labii superioris.
    - Zygomaticus major.
    - Levator anguli oris.
  - Elevators of lower lip—Paired mentalis muscle (elevates and protrudes central lower lip).
  - Depressor of lower Lip—Depressor labii inferioris.
  - Depressor of angle of mouth—Depressor anguli oris.
- **Vascular supply:**
  - Facial artery gives superior and inferior labial arteries which run within the orbicularis oris muscle close to the mucosal margin.
- **Lymphatic drainage** to submandibular and submental nodes.
- **Nerve supply:**
  - Motor supply—from buccal branches (supplies orbicularis oris).
  - Sensory supply:

  - Upper lip from infraorbital nerve (V2) branch of trigeminal nerve (V).
  - Lower lip from mentor nerve (V3).

Q25. How will you reconstruct the defects of lip?

Algorithm for reconstruction of lip defects (Algorithm 3.1):

- **Vermilion reconstruction:**
  - **Horizontal loss**—Mucosal apron flap (by Gillies and Millard) in which buccal mucosa of the opposing lip can be used as a donor flap and the donor defect can be skin grafted.
  - **Total vermilionectomy** (lip-shaving procedure):
    - Bipedicled mucosal advancement flap.
    - Tongue flaps.
    - Palatal mucosal full-thickness grafts.
  - **FAMM (facial artery myomucosal flap)** includes buccinator muscle and buccal mucosa based on facial artery,

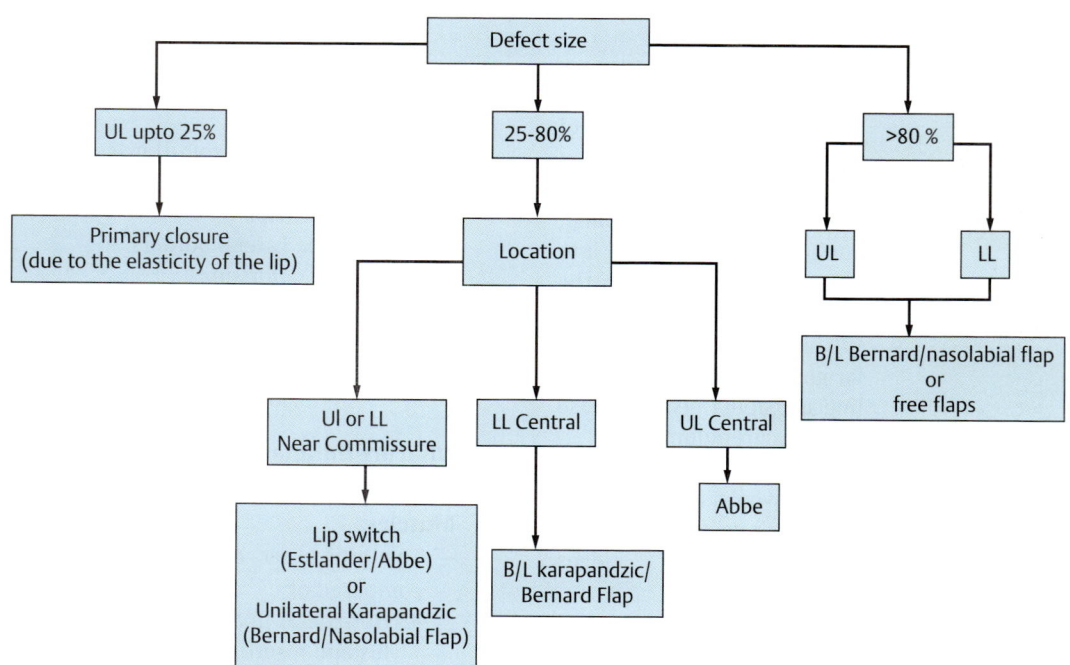

Algorithm 3.1 Algorithm for reconstruction of lip defects.

can be based either superiorly or inferiorly depending upon the location of the defect.

- **Less than 30% horizontal defect:**
  - Johanson staircase technique:
    - Used for central and lateral defects of lower lip.
  - Shuchardt rotation—advancement of cheek and lip tissues.
  - Opposing lip flap (Abbe flap) **(Fig. 3.14)**.
    - For upper lip central defects.
    - For lower lip, lateral part of upper lip is used as donor.
  - Estlander flap **(Fig. 3.15)**:
    - For defects of lateral lower lip.
    - Commissuroplasty is required at a later stage.

- Gillies fan flap (**Fig. 3.16**):
  - Is a combination of rotation at the commissure along with tissues of nasolabial fold
- Karapandzic (**Fig. 3.17**):
  - Mainly for central defects of lower lip.
  - Same as Gillies but leaves the neurovascular supply intact.
  - May be U/L or B/L and causes microstomia.
- **Commissure reconstruction:**
  - May be done by three-flap mucosal advancement and using the upper lip vermilion to reconstruct the commissure.

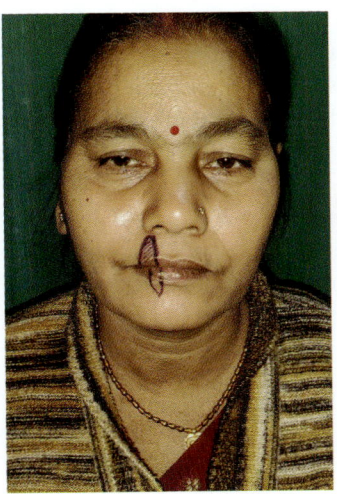
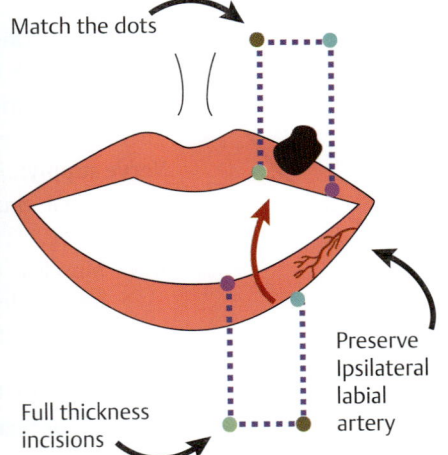

Match the dots

Preserve Ipsilateral labial artery

Full thickness incisions

Fig. 3.14 Abbe flap.

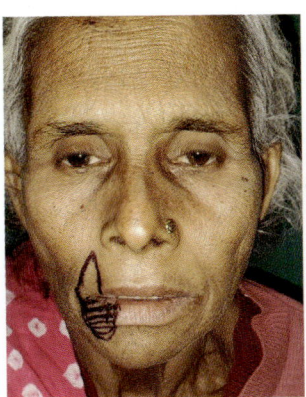
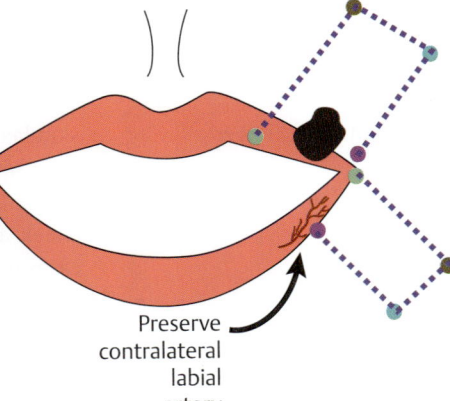

Preserve contralateral labial artery

Fig. 3.15 Estandler flap.

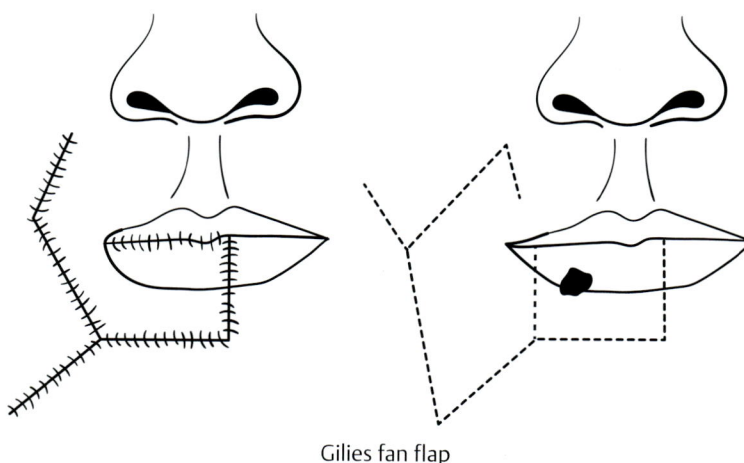

Fig. 3.16 Gillies fan flap.

Gilies fan flap

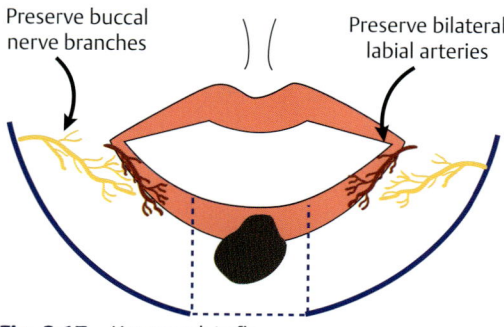

Preserve buccal nerve branches

Preserve bilateral labial arteries

Fig. 3.17 Karapandzic flap.

Vascular supply:
- Branches of external carotid artery: facial artery, superficial temporal artery, and transverse facial artery.

Lymphatic drainage:
- Of cheek is by lymphatic channels within the parotid nodes and along the facial vessels to the submandibular nodes.

Nerve supply:
- Facial muscles are innervated by facial nerve.
- Muscles of mastication, masseter and temporalis muscles are innervated by the trigeminal nerve.

- **Total lip defect:**
  - Bernard.
  - Nasolabial flap.

Q26. What are the anatomical considerations in cheek reconstruction?

Cheek is bounded by:
- Laterally: Preauricular crease.
- Superiorly: Zygomatic arch and lower eyelids.
- Medially: Nasal side-wall and nasolabial fold.
- Inferiorly: Mandibular border.

The cheek is divided into three zones:
- Suborbital.
- Preauricular.
- Buccal mandibular border.

Q27. What are the options for reconstruction of cheek defect?

Algorithm showing reconstructive options for cheek defects (Algorithm 3.2).

Options:
- **Advancement flaps:**
  - Useful for superomedial defects especially in elderly patients with available skin laxity.
  - V-Y advancement flaps are excellent choice for defects along the medial cheek and alar base. Excision in these cases is done as a square or a rectangle.
- **Transposition flaps:**
  - Banner flaps, bilobed flaps, and Limberg flaps are the options in medium-sized defect where skin laxity is present.

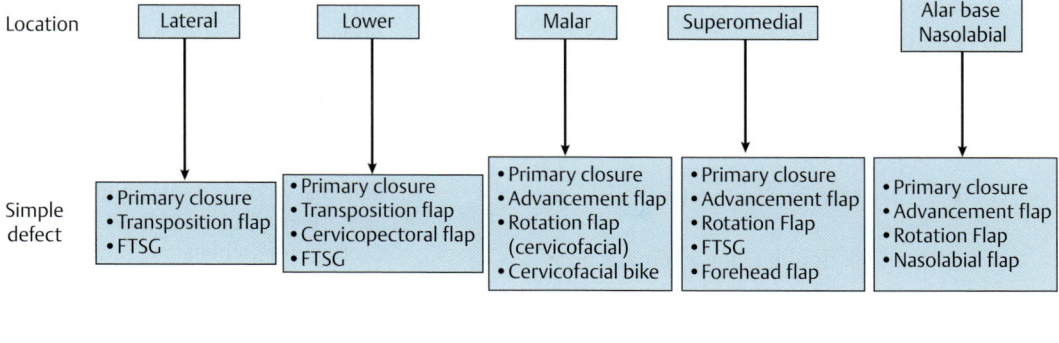

Location	Lateral	Lower	Malar	Superomedial	Alar base Nasolabial
Simple defect	• Primary closure • Transposition flap • FTSG	• Primary closure • Transposition flap • Cervicopectoral flap • FTSG	• Primary closure • Advancement flap • Rotation flap (cervicofacial) • Cervicofacial bike	• Primary closure • Advancement flap • Rotation Flap • FTSG • Forehead flap	• Primary closure • Advancement flap • Rotation Flap • Nasolabial flap
Complex Defect	• Free tissue transfer • Trapezius flap • Pectoralis flap	• Free tissue transfer • Trapezius flap • Pectoralis flap	• Free tissue transfer	• Free tissue transfer	• Free tissue transfer

Algorithm 3.2   Algorithm showing reconstructive options for cheek defects.

– Banner flaps from preauricular or nasolabial area are taken.
– Bilobed flaps uses a secondary flap to close the defect created by a primary flap.
– Rhomboid/Limberg flaps for defects primarily over lateral, lower cheek, and temporal areas.

• **Rotation flaps:**
  – **Cervicofacial flap** (**Fig. 3.18**):
    ▪ For moderate to large defects and upper medial region.
    ▪ Uses the loose skin of preauricular and neck skin.
    ▪ Juri and Juri popularized the inferomedially based rotation flap. The incision starts at the superior margin of the defect, extends along the zygomatic arch, then preauricular fold and then goes below the ear and retroauricular hairline to the mid-posterior line of the neck. The flap is anchored to the underlying periosteum of zygoma and lateral orbital wall so that there is no tension on the lower eyelid.
    ▪ The disadvantage of such flaps is necrosis at the distal end, particularly in inferomedially based flaps as compared to inferolaterally based ones.

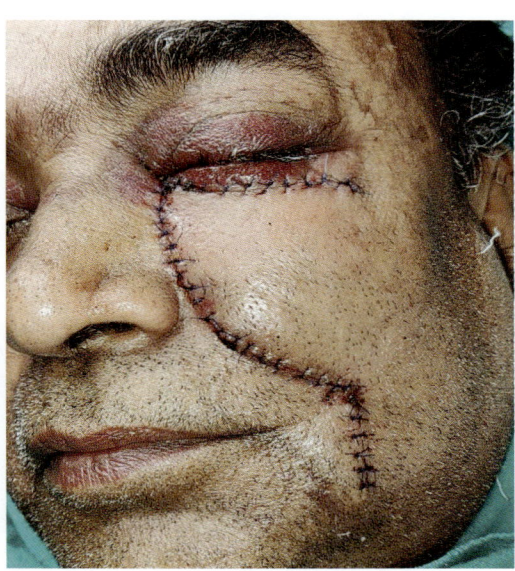

Fig. 3.18   Cervicofacial flap.

  – **Cervicopectoral flaps:**
    ▪ Ideal for defects in lower lateral areas of cheek, below an imaginary line joining the tragus and oral commissure.
    ▪ Incision goes from posterior aspect of defect, around the ear lobe, along the retroauricular hairline and then continued in the neck 2 to 3 cm behind the anterior border of trapezius and across the clavicle at deltopectoral groove.

- **Local composite flaps:**
  - **Pectoralis major flap** (Fig. 3.19a, b):
    - For lower lateral cheek defects, either for intraoral lining or skin cover or through and through cheek defects.
    - It is Mathes and Nahai type V muscle.
    - A line is drawn from acromion process to the xiphoid process and another line drawn from midclavicle meets the previous line perpendicular to the previous line.
    - The line from midclavicle to the xiphisternum represents the course of thoracoacromial vessels.
    - Skin paddle can be located medial or below the nipple and the pectoralis major muscle along with the overlying skin paddle is tunneled through the neck to reach the defect.
  - **Trapezius flap:**
    - Similar to pectoralis major flap, trapezius myocutaneous flap is also useful for lower lateral cheek defects.
    - It is a Mathes and Nahai type II muscle with dominant pedicle as transverse cervical artery and minor pedicles form dorsal scapular artery.
    - The lower and lateral flaps are more useful for cheek reconstruction because of long arc of rotation.
  - **Deltopectoral (DP) flap** (Fig. 3.20a, b):
    - Axial pattern skin flap based on the second, third, and fourth anterior perforating branches of internal mammary arteries.
- **Free tissue reconstructive options:**
  - Free radial artery forearm flap (FRAFF).
  - Parascapular flap.
  - Rectus abdominis flap.
  - Anterolateral thigh flap.
  - MSAP flap.
  - Fibula osteocutaneous flap.

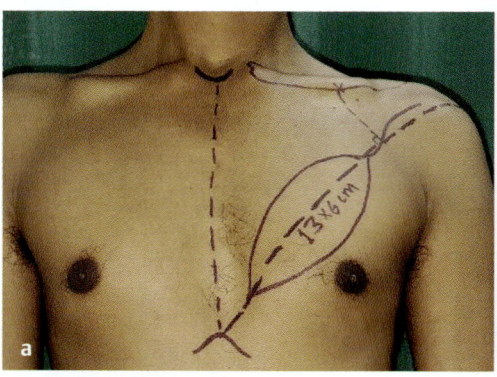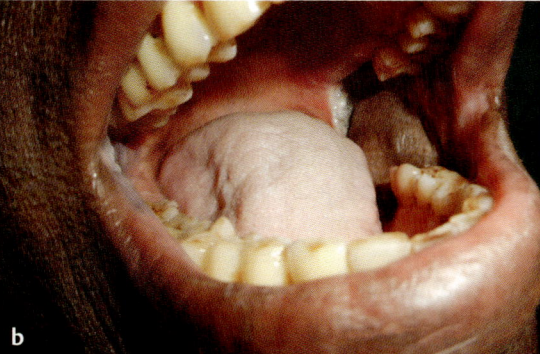

Fig. 3.19 (a, b) Pectoralis major myocutaneous (PMMC) flap.

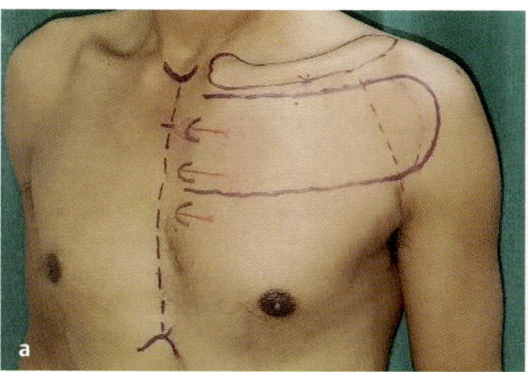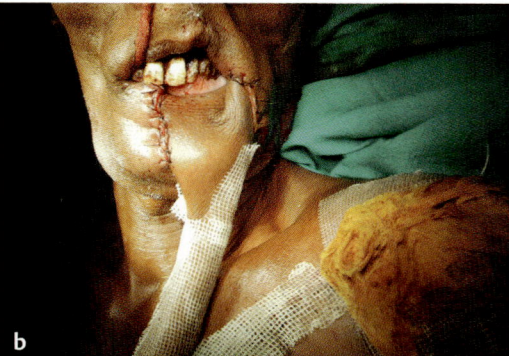

Fig. 3.20 (a, b) Deltopectoral (DP) flap.

Q28. What are the anatomical considerations in tongue reconstruction?

Anterior two-thirds defect → <10–20% → Primary closure

→ + Skin grafts

≥30% of native tongue remaining after resection → Radial artery forearm flap

→ Pedicled PMMC

Total /Near-total glossectomy → Rectus abdominis myocutaneous flap (VRAM)

→ Anterolateral thigh flap (ALT)

- In total glossectomy, the neo tongue must act as an obturator to prevent aspiration. So, when the flap is made convex into the oral cavity, swallowing and speech outcomes are better.

Q29. What are the anatomical considerations in mandible reconstruction?

Mandible defects are broadly classified into two groups based on the location of defect (**Fig. 3.21**):
- Anterior/Central.
- Lateral.
- Central segment: designated by "C."
  - Represents the segment lying between the two canine teeth.
- Lateral segment: designated by "L."
  - Represents the lateral segment of any length which do not include condyle.

- Hemimandible segment: designated by "H."
  - Same as "L" except that it includes the condyle.
- A defect may be a combination of one or more segments, (e.g., LC, HC, or LCL).
- To this bone defect, the letters "M," "S," or "MS" can be added to indicate the additional requirement of mucosa, skin, or both, respectively.

Algorithm for reconstruction of mandible defects (Algorithm 3.3):
- For smaller bone defects <3 cm—from non-vascularized iliac bone graft crest.
- For smaller bone defects—pedicled flaps like trapezius (with spine of scapula or with soft tissue defect pectoralis osteomyocutaneous flap may be used [with rib]).

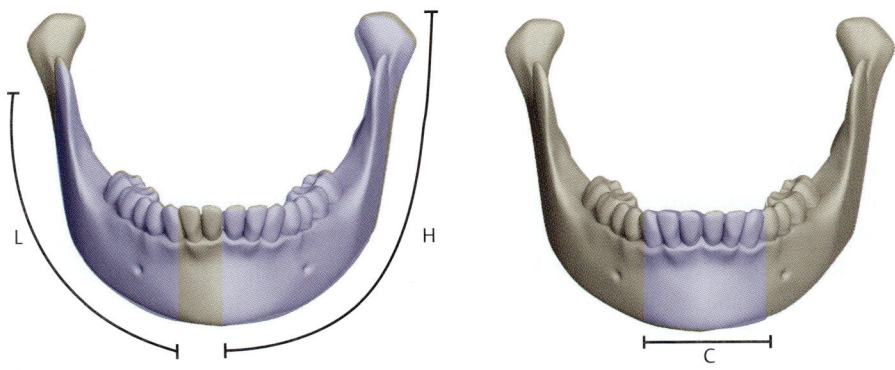

Fig. 3.21 HCL classification system of mandible defect.

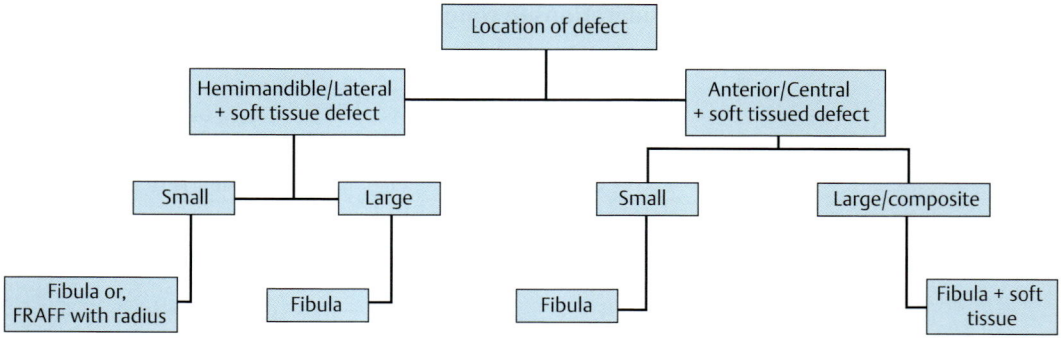

Algorithm 3.3 Algorithm for reconstruction of mandible defects.

Q30. What are the indications of nonvascularized bone grafts in mandible defects?

- Small defects <3 cm (of ramus/body).
- After resection of benign lesions (where radiation will not be used).
- No requirement of soft tissue reconstruction.
- In cases of nonunion of mandible fractures.

Q31. What are the indications of reconstruction plate use?

- AO reconstruction plates or titanium hollow screw reconstructive plate (THORP) are used.
- Plate thickness is usually >2.5 mm.
- Three to four screws on either side of native mandible are necessary for rigid fixation and plate is aligned along the lower border.
- **Indications:**
  - Lateral or posterior defects.
  - Debilitated, elderly patients.
  - Patients with poor prognosis.
- **Advantages:**
  - Decreased operating time.
  - Avoidance of a bone graft donor site.
- **Disadvantages:**
  - Risk of plate exposure or infection.
  - Risk of plate fracture.
  - No dental reconstruction can be done.
  - Due to thin shape, may not provide adequate bulk for reconstruction.

  - Occlusion is poorly maintained with a metal plate that includes a condyle.

Q32. What are the indications of a vascularized bone graft/flap in mandible defects?

- In any defect >3 cm.
- Requirement of both soft tissue and bone components.
- Requirement of postoperative radiation.
- Central defect of mandible.
- Young patients who will later require dental reconstruction.

Q33. What are the preoperative preparations in a case of free fibula reconstruction of mandible defects?

- **Systemic risk factor assessment:**
  - Screening tests to detect underlying cardiopulmonary and liver diseases.
- **Dental consultations** for preoperative impressions and models to be made.
- **Radiologic studies** which include CT or MRI, chest X-ray.
  - These scans define the anatomic boundaries of the local disease, assess the regional lymph node status, and serve as an important guide for planning surgical resection.
- **Donor site studies:**
  - Peripheral pulses must be looked for in cases where fibula is being used.
  - In cases of suspicion where pulses are abnormal in either a healthy young

patient or an older patient without other evidence of peripheral vascular disease.
- There may be peroneal arterial magna in which peroneal artery is dominant and both anterior and posterior tibial arteries are vestigial structures.
- Harvest of fibula in a peroneal artery dominant patient can lead to distal ischemia.
- Angiography must be performed in case this condition is suspected.
- **Fabrication of mandible template:**
  - To minimize the graft ischemia time during surgery, mandible templates are used for helping in graft shaping.
  - **Sources for fabricating mandible template:**
    - **Surgical specimen.**
    - **1:1 CT or MRI of mandible** in a transverse plane at a level just below the tooth roots allows fabrication of a template showing the curve of the inferior border of the mandible.
    - **Lateral cephalogram** provides a replica of the lateral view of the mandible.
      - These images can be transferred on a thin piece of acrylic plastic which is then cut out and used as a more durable template. And in combination with the surgical specimen as reference, fibula can be shaped at donor site with vascular pedicle remaining intact.
    - **Computer-aided designing and manufacturing (CAD-CAM) technique.**
      - Virtual surgery can be done in advance.
      - First step is osteotomy design, based on native mandible DICOM images of 3D CT.
      - ↓
      - CT images of patient fibula is used to do virtual osteotomies and bone opposition to

reconstruct the contour of the excised mandible.
↓
- Using CAM technique, cutting jigs for native mandible and fibula and a contoured reconstruction plate are generated.
↓
- During surgery, the cutting jig is shifted along the fibula to locate the skin paddle and pedicle length in the appropriate way.
↓
- Closed wedge osteotomies are made through cutting slots and remaining surgery proceeds in a standard fashion.

Q34. How will you shape the fibula graft?
- **Anterior grafts** (**Fig. 3.22a–e**):
  - Consists of a central segment attached to a lateral segment on each side. In the central segment, no extra osteotomies for mandible symphysis as the small loss in projection has no clinical significance.
  - First step is proper location of anterior segment on the donor bone so that pedicle reaches the region of angle of mandible easily.
  ↓
  - Osteotomy on either ends of anterior segment must be angled correctly and symmetrically in two planes because the body segment diverges away in both backward and upward direction from the anterior segment.
  ↓
  - Grafts' segment is fixed with miniplates in perpendicular planes at each osteotomy site. Contour of inferior surface is checked with the template for accuracy.
  ↓

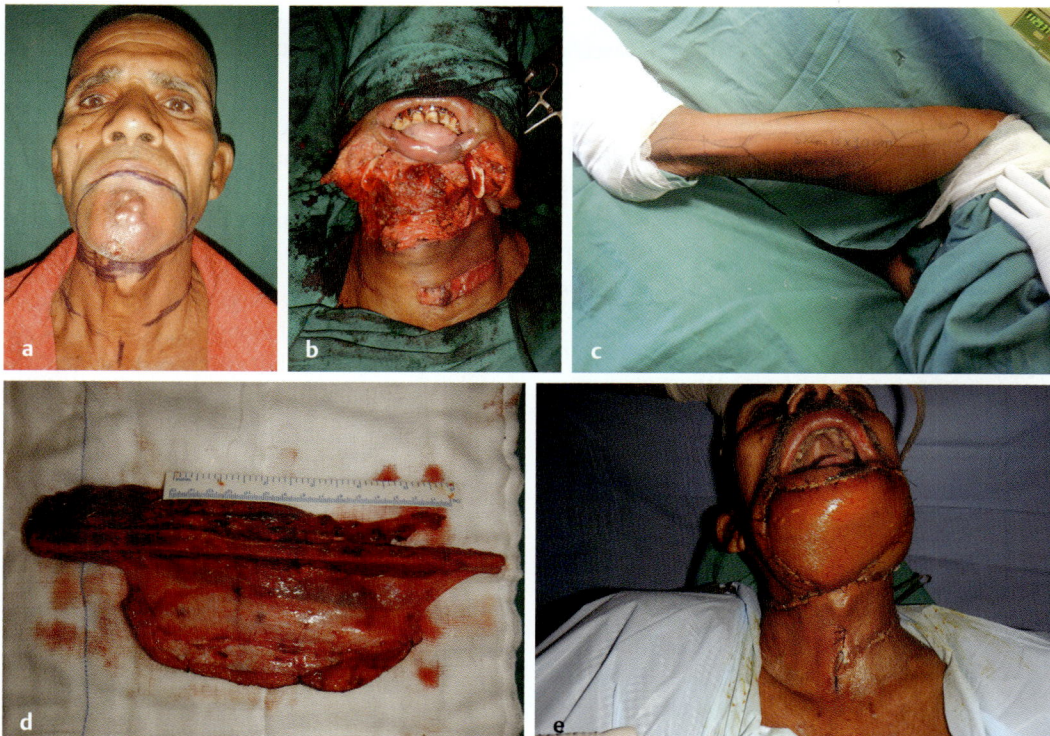

Fig. 3.22 (a–e) Anterior fibular graft.

- A long plate is then placed along the inferior border of anterior segment spanning both osteotomies.

$\downarrow$

- In setting of anterior grafts is often more challenging than in setting of lateral grafts because remaining mandible is a less stable platform. Only stable landmarks are midline and curve of maxillary arch.

- **Lateral grafts** (**Fig. 3.23**):
  - Grafts' design is shifted distally to allow the pedicle length to be maximized.
  - Body segment is located proximal to ramus segment on fibula bone which is angled anteriorly so that associated flap soft tissues will come to lie in submental area.
  - First step is to locate the angle on donor bone.

$\downarrow$

- Lateral template is used to help determine the angle of the two osteotomies needed to form the correct angle between the ramus and body segments of the graft. Dissecting its angle marks the template.

$\downarrow$

- Template is then aligned with graft along its ramus component and then along its body component marking the bone in reference to mark on template each time.

$\downarrow$

- This method defines a wedge-shaped piece of bone which when removed establishes the correct angle on the graft.
- Insetting of the lateral graft is generally assisted by first stabilizing the remaining native mandible with intermaxillary fixation.

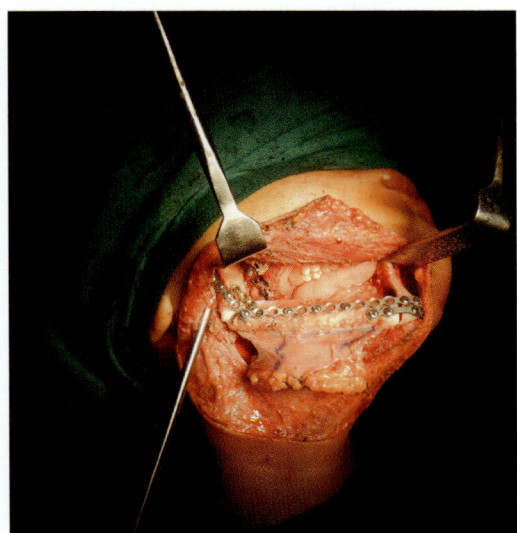

Fig. 3.23   Lateral fibular graft.

– General guideline is that for:
  ■ Posterior mandible reconstruction: Proximal fibula is used.
  ■ Anterior mandible reconstruction: Distal fibula is used.

Q35. What are the options for condyle reconstruction?

There are various options:
- The ramus of the bone graft can be left short, leaving a gap at the location of the condyle.
- The total length of the ramus with condyle can be taken as graft and its end can be rounded to make the shape of a condyle.
- If native condyle is available even if as a small part, it can be transplanted as a more vascularized graft onto the proximal end of the mandible graft.
- Prosthetic condyles are also available but the complication rates associated with them are high.

Q36. How will you do dental reconstruction?

Osseointegrated implants are used along with dental prosthesis for optimal dental reconstruction.

Q37. How does a vascularized graft heal? How it is different from that of a nonvascularized one?

The vascularized bone with its intact intrinsic blood supply maintains the viability of bone cells and bone matrix, leading to more rapid and complete bone union.

In this setting, it avoids the need for creeping substitution as in nonvascularized bone grafts repair.

Creeping substitution: Shortly, after transplantation of a free bone graft, most cells in the bone grafts are necrotic. Osseous regeneration in the bone graft occurs by gradual resorption and replacement of the necrotic bone graft by the surrounding host bone. This process is called creeping substitution.

Q38. What is the chemotherapy regimen in head and neck cancers?

A combination of paclitaxel, cisplatin, and 5-fluorouracil is used (PCF/PPF regimen).

Day 1: Paclitaxel   Dose: 175 mg/m² over 3 hours.

Day 2: Cisplatin   Dose: 100 mg/m².

Day 2–6: 5-Fluorouracil   500 mg/m²/d as continuous IV infusion. Repeat every 3 weeks.

Q39. What is the mechanism of action of chemotherapeutic agents?

- **Cisplatin**: It binds to DNA to form cisplatin-DNA adducts and causes cross-linking of DNA which triggers apoptosis.
- **Side effects:** ENT problem (ototoxicity), nephrotoxicity.
- **Paclitaxel**: Stabilizes the microtubules and prevents breakdown of microtubules during tumor cell division.
- **Side effects:** Neutropenia, painful muscles and joints.
- **5-Fluorouracil (5-FU):** It forms a metabolite 5-fluorodeoxyuridine monophosphate (FdUMP) which inhibits thymidylate

synthetize leading to DNA synthesis arrest in S phase.

- **Side effects:** Soreness and peeling of palms and soles (hand foot syndrome).

Q40. What is the radiation therapy (RT) protocol in CA oral cavity?

- **Definitive RT:**
  - Primary or gross adenopathy:
    - ≥70 Gy (2.0 Gy/d).
    - External beam RT > 50 Gy ± Brachytherapy.
  - Neck (low-risk nodal stations):
    - ≥50 Gy (2.0 Gy/d).
- **Adjuvant RT:**
  - Primary:
    - ≥60 Gy (2.0 Gy/d).
  - Neck:
    - High risk ≥60 Gy (2.0 Gy/d).
    - Low risk ≥50 Gy (2.0 Gy/d).

Q41. What are the indications of radiotherapy in head and neck cancers?

The indications are:

- Multiple levels of positive neck nodes.
- Extracapsular extension of the neck nodes.
- Deep invasion of primary tumor.
- Neurovascular invasion of the tumor.
- Tumor margins <5 mm.

Q42. What are the contraindications of radiotherapy?

- Collagen vascular disease.
- Previous radiotherapy (RT).

Q43. Why a previous RT is a contraindication to present RT?

- Tumor is radioresistant.
- Cancer has not been eradicated completely.

Q44. How does metastasis take place in head and neck cancers?

There are various routes through which metastasis takes place:

- Direct extension of the tumor.
- Tumor cells tracking along the nerves.
- Vascular invasion and spread via blood vessels.
- Lymphatic spread (1 cm² of a completely replaced lymph node contains approximately 10^9 cancer cells).

Q45. What is verrucous carcinoma?

- It is an exophytic cancer of buccal mucosa in elderly who do not have history of smoking/drinking.
- It is a slow growing lesion and does not metastasize to the regional lymph nodes.
- Surgery is the treatment of choice as it is radioresistant.

Q46. What is panendoscopy?

Panendoscopy is the endoscopic evaluation of:

- Nasopharynx.
- Oropharynx.
- Hypopharynx.
- Larynx.

Q47. What is the most common site in CA tongue?

Most common site of carcinoma tongue is anterior two-thirds, particularly on lateral margin.

Suggested Readings

1. Christiano JG, Bastidas N, Lanstein HN, Thorne CH, eds. Grabb and Smith's plastic surgery: head and neck cancer and salivary glands. 7th ed. Wolters Kluwer; 2014:327–341
2. Larson DL, Mathes SJ, eds. Plastic surgery: tumors of the head, neck and skin. Vol. 5. 2nd ed. Canada: Elsevier; 2006:159–188

Pressure Sores
Rimpi Jain

Introduction

Pressure sore is a chronic resistant wound developed from tissue loss due to ischemia caused by excessive and prolonged pressure against a bony prominence. But pressure sores are preventable if best efforts are taken regarding care of posture change, nutrition, muscle spasticity, bladder, and bowel. Grade I and II pressure sores can be managed by conservative measures but Grade III and IV sores require flap reconstruction. Principles described later must be followed to prevent recurrence which is vital in the management of pressure sores.

History

Particulars of the patient (name, age, sex, residence, occupation).

Chief Complaints

- Wound over buttock/back.
- Weakness in both lower limbs.
- Decreased/Loss of sensation in lower limbs.
- Leakage of urine and stool.

History of Present Illness

- Ask about the mode of onset: In most cases, the onset is gradual. Usually there is a history of some chronic diseases like cardiovascular accident (CVA), stroke or quadriplegia/paraplegia following road traffic accidents which led to bed-ridden condition of the patient and ultimately causes pressure sores.
- Ask about the duration of illness and when did the bedsore develop.
- Check the progression/recovery in the wound, if any.
- Ask about the loss of sensation.
- Ask about the weight loss and loss of appetite.
- Ask about the incontinence of urine and stool to know about the condition of bladder and bowel.
- Ask for the details of dressings.
- Take history of any surgical intervention and physiotherapy.
- Enquire about the nutritional condition of the patient—usually these patients are malnourished.

Past History

History of diabetes mellitus, tuberculosis, and hypertension.

Personal History

History of smoking, tobacco, and alcohol intake.

Family History

Same as in other cases.

Treatment History

Enquire about the treatment that the patient has received for the other/current bedsores, either medical or surgical. Also ask about any recurrence of bedsore.

History of Allergy

To any food or medication.

General Physical Examination

- Evaluate the patient's posture. Usually these patients are bed-ridden so their decubitus has to be noticed carefully.
- Check the temperature—whether febrile or not.
- Evaluate the general build-up of the patient—whether patient is of normal built or cachectic.
- Look for pallor, icterus, and pedal edema. These patients may have pallor and pedal edema.
- Check the nutritional status of the patient. Usually patients are malnourished. Measure skin-pinch thickness and mid-arm circumference.
- Look for pressure sores at any other site.

Local Examination of Bedsore

Inspection

1. **Attitude of the limb.**
2. **Examination of the ulcer** (all sub headings in a standard examination of ulcer needs to be mentioned):
   - **Site:** The location of bedsore has to be carefully checked at all probable sites.
   - Most common site is ischial tuberosity 28%
   - Trochanter   19%
   - Sacrum   17%
   - Heel   9%
   - Malleolus   5%
   - **Size:** Measure the size in both transverse and vertical dimensions.
   - **Shape:** Identify the shape: oval, circular, irregular, etc.
   - **Margins:** Check whether the margins are ill-defined or well-defined.
   - **Floor:** Check whether slough or dirty granulation tissue or healthy granulation tissue is present.
   - **Discharge from wound:** Check whether the discharge is minimal, moderate, or copious in amount.
   - **Odor:** Check whether the odor is foul or odorless.
   - **Surrounding skin:** Check whether healed margins or pigmentation is present.
   - **Bone is exposed or not:** If exposed, find the approximate size.
   - **Healed scars:** Check whether healed scars are present from previous pressure sores; these must be looked for at all probable sites.
   - **Fungal infection:** Look for any evidence of healed or ongoing fungal infection on the back or gluteal region.

Palpation

1. **Temperature:** Using a gloved hand feel for the local rise in temperature over the ulcer or surrounding skin. Compare with the normal areas.
2. **Tenderness:** Feel for the tenderness on touching the ulcer and its margins. In most of the cases, it is nontender due to loss of sensation in paraplegia or quadriplegia.
3. **Measure the exact size** of the ulcer. Also measure its distance from the specific bony landmarks like Greater trochanter, ischial tuberosity, and coccyx.
4. **Base of ulcer** must be felt to confirm the grading of the pressure sore. It is especially important in apparently small ulcers as on the surface, they look small but in deeper plane, they extend to a wider area (Iceberg's phenomenon). This can be done using a gloved digit (**Fig. 4.1**).
5. **Grading of bedsore:** SHEA pressure sore grading system is widely used. (It was developed by Darrell Shea, an orthopaedic surgeon.)
   - Grade I: Ulcer confined to epidermis and superficial dermis.
   - Grade II: Ulcer extends through skin and into subcutaneous fat.
   - Grade III: Ulcer extends into the underlying muscle.
   - Grade IV: Ulcer has invaded bone or joint structures.

Systemic Examination

Neurological Examination

It is very important in a case of pressure sore.
- **Mental status:**
  - Check whether the patient is conscious, oriented to time, place, and person.
  - Examine memory by asking simple questions related to present and past incidences, (e.g., what did you eat in the breakfast? What time is it?).
  - **Motor system:** Examine both lower limbs and both upper limbs, proximal to distal and look for:
    - Muscle bulk.
    - Muscle tone.
    - Muscle power, which is graded as follows:
      0—No muscular contraction.
      1—Visible muscle contraction, but no movement at joint.
      2—Movement at the joint but not against the gravity.
      3—Movement against gravity, but not against resistance.
      4—Movement against some resistance, but less than normal.
      5—Movement against full resistance, normal strength.
- **Reflexes:** Deep tendon reflexes are examined to check the level of impairment of neurological function.
  - **Biceps:** Elicited by striking just anterior to the elbow (C5–C6, musculocutaneous).

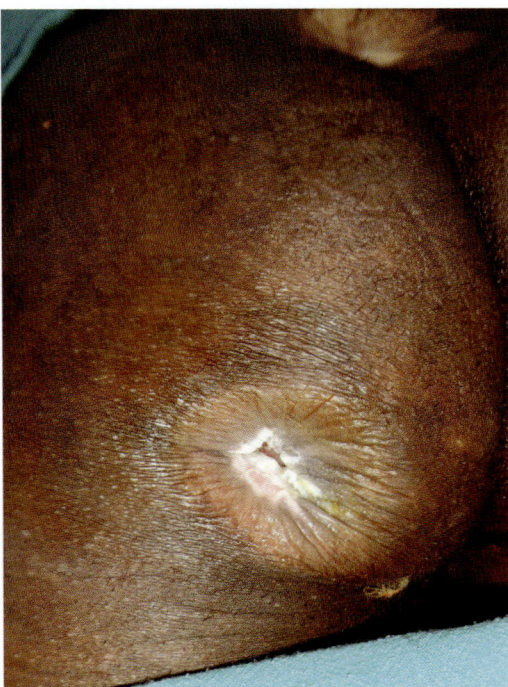

Fig. 4.1 Iceberg phenomenon in an ischial pressure sore.

- **Triceps:** Elicited by striking just posterior to the elbow (C6–C7, radial).
- **Patellar:** Elicited by striking just inferior to patella (L2–L4, femoral).
- **Ankle:** Elicited by striking just posterior to ankle joint on the Achilles tendon (S1–S2, tibial).
- There are other reflexes also, such as brachioradialis and jaw jerk.
- **Grading of reflexes:**
  0—Absent.
  1—Hypoactive.
  2—Normal.
  3—Brisk/Hyperactive.
  4—Markedly hyperactive with clonus.
- **Sensory examination:**
  - Before any test explain it to the patient.
  - Keep patient's eyes closed during examination.
  - Test all four extremities.
  - Examine pain, crude touch, light touch and pressure, vibration, proprioception (read sensory examination in "brachial plexus injury"). (Chapter 5)

Cardiovascular System

Auscultate for any added heart sounds present or not as these patients may have chronic diseases like hypertension and heart failure. Blood pressure must be taken.

Respiratory System

Auscultate for breath sounds and air entry. Due to bed-ridden status, they might have basal collapse pneumonia.

Abdomen

Look for organomegaly, if any.

Genitourinary System

Examine carefully for catheter in situ, type of catheter, whether any evidence of fungal infection in the inguinal or penoscrotal folds or gluteal cleft which is common in such patients.

Provisional Diagnosis

This is a case of 1-year-old traumatic paraplegia with sacral pressure sore, Grade IV, with bladder and bowel incontinence.

Questions

Q1. How will you proceed?
- Investigate the patient to get information about the general condition of the patient and build up the deficits.
- Explain to the family members about the routine care of the patient with pressure sore while waiting for surgery.
- Determine anesthetic fitness for surgery.
- Plan the optimum coverage of the wound.

Q2. How will you manage this case?
- This is a case of Grade IV pressure sore so for preparation of the patient and wound, go for aggressive wound care and optimization of nutrition.
- If facilities are available, go for bone biopsy and culture. If the result is positive, then go for a 6 weeks course of antibiotics following which plan for flap reconstruction after obtaining anesthetic fitness.
- In cases where bone biopsy is positive, a partial osteotomy of the bony prominence is done at the time of flap reconstruction.

Q3. What investigations you would like to write for the patient?
- Baseline investigation to assess the general status and anesthetic fitness of the patient for surgery:
  - Complete blood count, ESR, PT/INR
  - Renal function tests: Serum creatinine, blood urea.
  - Liver function tests: As most of these patients are malnourished.
  - Total protein, serum albumin, A/G ratio.
  - Chest X-ray—Posteroanterior (PA) view (to rule out any consolidation).
  - Electrocardiography—In all 12 leads.
  - Viral markers—HbsAg, HCV, HIV 1 & 2.

Q4. Is there any role of MRI in pressure sore?

- MRI is helpful in diagnosing the underlying osteomyelitis of the bone. It has an overall accuracy of 97% with sensitivity of 98% and specificity of 89%.
- It also helps in defining the extent of infection, which helps in guiding the surgical resection.

Q5. What is the role of bone biopsy in pressure sore?

- It is helpful in directing the antibiotic therapy.

Q6. What is decubitus ulcer and from where is the word decubitus derived?

- *Decubitus ulcer* is used as a substitute for *pressure sore*. The word *decubitus* is derived from the Latin word "decumbere" which means "to lie down." This word is used as a synonym for pressure sore as it occurs over areas that have underlying bony prominences when the subject is recumbent, (e.g., the sacrum, trochanter, heel, and occiput).

Q7. What are the causes of pressure sores?

The causes of pressure sores are:

- **Pressure:**
  - Persistent pressure is the most common cause of pressure sore.
  - Pressure sores result from pressure applied to soft tissue at a level higher than that found in the blood vessels supplying that area for an extended time period.
  - Tissue ischemia and necrosis of intervening tissues develop first at the deepest tissue, next to the bone. Therefore, pressure sores are typically sizable by the time skin breakdown is apparent.
    - **In supine position:** Greatest pressure at the sacrum, heels, and occiput ranging from 40 to 60 mm Hg.
    - **In the prone position:** Knees and chest develop approximately 50 mm Hg of pressure.
    - **In the sitting position:** Pressures up to 75 mm Hg develop over the ischial tuberosities.
- **Friction:**
  - Friction is the force resisting relative motion between two surfaces and is the precursor to shear.
  - It usually develops between the patient's skin and any contact surfaces like patient's bedding, transfer devices such as sheets, rollers, or slide boards, various appliances and orthotics, and wheelchair cushions.
  - Excess friction causes superficial skin injury such as abrasions and blisters which lead to further damage.

    $\downarrow$

  - It compromises the integrity of the skin which leads to loss of transepidermal water and allows moisture to accumulate.

    $\downarrow$

  - Moisture in turn increases the coefficient of friction and promotes adherence to sheets and other contact surfaces.
- **Shear:**
  - Shear develops when there is adherence of the skin and superficial tissues to sheets or bedding due to friction, which are then stretched tightly over deeper structures.
  - This causes underlying blood vessels to stretch and angulate, leading to injury of vessels.
- **Moisture:** Moist skin has a higher coefficient of friction and is prone to maceration and excoriation.
- **Malnutrition:** It decreases the chances of wound healing.
- **Neurological injury:** Immobility, either in bed or in a wheelchair, leads to increased pressure, friction, and shear that is a causative factor in all pressure sores.

Q8. What are the preoperative preparations for these patients?

The preoperative preparation of these patients is of utmost importance as it will influence the wound healing and surgical outcome.

- **Improve nutrition:**
  - The target serum albumin should be >3 mg/dL.
  - 1.5 to 3 g/kg/d of protein is required in these patients to restore lost lean body mass and 25 to 35 g/kg/d of non-protein calories.
- **Improve hemoglobin:**
  - Hemoglobin should be built up before surgery, preferably >12 g%.
  - Ferrous iron and copper help in normal collagen metabolism.
  - Zinc helps in epithelialization and fibroblasts proliferation.
  - Calcium is a cofactor for many enzymatic pathways.
- **Treatment of infection:**
  - Preoperative antibiotics are given to cover gram-positive, gram-negative, and anaerobic infections.
  - Most common organism found in wound culture are *Staphylococcus*, *Streptococcus*, *Corynebacteria*, *Proteus*, *E. coli*, and *Pseudomonas*.
- **Relief of pressure:**
  - Most important factor in the development of pressure sores is excessive and prolonged pressure.
  - If external pressure is greater than end capillary bed pressure (32 mm Hg), tissue perfusion will be impaired and ischemia will result.
  - Posture should be changed every 2 hourly for bed-ridden patients and weight bearing should be shifted every 15 minutes in wheelchair-bound patients.
- **Correction of spasm:**
  - One of the causes of pressure sore is muscle spasm. More proximal the lesions, more the chances of pressure

sore. Various options to relieve the muscle spasm are:
  - Valium (diazepam), baclofen, and dantrolene are the drugs used. The drug of choice is baclofen, a gamma-amino butyric acid receptor agonist; however, diazepam and dantrolene are effective alternatives.
  - Rhizotomy (interruption of spinal roots in spinal canal).
  - Phenol rhizotomy.
- **Release of contracture:** Bed-ridden patients are prone to develop joint contractures. Contractures occur due to tightening of both muscles and joint capsules and are common in hip flexors. If physical therapy is unsuccessful then tenotomies are performed.
- Respiratory and neurologic functions should be stable.

Q9. What are the risk assessment scales for pressure sore?

There are multiple risk assessment scales:
- **Braden:** It is the most widely used pressure sore assessment tool. The Braden scale incorporates six subscales:
  - Sensory perception.
  - Skin moisture.
  - Activity.
  - Mobility.
  - Friction and shear.
  - Nutrition.

Note: Scores range from 6 to 23, with higher scores associated with an increased risk of developing pressure sores.

- **Norton:** It is used in geriatric patients. The scale incorporates general physical condition, mental status, activity, mobility, and incontinence. It ranges from 5 to 20, with lower scores associated with greater risk.
  - Score of 11 or less had a 48% incidence of pressure sores.
  - Score of 18 or greater had a 5% incidence.
- Gosnell.
- Waterlow.
- Douglas.

Q10. What are the measures to be taken by the family members when the patient is at home or the nursing officers in the hospital to prevent pressure sore?

- **Frequent posture change:** Most important in preventing pressure sore. Position should be changed every 2 hours for at least 10 minutes.
- **Support surfaces:** Two types of support surfaces exist:
  - **Constant low-pressure (CLP) devices:** They distribute pressure over a large area, (e.g., static air, water, gel, bead, silicone, foam, and sheepskin supports).
  - **Alternating-pressure (AP) devices:** pressure vary under the patient; avoid prolonged pressure over a single anatomic point.
    - **Types of CLP devices:**
      - **Low air loss (LAL) beds:**
        i. The bed has air-filled cells through which warm air circulates.
        ii. The circulating air both equalizes pressure exerted on the patient and keeps the skin dry.
        iii. LAL surfaces exert less than 25 mm Hg pressure on any part of the body.
      - **Air-fluidized (AF) beds** (Clinitron or Kin air bed):
        i. Circulate warm air through fine ceramic beads and has drying effect similar to LAL beds.
        ii. These beds exert less than 20 mm Hg pressure on the patient, but are expensive, heavy, and cumbersome.
        iii. The fluid supporting the body consists of air and ceramic spheres.
        iv. By use of numerous spheres, the density of the supporting medium is increased and the volume of air necessary to support the body is markedly decreased.

- **Skin care:**
  - Ideal skin care encompasses cleaning, hydrating, protecting, and replenishing the skin as needed.
    - Assess the patient's skin daily, especially on the back.
    - Cleanse skin when indicated using a pH-balanced cleanser.
    - Avoid soap and hot water.
    - Avoid friction and scrubbing.
    - Minimize exposure to moisture (e.g., leakage due to incontinence, wound discharge).
    - Use skin barrier product to protect vulnerable skin.
    - Use emollients to maintain skin hydration.
- **Relief from spasm:** Both medical and surgical measure can be considered.
- **Incontinence:**
  - Use diapers in conjunction with meticulous skin care as prolonged use of urinary catheter is associated with multiple risks.
  - Fecal incontinence is a risk factor for pressure sores. Possibly the most common predisposing condition to fecal incontinence is fecal impaction, which is common in older adults and may lead to overflow incontinence. Conservative measures include diet modification and a wide variety of anti-motility agents.
- **Improve nutrition** by prescribing high protein diet.

Q11. What are the goals of reconstruction?
- **Reliable soft tissue coverage:**
  - The ideal coverage for a pressure sore should not be just a skin flap as bulk is also required to provide the cushion effect.
  - Muscle flaps are preferred whenever plausible as they eliminate the dead space and improves the vascularity of

the wound, in spite of being more sensitive to pressure necrosis than skin.

- **Form and function:** When pressure sores develop in ambulatory patients, both postoperative function and body contour need to be considered in planning the reconstruction. So, the choice of flap coverage must not hamper the functional status of the patient.

Q12. What are the treatment options for pressure sore?

- **Nonsurgical treatment** is done for Grade I and Grade II.
  - **Pressure relief:** This continues to be critical in the treatment of pressure sores.
  - **Spasticity correction:** Spasticity should be addressed not only to improve patient positioning, weight distribution, and hygiene but also to prevent tension on the healing wound, particularly if surgical intervention is planned.
  - **Correction of malnutrition:** Albumin levels below 3.5 g/dL are associated with ulcer recurrence within 1 year.
  - **Control of infection:** Osteomyelitis is a common complication of deep pressure sores. So, biopsy-directed antibiotic therapy is advised.
  - **Wound care:** Appropriate dressing should be used like micronized silver-containing dressing materials, etc.

- **Negative-pressure wound therapy** (NPWT) entails applying local negative pressure to a wound (**Fig. 4.2**).
  - The foam sponge used in NPWT consists of an open-cell polyurethane or polyvinyl alcohol with a pore size ranging from 400 to 600 µm in diameter.
  - Negative pressure can be adjusted around 125 mm Hg in either continuous or intermittent mode.
- **Manipulating the local wound milieu:** Use of biologic and recombinant growth factors as possible modalities for the nonsurgical treatment of pressure sores.

- **Surgical treatment:** Principles of surgical management of pressure sore:
  - Debride the ulcer and underlying bursa.
  - Use radical removal of underlying bone and any heterotopic ossification.
  - Pad bone stumps and fill dead space.
  - For coverage use a flap as large as possible. Keep the suture line away from the area of direct pressure.
  - Preserve all future options for coverage.
  - Use flap design that does not violate adjacent flap territories.
  - In ambulatory patients, consider both postoperative functions and body contour in planning and reconstruction.
  - Resurface with large regional pedicled flaps.

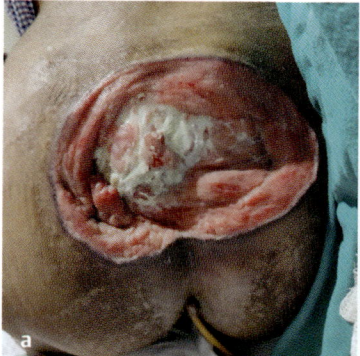 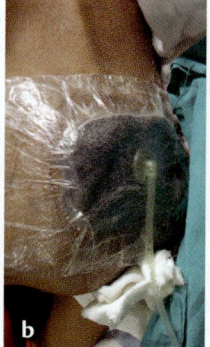 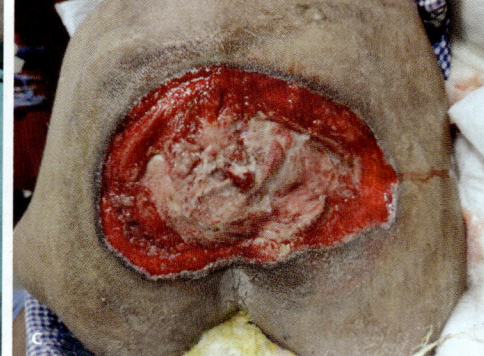

Fig. 4.2 **(a–c)** Improvement in wound after negative-pressure wound therapy (NPWT).

– Graft the donor site of the flap, if necessary.

Q13. What are the local flap options for pressure sore?

- Limberg flap (**Fig. 4.3**).
- Transposition flap (**Fig. 4.4**).
- Rotation flap.

Avoid primary closure of the wound.

Q14. How can Limberg flap be used in pressure sore?

- The design of Limberg flap for sacral pressure sore can vary depending upon the dimensions of the defect.
- If a single Limberg flap is not adequate enough to cover the defect, two-flap or three-flap Limberg may be planned (**Fig. 4.5a, b**).

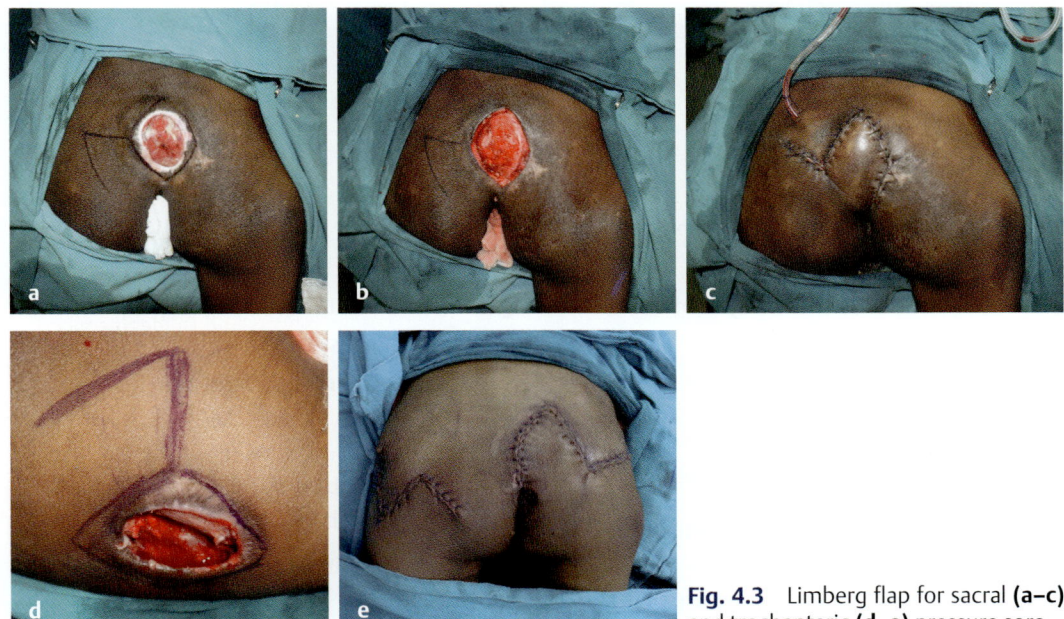

Fig. 4.3 Limberg flap for sacral **(a–c)** and trochanteric **(d, e)** pressure sore.

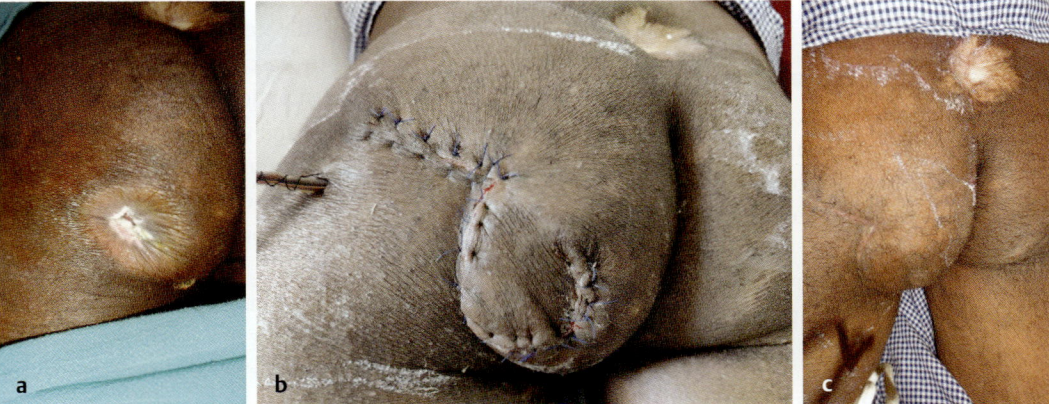

Fig. 4.4 **(a–c)** Transposition flap for ischial pressure sore.

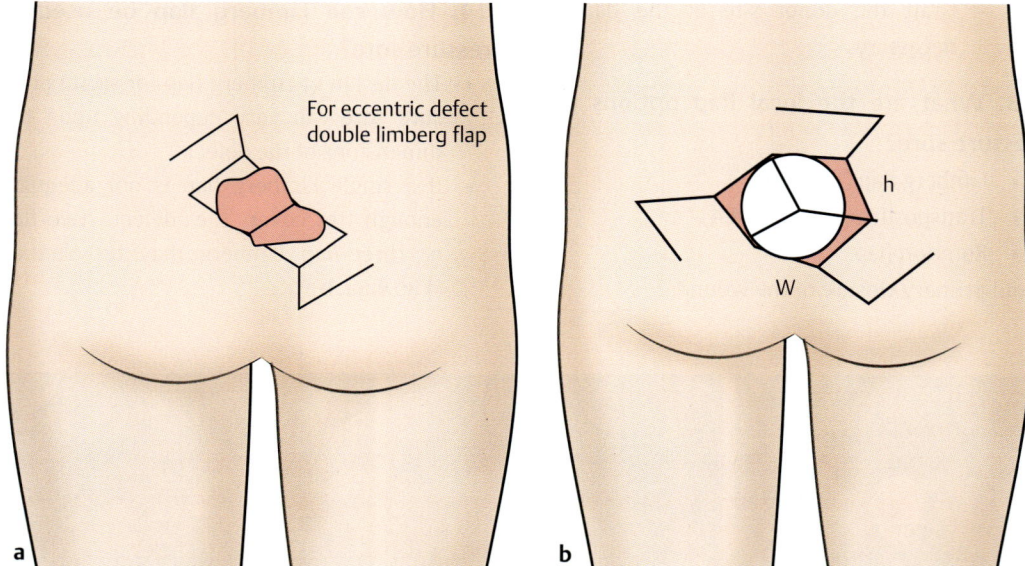

For eccentric defect
double limberg flap

h

W

a

b

Fig. 4.5 **(a, b)** Various designs of Limberg flap for sacral pressure sore.

Q15. What are the advantages of musculo-cutaneous flap for pressure sore?

- Maintains adequate blood supply as its vascularity is good.
- Provides bulky padding in pressure sores.
- Is very effective in infected wound.

Q16. What are the disadvantages of musculocutaneous flap?

- Is sensitive to external pressure.
- Leads to functional deformity in ambulatory patients.
- Lack of bulk in elderly patients and spinal cord patients.

Q17. What are the advantages of fascio-cutaneous flap?

- Maintains adequate blood supply.
- Provides durable coverage.
- Has minimal potential for functional deformity.
- Reconstructs more closely the normal anatomic arrangement over bony prominences.

Q18. What is the disadvantage of fascio-cutaneous flap

Provides limited bulk for large pressure sores.

Q19. What are the various flap options for sacral pressure sore?

Flaps for sacral pressure sore are:
- V-Y gluteus maximus.
- V-Y gluteus maximus (contralateral).
- Readvance bilateral V-Y gluteus maximus.
- Transverse back flap.

V-Y gluteus maximus advancement flap
- **Origin:**
  - The origin of the gluteus maximus is the gluteal line of ilium and sacrum.
  - The insertion point is the greater tuberosity of the femur and the iliotibial band of the fascia lata.
  - Blood is supplied by the superior gluteal artery and venae comitantes.
  - The pedicle courses along the deep surface of the gluteus muscle after emerging above the piriformis muscle.
- **Landmarks:**
  - The bony landmarks-lateral edge of the sacrum and greater trochanter identify the origin and insertion, respectively, of the muscle.
  - The posterior superior iliac crest and the ischial tuberosity mark the superior

and inferior margins of the muscle, respectively.

- **Arc of rotation:**
  - The point of rotation is at the lateral border of the sacrum where the dominant vascular pedicle enters the muscle.
- **Flap design:**
  - The skin island is centered over the medial muscle, adjacent to the sacral wound.
  - It can be designed as bilateral V-Y advancement flap in cases of large sacral wound (**Fig. 4.6a, b**) or superior gluteal artery perforator flap (**Fig. 4.7a–d**). The entrance of superior gluteal artery (SGA) is marked at the junction of proximal and middle thirds on a line drawn from posterior superior iliac spine (PSIS) to the apex of the greater trochanter. Another line is drawn connecting PSIS and coccyx and piriformis muscle is marked midway on this line. SGA emerges superior to the piriformis muscle. The flap is then drawn as centered over the SGA.
  - In patients with an increased risk of pressure sore recurrence (e.g., paraplegics, quadriplegics, patients with altered mental status or decreased local sensation), it is important to design the skin island as large as possible so that readvancement is an option in the future (**Fig. 4.8**).
  - For patients who are ambulatory and with normal sensation, the flap needs to be only as large as the defect.

Q20. What are the various flap options for ischial pressure sore?

Flaps for ischial pressure sore:
- Inferior gluteus maximus island flap.
- Inferior gluteus thigh (IGT) flap.
- Readvance IGT.
- V-Y hamstring.
- Gracilis.
- TFL (tensor fascia lata): expanded or delayed.
- Rectus abdominis.

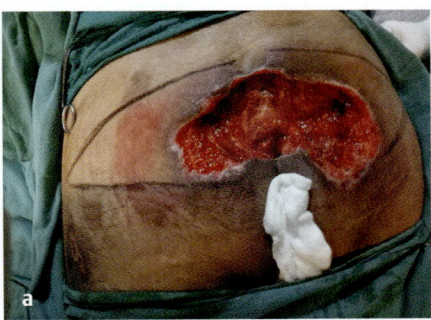
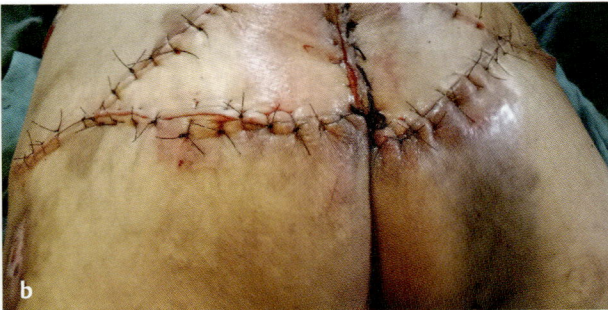

Fig. 4.6 (**a, b**) Bilateral V-Y gluteus maximus advancement flap.

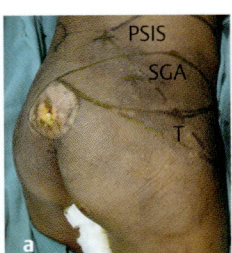
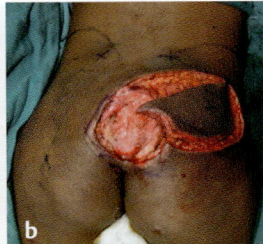
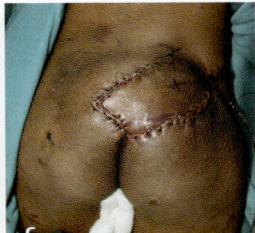
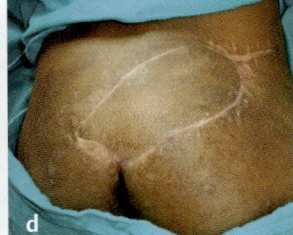

Fig. 4.7 Superior gluteal artery perforator (SGAP) flap: (**a**) markings, (**b**) flap elevation, (**c**) insetting of flap, (**d**) postoperative follow-up.

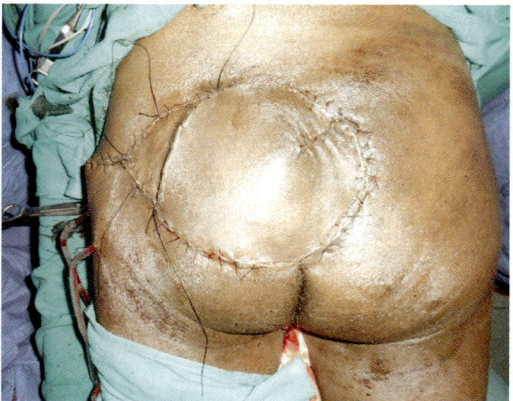

Fig. 4.8 Large gluteus maximus advancement flap.

Inferior gluteus maximus island flap (Fig. 4.9)
- **Origin:**
  - The origin of the inferior gluteus maximus is from the gluteal line of ilium and sacrum. Its insertion is at the greater tuberosity of the femur and iliotibial band of the fascia lata.
  - Blood supply is from the inferior gluteal artery.
- **Landmarks:**
  - Inferior gluteal artery (IGA) emerges from the greater sciatic foramen at a point marked at the junction of middle and lower thirds on a line drawn from PSIS to the ischial tuberosity.
  - The skin island should be centered over the gluteal crease between the ischial tuberosity medially and greater trochanter laterally.
- **Flap design:**
  - The medial edge of the skin island usually abuts the lateral edge of the ischial sore; therefore, no skin bridge is necessary.
  - The skin island should be as large as possible.
  - The skin island should also be positioned slightly distal to the ischial sore to compensate for the shortening of the axis of the flap as the muscle is rotated medially.

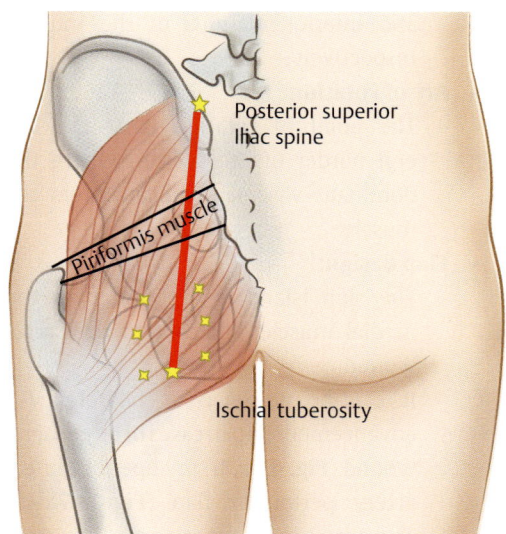

Fig. 4.9 Markings of inferior gluteus maximus island flap.

Gluteal thigh flap (Fig. 4.10)
- **Origin:**
  - The gluteal thigh flap receives its blood supply from the descending terminal branch of the inferior gluteal artery.
- **Landmarks:**
  - A line drawn vertically, midway between the greater trochanter and ischial tuberosity and perpendicular to the gluteal crease, represents the central axis of the flap as well as the course of the inferior gluteal artery as it continues on to the posterior thigh.
- **Flap design:**
  - The flap is centered over the posterior thigh and designed less than 12 cm in width to allow direct donor site closure.
  - The distal tip of the flap can extend to within 8 cm of the popliteal fossa.
  - The key anatomic structures during the dissection are the sciatic nerve, the posterior cutaneous nerve, and the inferior gluteal artery.
  - Flap elevation should begin with the distal skin incision to confirm that the flap is centered over the vascular pedicle.

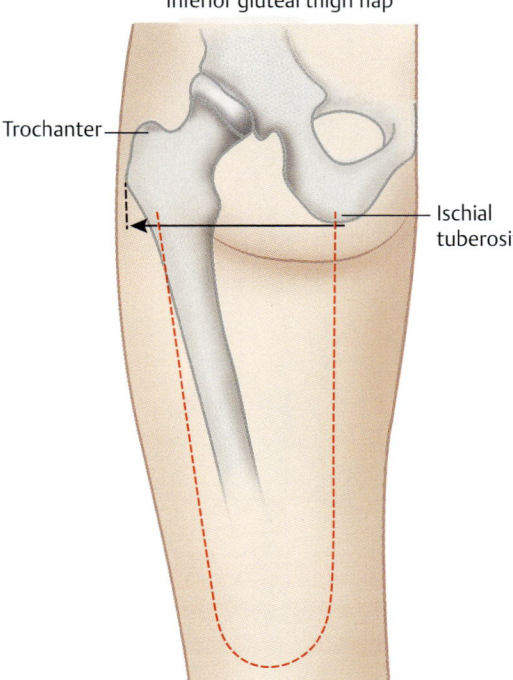

Inferior gluteal thigh flap

Trochanter

Ischial tuberosity

Fig. 4.10   Markings of posterior gluteal thigh flap.

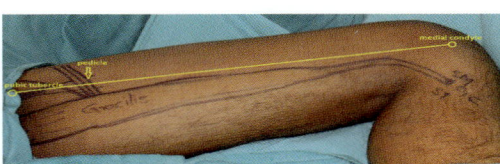

Fig. 4.11   Pressure sore (Gracilis).

Gracilis flap (Fig. 4.11)
- **Origin:**
  - The origin of the gracilis flap is pubic symphysis.
  - The insertion point is the medial condyle of the tibia.
  - The blood supply is derived from the ascending branch of the medial circumflex femoral artery and venae comitantes.
  - The anterior femoral cutaneous nerve provides sensory innervation to the majority of the anterior medial thigh.
  - A small cutaneous branch of the anterior obturator nerve provides sensory

innervation to the superior skin territory of the gracilis muscle.
- **Landmarks:**
  - Dominant pedicle enters the posterior medial muscle belly approximately 10 cm inferior to the pubic tubercle.
- **Flap design:**
  - A line is drawn between the pubic tubercle and the medial condyle of the femur.
  - The muscle is located 2 to 3 cm posterior and parallel to this line.
  - The skin island (8×15 cm) is centered over the proximal third of the muscle, but it can extend over the middle third of the muscle.
  - The skin island over the distal Gracilis is not reliable.

Q21. What are the various flap options for trochanteric pressure sore?
Flaps for trochanteric pressure sore:
- Tensor fascia lata (TFL) ± V-Y.
- Readvance TFL.
- Vastus lateralis.
- Rectus femoris.
- IGT.
- Rectus abdominis.

V-Y modification of TFL flap provides more proximal and better vascularized tissue than the classic TFL flap, as well as more muscular portion of the flap to fill the area.

Tensor fascia lata flap (Fig. 4.12)
- **Origin:**
  - Origin of the tensor fascia lata is at the anterior superior iliac spine.
  - The insertion point is the iliotibial tract of the fascia lata.
  - The dominant blood supply is via the ascending branch of the lateral circumflex femoral artery and venae comitantes, a branch of the femoris vessels.
  - T_{12} innervates the upper skin territory over the muscle origin.
  - The lateral femoral cutaneous nerve of the thigh (L2–L3) innervates the remaining skin territory.

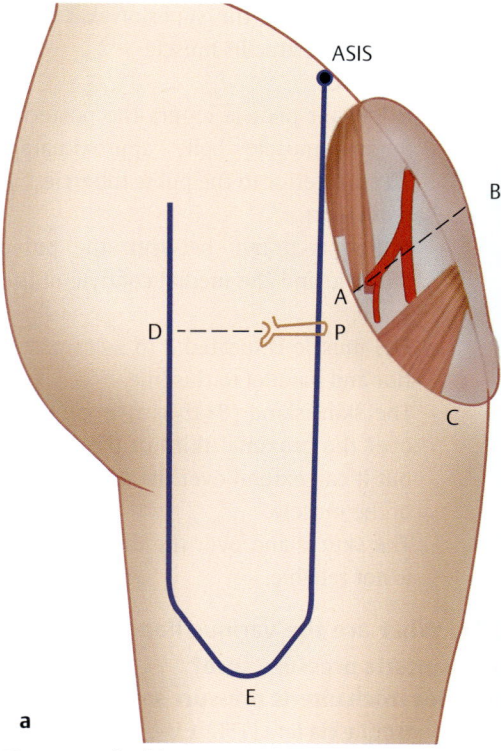

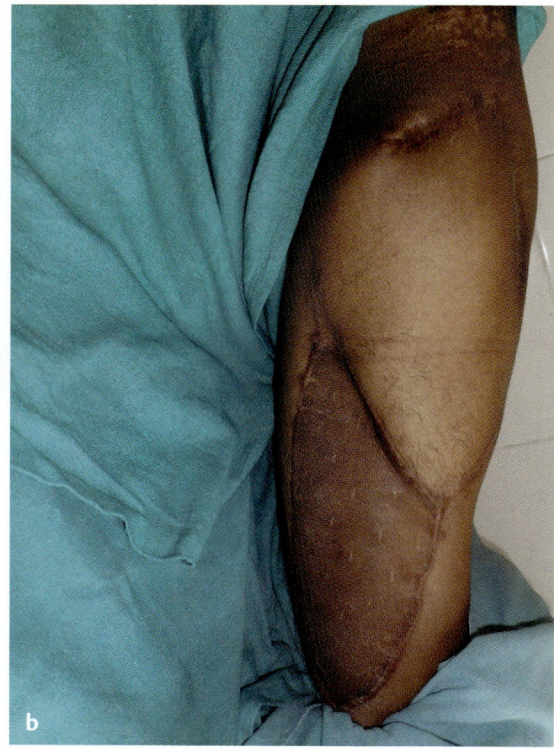

Fig. 4.12 **(a, b)** V-Y tensor fascia lata flap.

- **Landmarks:**
  - A line drawn from the anterior superior iliac spine to the knee represents the anterior extent of the skin island of the flap that can be designed.
  - A second line 'AB' (width of the defect) distance away from the first line so that AB=DP.
  - 'P' is the pivot point, 10 cm below ASIS at which the pedicle enters the flap.
  - 'D' is the posterior extent of the skin paddle.
  - 'E' is the distal limit of the flap
- **Flap design:**
  - A line is drawn from the anterior superior iliac spine to the midportion of the lateral thigh, at least two thirds of the length of the thigh.

  - The flap can be designed up to 15 cm in width to allow primary closure of the skin.
  - The distal limit of the flap extends to 10 cm above the knee. Beyond this, the flap is best delayed.

It can be used as rotation or V-Y advancement flap.

Vastus lateralis flap

- **Origin:**
  - The origin of the vastus lateralis flap is the intertrochanteric line, greater trochanter, gluteal tuberosity of the femur, and intramuscular septum.
  - The insertion point is at the patella.
  - The main blood supply is provided by the descending and transverse branches of the lateral circumflex femoral artery and venae comitantes.

- Both branches of the lateral circumflex femoral artery enter the deep surface of the muscle within its superior third (10-15 cm below the anterior superior iliac spine).
- The descending branch courses inferiorly along the medial border of the muscle.

- **Landmarks:**
  - A line is drawn from the point 10 cm below the anterior superior ilias spine at the level of the greater trochanter to the lateral condyle of the femur.

- **Flap design:**
  - Most commonly, the vastus lateralis flap is elevated without a skin island.
  - The skin incision is made along the line drawn from the level of the greater trochanter to the lateral condyle of the femur.
  - A skin island can be incorporated and de-epithelialized if further tissue bulk is necessary to obliterate the wound cavity or if stable cutaneous coverage is required.

Q22. What are the options for heel pressure sore?

- Lateral calcaneal artery flap.
- Medial plantar flap.
- Reverse sural artery flap.

Q23. Which is the sensate flap for sacral pressure sore?

- Gluteal thigh flap.

Q24. What are the other options for sensate flap?

- Gracilis.
- Posterior thigh flap.
- TFL flap.

Q25. Why overhanging margins are excised?

- As pressure sore is an ice berg, for radical debridement overhanging margins are excised.

Q26. What postoperative care should be taken for this patient?

The measures used to address pressure relief, shear, friction, moisture, skin care, incontinence, spasticity, and nutrition should be continued aggressively throughout the postoperative period.

- **Positioning:** Pressure on the flap should be avoided. Patient should be placed in prone or lateral decubitus position depending on the flap. Frequent repositioning and turning is required.
- **Dressing:** Constrictive bandages are avoided.
- **Suction drains:** Drains should be left in place until serous fluid drainage decreases to 20 mL in 24 hours.
- **Antibiotics:** Should be continued for 7 to 10 days or longer if signs of infection are there.
- **Mobilization:** Weight bearing at the site of flap inset is avoided for 3 to 4 weeks, followed by a program of gradually increased weight bearing on the flap site.
- **Hospital stay:** Usually up to 3 weeks.
- **Rehabilitation:**
  - Because of the significant risk of pressure sore recurrence, regardless of how long patients are kept in bed, they should begin active and passive range-of-motion exercises of the uninvolved extremity early in the postoperative course.
  - The affected extremity can be started on exercises just prior to the initiation of sitting protocol.

Q27. What are the associated complications after surgery?

- **Wound Dehiscence:**
  - Causes of wound dehiscence:
    - When the flap is sutured under pressure (**Fig. 4.13a, b**).
    - When the patient is noncompliant with postoperative body positioning.

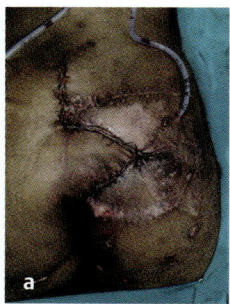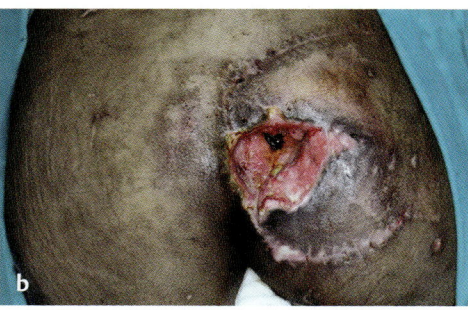

Fig. 4.13 (a, b) Wound dehiscence in flap reconstruction for sacral pressure sore.

– Should be promptly treated with operative debridement and flap readvancement.

• **Hematoma:**
– Hematomas predispose to other complications such as wound infection, bursa formation, flap necrosis, and subsequent pressure sore recurrence.
– Once recognized, they should be immediately evacuated.

• **Seroma:**
– Causes of seroma formation:
  ▪ Residual dead space.
  ▪ Inadequate immobilization of the patient postoperatively with resultant shearing forces.
  ▪ Inadequate resection of the bursae.
– Suction drainage should be used for all patients undergoing pressure sore reconstruction.
– If a seroma develops after removal of the drains, percutaneous drainage may be performed.

• **Wound infection:**
– Most often it is due to inadequate wound debridement.

– When present, drainage should be done along with appropriate antibiotics.

• **Partial flap necrosis:**
– It is usually related to incorrect flap design.
– Certain flaps are more susceptible to partial flap loss from a tenuous blood supply to a portion of the flap, e.g., the distal edge of the tensor fascia lata. Modifications like delay of the flap or use of tissue expansion can prevent this complication.
– If there is small necrosis, healing by secondary intention is done by conservative measures.

• **Recurrence.**

Suggested Readings

1. Foster RD. Mathes text book of plastic surgery. Pressure Sores. Vol. 6. 2nd ed. Elsevier; 2006: 157, 1317–1353
2. Kwon R, Rendon JL, Janis JE. In: Neligan PC, ed. Plastic surgery: pressure sores. Vol. 4. 4th ed. Canada: Elsevier; 2018:350–380

5 Traumatic Brachial Plexus Injury (BPI)

Veena K. Singh and Ansarul Haq

Learning Objectives

At the end of this chapter, the student will be able to:
1. Understand the anatomy of brachial plexus.
2. Describe the clinical presentation of the case.
3. Demonstrate the motor and sensory examination of upper extremity.
4. Describe the clinical presentation of the case.
5. Understand the planning of brachial plexus injury management.
6. Understand the type of surgery according to the stage and type of injury.

Introduction

The management of brachial plexus injury (BPI) is entirely dependent on a thorough understanding of its three-dimensional intricate anatomy. The detailed history of the relative position of head and neck at the time of trauma provides important clues regarding the type of BPI. Examination of brachial plexus is an exhaustive task as it requires examination of more than 50 muscles. A good way of examination is to go in a sequence from the origin (roots) to the distal individual nerves, with examining all muscles supplied by the intermediate branches. Proper diagnosis, meticulously performed surgical procedure, physiotherapy, and over all patient's own motivation influence the surgical outcomes to a varying extent.

Anatomy of Brachial Plexus

Brachial plexus is a complex structure formed by the contributions from ventral spinal nerve roots of C5–T1 and located in the posterior triangle of neck between anterior and middle scalene muscles. Once the three trunks—anterior (C5 and C6), middle (C7), and posterior (C8 and T1)—are formed, each divide into anterior and posterior divisions. The anterior divisions of upper and middle trunk form the lateral cord, anterior division of lower trunk forms the medial cord, and the posterior divisions of all trunks join to form the posterior cord. The plexus passes above the first rib and deep to clavicle, thus getting divided into supraclavicular and infraclavicular parts. As it descends into the axilla, the relationship of the cords with the axillary artery gives the names of lateral, medial, and posterior cords. The terminal branches of the cords give major nerves to the muscles of upper extremity (**Fig. 5.1, Flowchart 5.1**). When additional contribution from C4 is there, it is called pre-fixed brachial plexus and when contribution from T2 is received, it is called post-fixed brachial plexus.

Chief Complaints of the Patient

- Inability to elevate the shoulder/arm.
- Inability to bend the elbow.
- Inability to straighten the elbow.
- Inability to extend/flex the wrist and fingers.

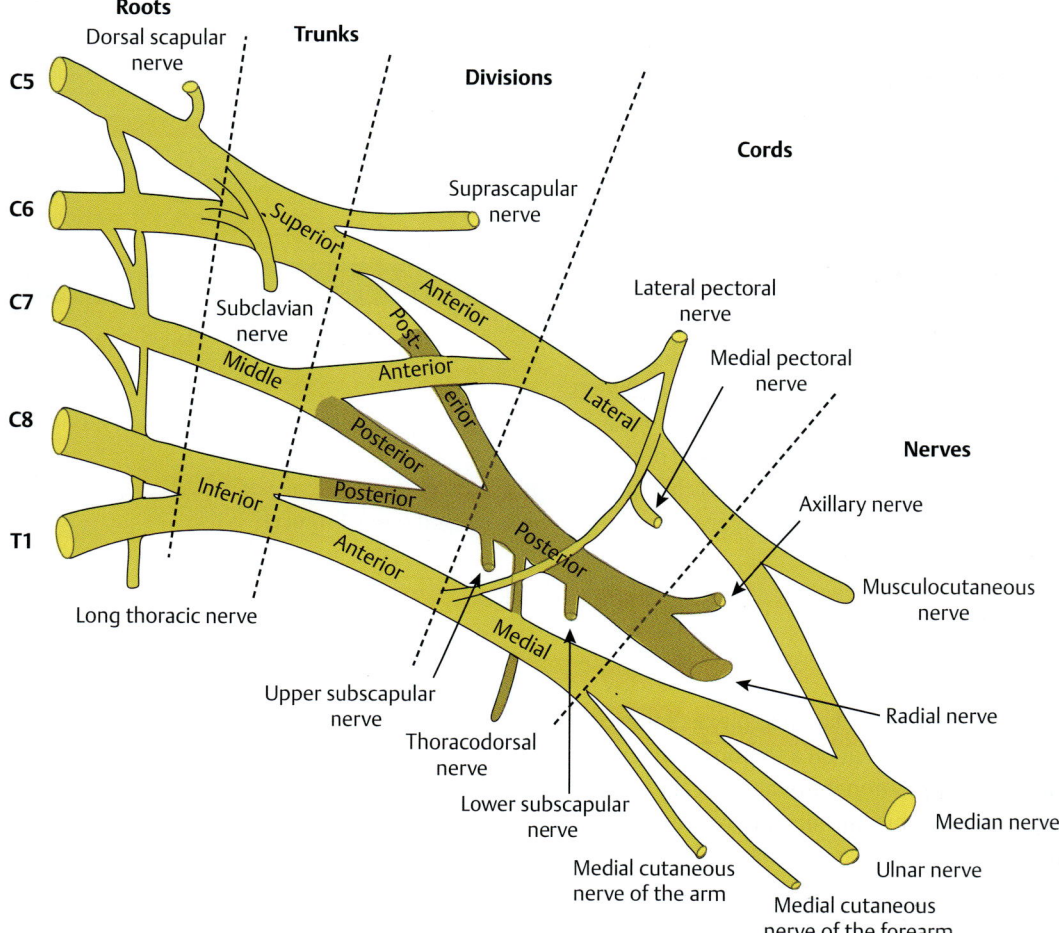

Fig. 5.1 Anatomy of brachial plexus.

- Complete loss of/decreased sensation.
- Heaviness/pain in the affected limb.

History of Present Illness

- Duration:
  - When was the injury sustained?
  - Exact date of injury (if the patient remembers).
- Mode of injury: Most common is accidental, sometimes assault (blunt trauma with lathi, etc.) or homicidal or birth injury. Exact description of the accident or trauma is important to understand the relation between the position of upper limb and the presentation of nerve injury.

For example, when the patient presents with a history of trauma in which the head is shifted away from the injured side along with an evidence of denervation of paraspinous muscles, it strongly suggests severe nerve injury such as root avulsion. A history of shoulder dislocation or glenoid fracture is associated with a high incidence of infraclavicular BPI, whereas with a history of cervical spine injury, root injuries are more likely.

- Whether the patient was conscious/unconscious at the time of trauma.
- Any history of ear, nose, or oral bleeding or vomiting.
- Associated injuries such as fractures of clavicular or acromion process or humerus

fracture or fractures of clavicle in a case of polytrauma.

- Any history of surgical procedure.
- Pain over the limb—radiating, electric shock sensation, deafferentation pain, radiculopathy.
- Hand dominance.
- History of physiotherapy/muscle stimulation/splintage/use of arm pouch sling.
- Edema, especially over the hand and fingers, due to dangling of the limb (use of arm pouch sling prevents it) and stiffness of the joints.

Past History

- History of diabetes mellitus, hypertension, tuberculosis, or any other medical illness.
- Any surgery done in the past for nerve injury or intervention for fracture.

Personal History

History of addiction including alcoholism, smoking, marital status, number of kids, employment status.

Family History

Number of family members dependent on the patient.

Treatment History

Any physiotherapy or nerve stimulation since the injury.

History of Allergy

To food or medications.

General Physical Examination

- Level of consciousness: Whether oriented to time, place, and person.
- Whether cooperative/irritable.
- Build: The bony stature of the patient (whether small/medium/tall build).
- Nutrition: Whether well-nourished or malnourished.
- Facies: Look carefully for the features of Horner's syndrome.
- Pallor/cyanosis/jaundice/clubbing.
- Pedal edema.
- Pulse: Rate/min, rhythm, volume, any irregularity.
- BP: Must be measured in both SBP and DBP.
- Respiration: Rate/min, rhythm, thoracoabdominal.
- Body temperature: To exclude the febrile status of the patient.
- Neck veins: Look for external jugular and internal jugular veins, if they are engorged.
- Neck nodes: To be checked.
- Any other deformity/scar elsewhere in the body.
- Any skin abnormality/similar lesions in the body.

Systemic Examination

- Abdomen.
- Central nervous system (CNS).
- Cardiovascular system (CVS).
- Respiratory system,

Refer to chapter 3 on Carcinoma Oral Cavity.

Local Examination

Sequence of steps in clinical examination:

- Ensure proper exposure in adequate light with explained informed consent.
- Proper exposure: Patient is made to stand and the entire upper half of the trunk needs to be exposed completely. Ask the patient to remove any clothing on the upper torso including vest.
- Attitude of the limb: Carefully watch the posture of the affected limb from shoulder to the fingertips.
  - Total/pan/global BPI is characterized by high up shoulder and complete

paralysis of the upper limb giving it a flaccid appearance, with decreased sensation and pale extremity.

– In classic Erb's palsy which occurs at C5–C6, there is a Potter's/Waiter's tip deformity characterized by affected limb in adducted, internally rotated with extended elbow posture.

• Generalized muscle wasting of shoulder girdle, arm, forearm, and hand. Always compare with normal limb (**Fig. 5.2**).

• Scars, tattoos: There may be presence of scars from previous injuries or any previous surgery.

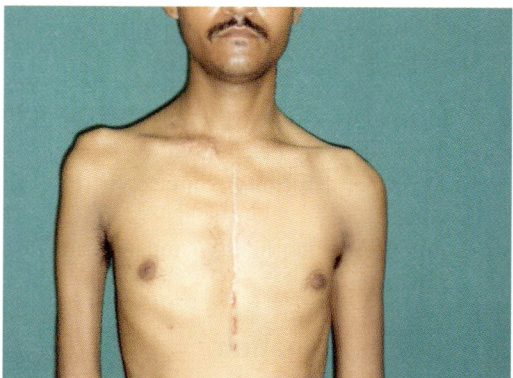

Fig. 5.2 Atrophy of muscles in the affected limb (right).

• Look for soft tissue loss and joint contracture, if any.
• Bony abnormalities: Clavicle, humerus.
• Palm: Dry.
• Nails: Dull, lusterless.
• Face: Look for ptosis, meiosis, anhidrosis, enophthalmos (Horner's sign) (**Fig. 5.3**).
• Sulcus sign: The depression between the acromion process of shoulder joint and the head of humerus (**Fig. 5.4**).

Palpation

Motor Examination

• Remember Medical Research Council (MRC) grading.
• If any muscle is weak, then again check the muscle with patient in lying position on a bed to eliminate the effect of gravity.
• Few things to be remembered while testing the muscle:
  – Look for the contraction of the muscles.
  – Feel for the bulk during contraction.
  – Move against resistance.
  – Normal side first followed by affected side.
  – Passive range of movements to be checked at all joints.

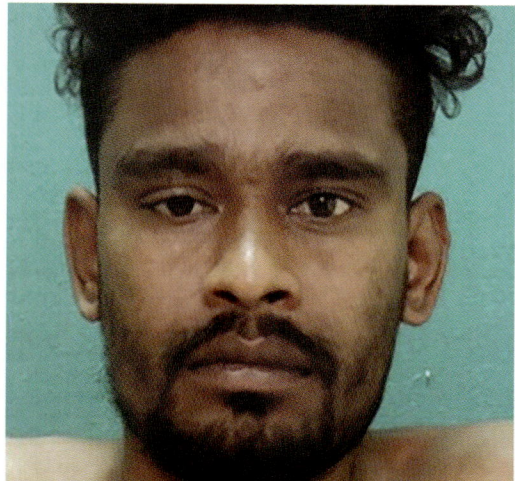

Fig. 5.3 Horner's sign.

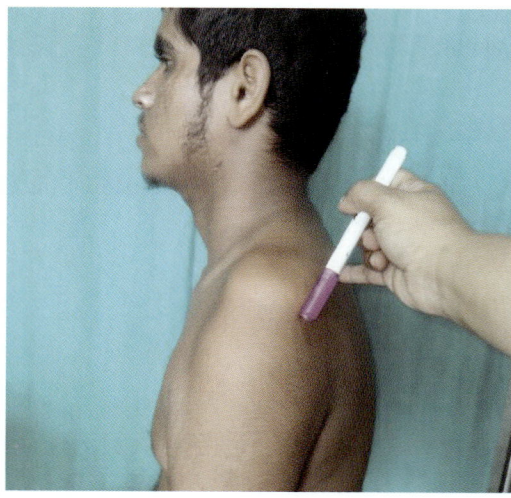

Fig. 5.4 Sulcus sign.

A. Sequence of examination must be targeted to localize the lesion.

Roots: Dorsal scapular nerve C5–C7 (rhomboids major and minor).

Long Thoracic Nerve C5–C7 (serratus anterior).

Trunk: Suprascapular Nerve C5–C6 (supra- and infraspinatus).

Cords: Medial pectoral nerve C6–T1 (pectoralis); lateral nerve C5–C6 (major/minor).

Upper and lower subscapularis C5–C6 (subscapularis muscle).

Thoracodorsal nerve C7–C8 (latissimus dorsi).

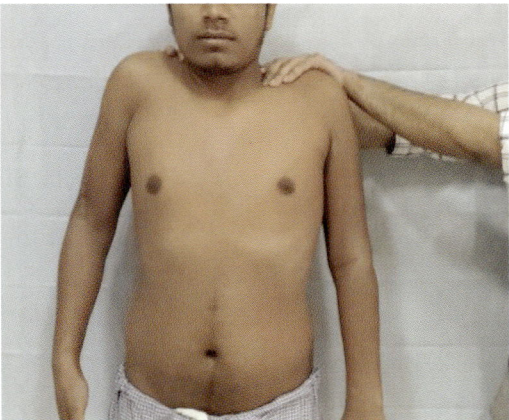

Fig. 5.5 Action of trapezius.

1. Start with trapezius (spinal accessory–XI, C3–C4) (**Fig. 5.5**):
   • Stand behind the patient and ask him to shrug his shoulder.
   • Check against resistance also.
2. Rhomboids (**Fig. 5.6**):
   • Rhomboids muscles are covered by trapezius so first relax the trapezius by placing the hand in the small of back.
   • Along the vertebral border, place the fingers between the two shoulder blades.
   • Ask the patient to lift the hand off the back and feel for the rhomboids pushing the fingers out.
3. Serratus anterior (**Fig. 5.7**):
   • Push-out test/wall-press test.
   • Ask the patient to stand in front of a wall and try to push with his hand, first on normal side and then on affected side. If required, the examiner will support the arm of the affected limb with one hand.
   • See and feel for the lower pole of the scapula winging laterally.
4. Suprascapular nerve (upper trunk):
   • Supraspinatus (**Fig. 5.8**):
     – Stand in front of the patient and ask him to abduct the shoulder to 90 degrees in forward flexion with the thumbs pointing downward.

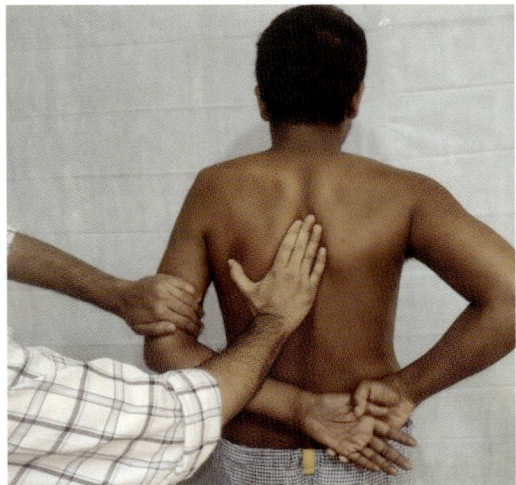

Fig. 5.6 Action of rhomboids.

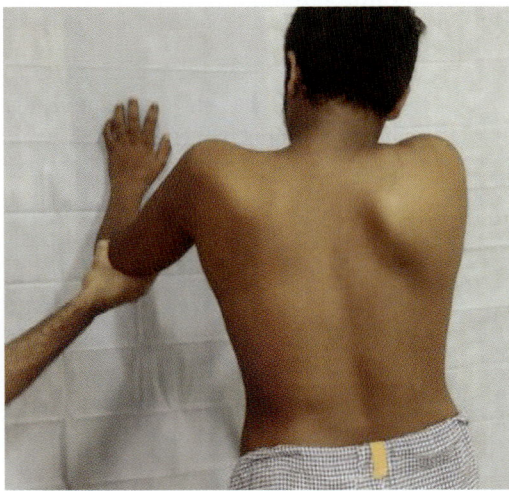

Fig. 5.7 Action of serratus anterior.

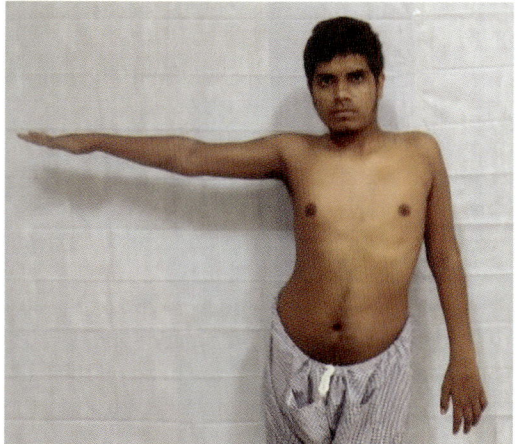

Fig. 5.8 Action of supraspinatus.

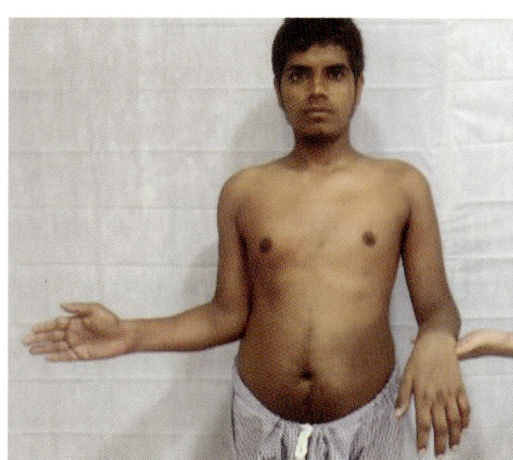

Fig. 5.9 Action of infraspinatus.

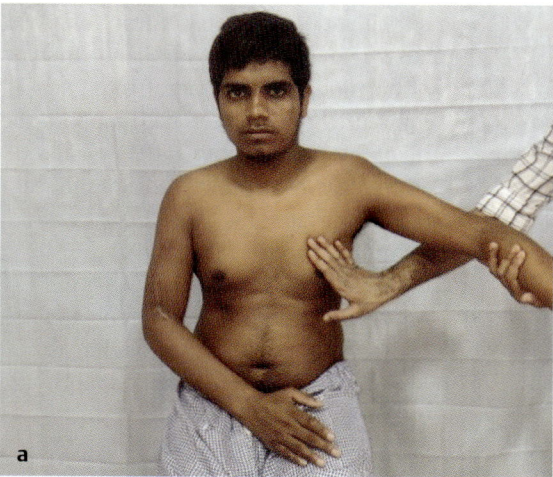

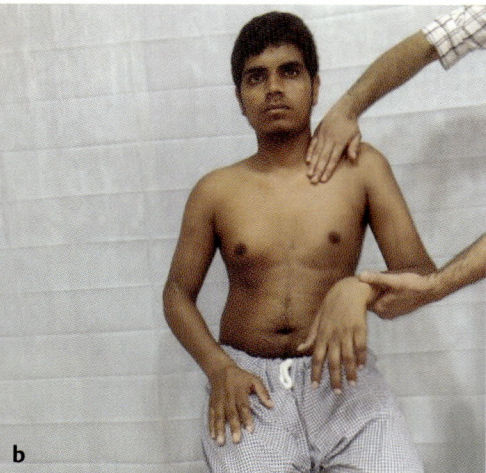

Fig. 5.10 **(a)** Action of sternocostal head of pectoralis major. **(b)** Action of clavicular head of pectoralis major.

- Apply resistance on the arm while patient attempts to elevate it.
- Infraspinatus (**Fig. 5.9**):
  - In standing position, the patient is asked to keep the arm in neutral position with elbow flexed to 90 degrees.
  - Ask the patient to externally rotate the arm while the examiner applies a medially directed force to the arm.

5. Medial cord (medial pectoral nerve) C6–T1 and lateral cord (lateral pectoral nerve) C5–C6:
   - Sternocostal head (**Fig. 5.10a**):
     - Stand in front of the patient.

- Ask the patient to rest his both hands on the hips and push hand.
- The examiner feels for the anterior axillary fold.
- Tests for medial cord injury.
- Clavicular head (**Fig. 5.10b**):
  - The patient is asked to touch the contralateral shoulder.
  - The examiner palpates for contraction of the muscle beneath the clavicle.
  - Tests for lateral cord injury.

6. Posterior cord (thoracodorsal nerve, C7); latissimus dorsi muscle (**Fig. 5.11**):
   - Stand behind the patient.

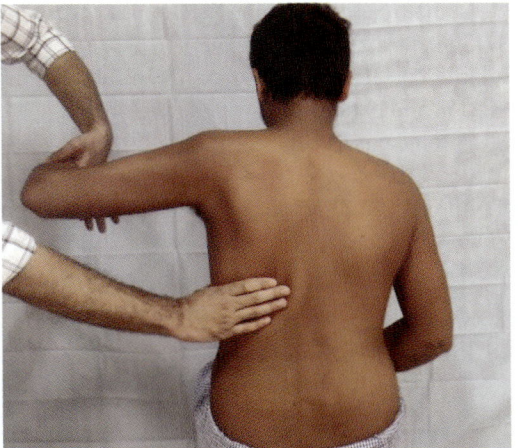

Fig. 5.11 Action of latissimus dorsi.

- Support the arm in a flexed position and ask the patient to push it down.
- Feel for contraction of muscle in posterior axillary fold.

7. Branches:
   - Axillary nerve C5–C6 (deltoid) (**Fig. 5.12a, b**):
     – Ask the patient to sit on a stool and rest the affected limb on an adjacent table.
     – Ask the patient to extend, abduct, and flex the shoulder so as to examine the posterior, middle, and anterior deltoid.
     – In isolated axillary nerve palsy, two signs must be elicited to confirm the diagnosis.
   - Swallow-tail sign: Ask the patient to extend the shoulder while moving the body forward—An extension lag of ≥20 degrees as compared to the normal side is a positive sign.
   - Abduction internal rotation:
     – Ask the patient to maximally abduct the shoulder while the arm is internally rotated and elbow in flexion.
     – Abduction lag as compared to the normal side is a positive sign.
     – Musculocutaneous nerve C5–C6 (biceps, brachialis)
       ▪ Biceps (**Fig. 5.13**): Check for flexion of elbow with hand in full supination.

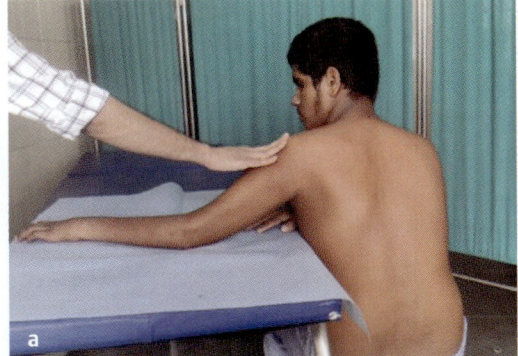

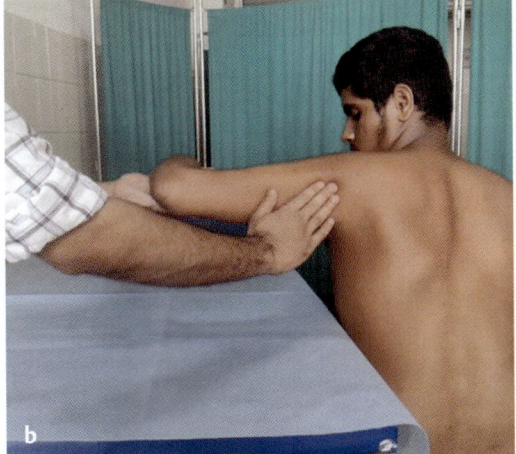

Fig. 5.12 **(a)** Action of deltoid (anterior fibers). **(b)** Action of deltoid (posterior fibers).

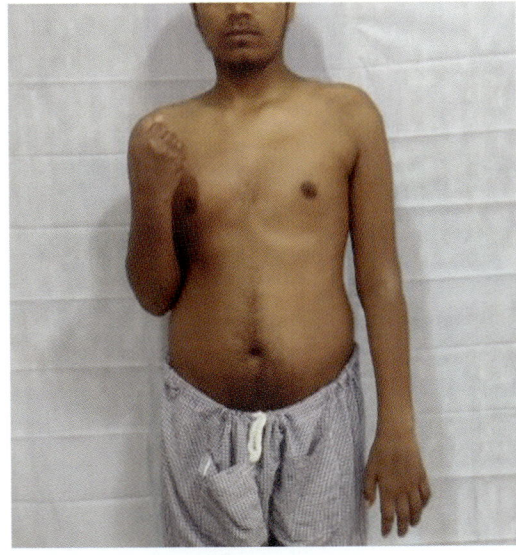

Fig. 5.13 Action of biceps.

○ Be cautious of brachioradialis which might cause some elbow flexion in upper trunk injury (**Fig. 5.14**).

– Radial nerve (**Figs. 5.15** and **5.16**).
– Median nerve (**Figs. 5.17**, **5.18**, and **5.19**).
– Ulnar nerve (**Figs. 5.20** and **5.21**).

B. Do not miss to examine the donor nerves.
1. Spinal accessory (trapezius).
2. Intercostal nerve (chest-X-ray in full inspiration and expiration).
3. Phrenic nerve (**Fig. 5.22**).
4. Contralateral C7 nerve.
C. All the findings have to be documented in a motor function assessment chart (**Fig. 5.23a, b**).

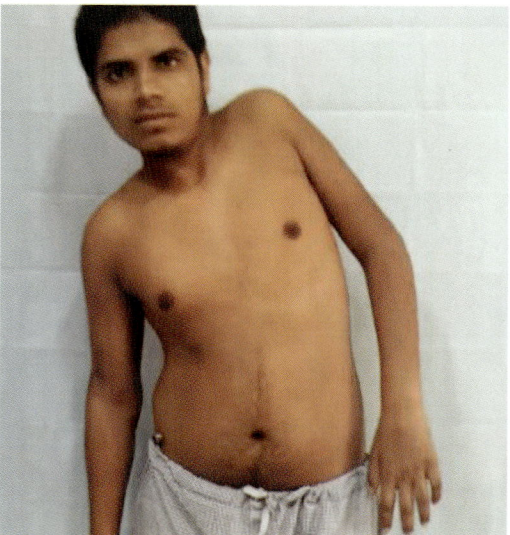

Fig. 5.14 Action of brachioradialis.

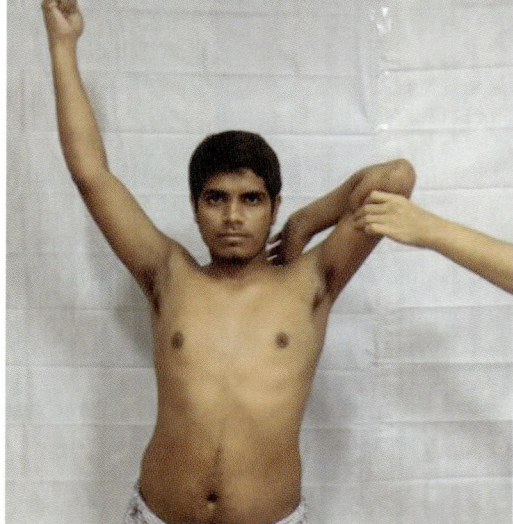

Fig. 5.15 Action of triceps.

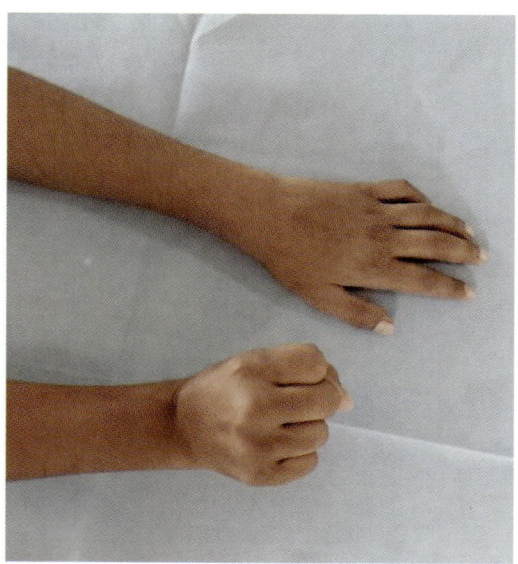

Fig. 5.16 Action of wrist extensors.

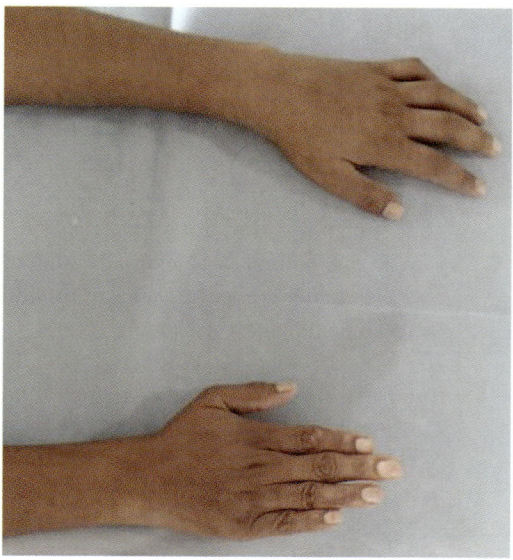

Fig. 5.17 Action of wrist flexors.

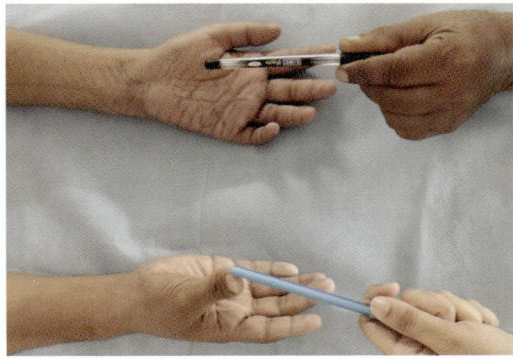

Fig. 5.18 Pen test for abductor pollicis brevis (median nerve).

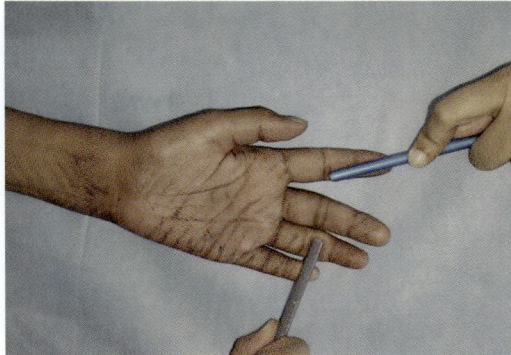

Fig. 5.19 Action of flexor digitorum superficialis (FDS).

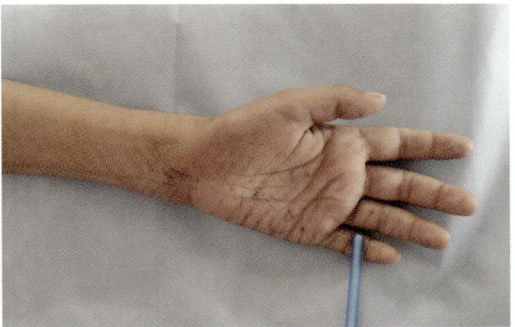

Fig. 5.20 Action of flexor digitorum profundus of little finger (ulnar nerve).

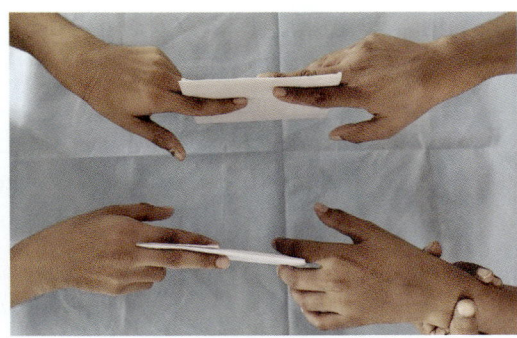

Fig. 5.21 Action of palmar interossei (card test).

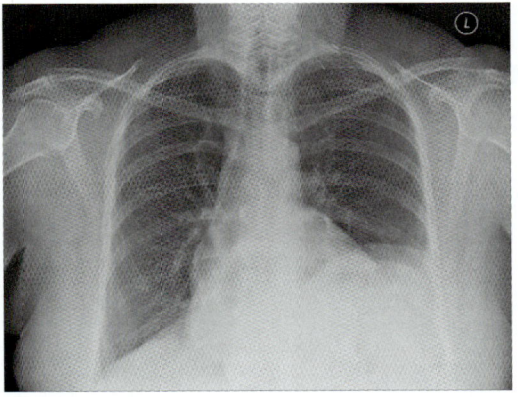

Fig. 5.22 Chest X-ray for excluding phrenic nerve palsy.

Sensory Examination

First assess the dermatomes and then according to the distribution of the terminal branches document the findings in a sensory function assessment chart (**Fig. 5.24a–d**).

Motor function assessment chart of Brachial plexus injury patients

Arc labels: C6, C7, C6, C5, T1

(CN XI, C3,C4)	Serratus Anterior			II III IV V	Opp. poll	APB
Trapez	Posterior	Biceps	Pronator teres	FDS		
	Lateral (DELTOID)		FCR	PL	FPB	
(C3,C4, C5)		Triceps			FPL	Add. Poll
Levator scapulae	Anterior	Brachialis	ECR	ECU	ADO	
	Supra-spinatus	Brachio-radialis	EDC/EIP	APL/EPB	Posterior interosseous nerve	
(C4,C5)		Supinator		EPL	FDP II III IV V	
Rhombus	Infra-spinatus	Teres major		FCU	Anterior interosseous nerve	
		Latissimus dorsi				
a	Pectoralis majorclavicular head		Pectoralis major sternal head		Right	Left

Right panel:
Name:
Birth date:
Date of trauma:
Date of exam:
Homer's syndrome
Tinel sign location:
EMG:
CXR:
MRI:

Branchial plexus injury - motor function assessment chart

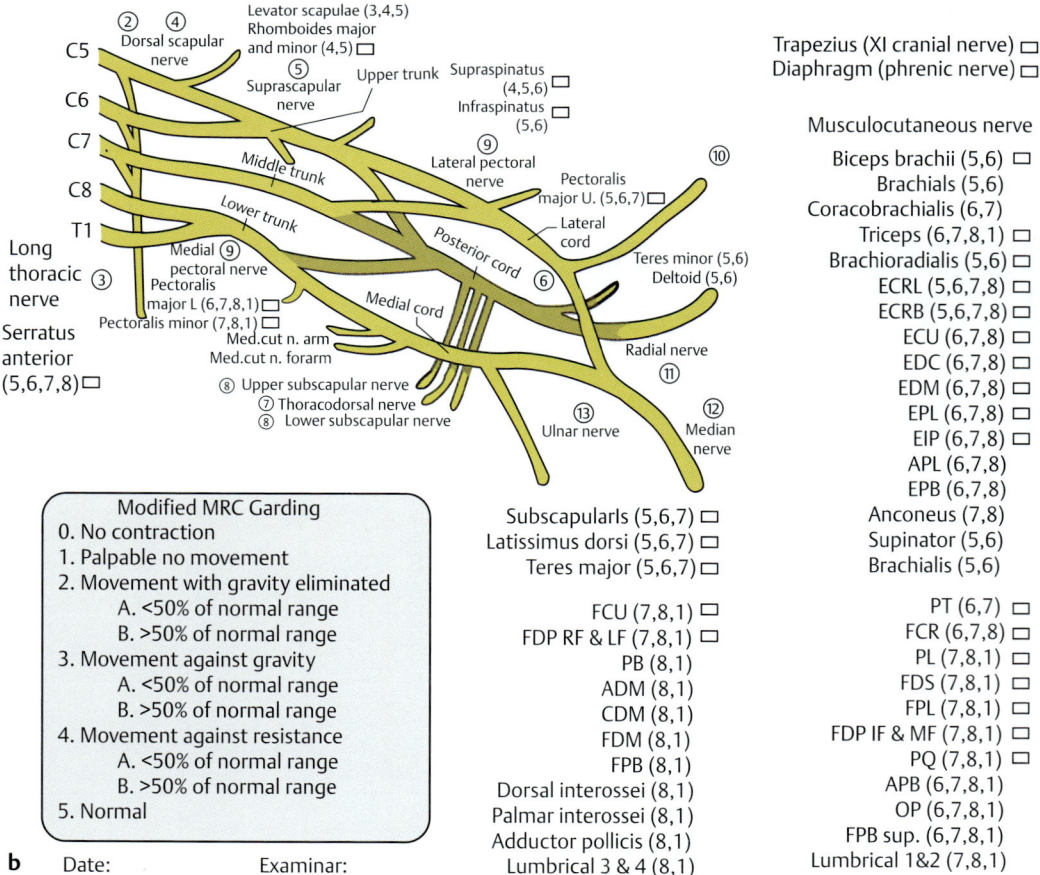

Levator scapulae (3,4,5)
Rhomboides major and minor (4,5)
Supraspinatus (4,5,6)
Infraspinatus (5,6)
Dorsal scapular nerve
Upper trunk
Suprascapular nerve
Middle trunk
Lower trunk
Lateral pectoral nerve
Pectoralis major U. (5,6,7)
Medial pectoral nerve
Pectoralis major L (6,7,8,1)
Pectoralis minor (7,8,1)
Posterior cord
Lateral cord
Medial cord
Med.cut n. arm
Med.cut n. forarm
⑧ Upper subscapular nerve
⑦ Thoracodorsal nerve
⑧ Lower subscapular nerve
Teres minor (5,6)
Deltoid (5,6)
Radial nerve
Ulnar nerve
Median nerve

C5, C6, C7, C8, T1
Long thoracic nerve ③
Serratus anterior (5,6,7,8)

Trapezius (XI cranial nerve)
Diaphragm (phrenic nerve)

Musculocutaneous nerve
Biceps brachii (5,6)
Brachials (5,6)
Coracobrachialis (6,7)
Triceps (6,7,8,1)
Brachioradialis (5,6)
ECRL (5,6,7,8)
ECRB (5,6,7,8)
ECU (6,7,8)
EDC (6,7,8)
EDM (6,7,8)
EPL (6,7,8)
EIP (6,7,8)
APL (6,7,8)
EPB (6,7,8)
Anconeus (7,8)
Supinator (5,6)
Brachialis (5,6)

PT (6,7)
FCR (6,7,8)
PL (7,8,1)
FDS (7,8,1)
FPL (7,8,1)
FDP IF & MF (7,8,1)
PQ (7,8,1)
APB (6,7,8,1)
OP (6,7,8,1)
FPB sup. (6,7,8,1)
Lumbrical 1&2 (7,8,1)

Subscapularls (5,6,7)
Latissimus dorsi (5,6,7)
Teres major (5,6,7)

FCU (7,8,1)
FDP RF & LF (7,8,1)
PB (8,1)
ADM (8,1)
CDM (8,1)
FDM (8,1)
FPB (8,1)
Dorsal interossei (8,1)
Palmar interossei (8,1)
Adductor pollicis (8,1)
Lumbrical 3 & 4 (8,1)

Modified MRC Garding
0. No contraction
1. Palpable no movement
2. Movement with gravity eliminated
   A. <50% of normal range
   B. >50% of normal range
3. Movement against gravity
   A. <50% of normal range
   B. >50% of normal range
4. Movement against resistance
   A. <50% of normal range
   B. >50% of normal range
5. Normal

b   Date: Examinar:

Fig. 5.23 **(a, b)** Motor grading chart.

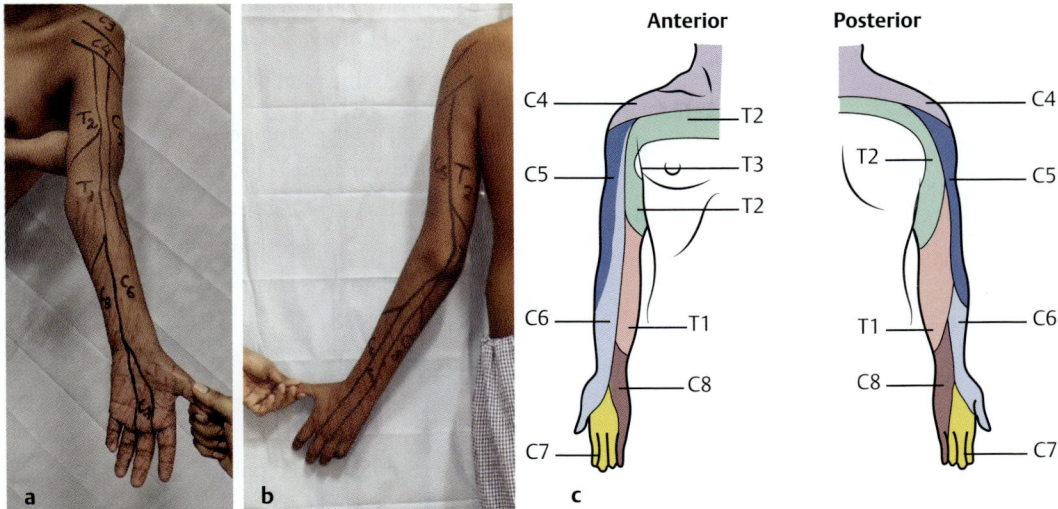

Brachial plexus injury - sensory assessment chart

Name:
No.:
Sex: Male/Female
Date of birth:
Date of injury:
Side injured: Right/Left

Horner's: Present/Absent
Tinels sign: Present/Absent
     Location
     Nature: Static/Advancing
Deep pain:
     Supraspinatus: Present/Absent
     Deltoid: Present/Absent
     Biceps: Present/Absent

MRC grading

S0: No sensation
S1: Deep pain
S2: Superficial pain and some touch
S3: S2 without over-response
S3+: S2 with some 2 PD
S4: Normal sensation

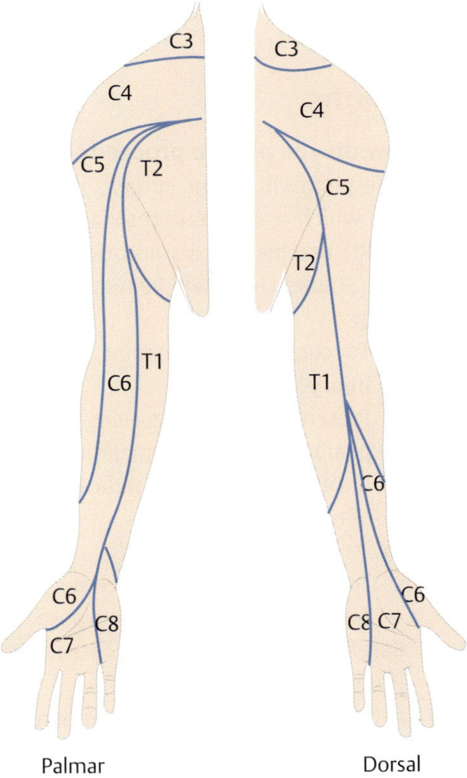

Date   Examiner

Fig. 5.24 (a–d) Sensory mapping of upper limb.

Reflexes and Vascularity

Three reflexes: biceps, triceps, supinator.

Elbow flexion	C5, C6
Elbow extension	C7, C8
Forearm supination	C6
Forearm pronation	C7, C8
Wrist flexion/extension	C6, C7
Metacarpophalangeal (MCP) joint flexion/extension	C7, C8
Grip	C8
Fingers abduction	T1

Provisional Diagnosis

This is a case of a 4-months old post–road traffic accident, left-sided global BPI in a 20-year-old male patient without any associated bony injury or vascular injury.

Questions

Q1. How do you plan to proceed?

- The plan will be for surgery in this case, for which a magnetic resonance imaging (MRI) brachial plexus and nerve conduction studies (NCS) will be required.
- MRI:
  - To confirm the location and type of injury.
  - Presence of meningoceles and disappearance of the ganglion from the intraforaminal space indicate avulsion of roots.
- NCSs:
  - To see the status of injured nerves.
  - Also for documentation purpose.
- Baseline investigations for preanesthetic fitness.
- Other radiological investigations required in this case to exclude the bony fractures would be:
  - X-ray cervical spine.
  - X-ray chest (CXR): Posteroanterior (PA) view in full inspiration and expiration (to exclude phrenic nerve injury).
  - X-ray shoulder joint.

- Other optional investigations can be: Myelography.

Nagano's classification of myelographic findings:

N	Normal root sleeve shadow
A1	Slightly abnormal sleeve shadow
A2	Obliteration of lip of root sleeve
A3	No root shadow visible
D	Complete defect instead of a root sleeve shadow
M	Traumatic meningocele

  - Computed tomography (CT) myelography.
  - Spinal evoked potentials.
    - Sensory-evoked potentials.
    - Corticosensory-evoked potentials.

Note: No single test can tell surgeon whether the injured patient requires surgical exploration and reconstruction. It has to be decided on the basis of clinical examination and duration of injury.

Q2. How to decide the timeline for surgery?

- Timing of surgery depends upon two factors:
  - Mode of injury sustained.
  - Presentation of the patient.
    - Immediate surgery:
      - Penetrating injury (e.g., stab wound).
      - Iatrogenic injury.
      - Vascular injury.
    - Early surgery (6 wk–3 mo after injury).
      - Global BPI.
      - High-energy injuries, high-velocity gunshot wounds.
    - Early surgery at 3 to 6 months:
      - Partial BPI.
      - Low-energy injuries, low-velocity gunshot wound.
    - Late delayed (after 6 mo):
      - Pseudomeningoceles at many levels.
      - Extensive cervical fractures.
      - Proximal plexus injury at multiple levels.
      - At 5 months; earlier in cases of root avulsions.

– Discussion with patient and family members at the first presentation is of utmost importance:
  ▪ What is brachial plexus and its work?
  ▪ Mechanism of injury.
  ▪ Timing of injury.
  ▪ Type of surgery and its stages.
  ▪ Requirement of compliance in pre- and postop physiotherapy.
  ▪ Finance involved.
- Standard treatment stages can be according to the following timeline:
  – Stabilization (1st month).
  – Diagnostic (2nd month).
  – Surgery (3–5 mo).
  – Rehabilitation (2 y).
  – Late reconstruction stage.

Q3. What are the cases which can be kept on conservative management?
Indications for conservative management:
- No disruptive lesion on MRI.
- Only generalized edema of brachial plexus.
- Progressive Tinel's sign.
- Postganglionic injury.

Q4. Which type of injury is common at what level of the plexus?

Roots:
- C8, T1—Avulsion more common
- C5, C6—Stretch/Rupture more common

Q5. How is BPI classified?
BPI is classified into the following:
- Preganglionic.
- Postganglionic.
- Preclavicular.
- Retroclavicular.
- Infraclavicular.

Q6. What are the features suggestive of preganglionic root injury?
- Proximal motor paralysis (rhomboids, serratus).
- Intolerable pain (root pain or deafferentiation).
- Horner's sign.
- Absent or weak Tinel's.
- Cervical spine.
- Elevation of hemidiaphragm.
- Pseudomeningocele.

Q7. How will you differentiate the supraclavicular and infraclavicular injuries?

	Supraclavicular	Infraclavicular
Location	Preganglionic root, Postganglionic nerve, Preclavicular nerve Retroclavicular nerve	Cord and branches
Inspection	Drop shoulder Winged scapular Flail arm Neck shift to unaffected side	Flail arm
Associated	Cervical spine First rib Clavicle	Scapula, humerus
Associated vessel injury	Less chances of subclavian artery injury	High chance of subclavian/axillary artery injury
Extent of nerve lesions	High chances of root injury	Low chances
Types of nerve injury	Avulsion > Rupture	Rupture > Avulsion
Tinel's	Variable	Below coracoid process
Surgery	Nerve transfer	Nerve grafts

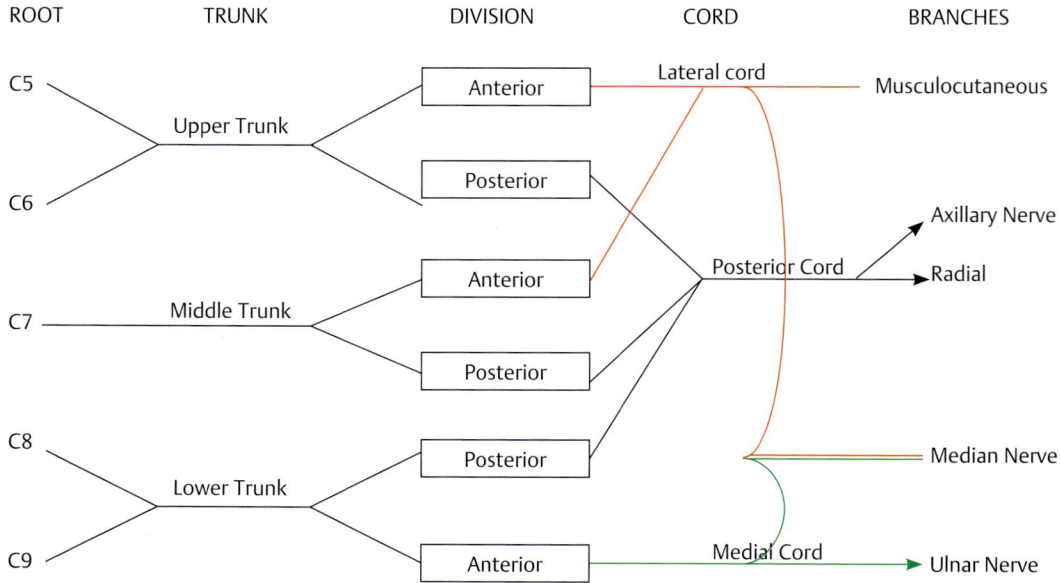

Flowchart 5.1 Anatomy of brachial plexus.

Q8. How will you classify nerve injuries?

Seddon and Sunderland's classification of nerve injuries:

Seddon	Sunderland	Injury	Spontaneous recovery	Nerve conduction study	Electromyography
Neurapraxia	Grade I	Focal segmental demyelination	Yes	Partial/complete conduction block proximally Preserved conduction block distally even after 2 weeks	Normal morphology and poor MUAP recruitment
Axonotmesis	Grade II	Damaged axon with intact endoneurium	Yes, slower than neurapraxia	Partial/complete conduction block proximally Preserved conduction block distally until Wallerian degeneration sets in	Abnormal activity
Axonotmesis	Grade III	Damaged axon and endoneurium with intact perineurium	Not very likely, surgical intervention may be needed		
Axonotmesis	Grade IV	Damaged axon, endoneurium, and perineurium with intact epineurium	Highly unlikely, surgical intervention is necessary		
Axonotmesis	Grade V	Complete nerve transection (disruption of myelin sheath, axon, endoneurium, perineurium and epineurium)	No, surgical intervention is necessary	Complete conduction block proximally and distally	Abnormal activity

McKinnon added a Grade 6 in the Sunderland classification to include mixed pattern of nerve injuries.

Q9. How will you elicit Tinel's sign?

Also known as **Hoffman-Tinel sign**.

- Gentle tapping with examiner's fingertip is done along the course of the nerve from distal to proximal.
- Ask the patient if he/she feels pins and needles' sensation or an electric shock sensation in the distal part of the hand.
- If the patient feels tingling sensation, Tinel is said to be positive.
- Progressive Tinel's sign indicates nerve regeneration.
- Nonprogressive Tinel's sign indicates no regeneration or a neuroma formation at the site of injury.

Q10. How will you perform sensory examination in any nerve injury?

The sensory examination includes tests for:

1.	Tactile sensation	Light touch, crude touch, pressure, and two-point discrimination
2.	Pain sensation	
3.	Temperature	
4.	Position sense	
5.	Stereognosis	

All sensory tests require patient cooperation and intelligence and patience on examiner's part.

- Light touch sensation:

Always explain the procedure to the patient before actually executing it.	The patient is asked to close the eyes and with a light cotton wisp, touch the affected limb from proximal to distal and compare with the normal side.
	Always compare with the normal limb and proceed from proximal to distal.

- Crude touch sensation:
  - Same as above, but using the tip of examiner's finger.

- Pressure sensation: Same as above, but using the broad tip of a pen or a pencil
- Two-point discrimination:
  - Take a caliper and touch the skin of the patient's fingertips at two points simultaneously.
  - Alternatively, a paper pin opened in the shape of an inverted "V" can also be used.
  - Ask the patient if he/she can feel two points simultaneously or only one point.
  - Keep doing this until a minimum distance is reached at which the patient is able to differentiate between two separate points.
  - Normal 2-PD:
    - 2 to 4 mm at finger tips.
    - 4 to 6 mm on volar surface of finger.
    - 8 to 12 mm on palm.
- Pain Sensation:
  - An object with a sharp end like a safety pin or a wooden toothpick with pin-point tip can be used.
  - Patient must be shown the object while explaining the procedure as to calm down his/her anxiety.
  - The skin **MUST NOT** be pricked.
  - Sequence from proximal to distal and comparison with the normal side is followed.
- Temperature:
  - Sensation to cold and hot temperature is tested.
  - To test sensation to cold and hot objects, two separate test tubes filled with hot and cold object can be tested one by one.
  - Alternatively, cold sensation can be checked by using the tines of a tuning fork.
- Position sense:
  - To check the position sense, the patient is first asked to close the eyes and then he/she identifies the direction in which a joint is moved by the examiner.

- Stereognosis:
  - The term "Stereognosis" refers to the ability to identify an object by its touch/ feel.
  - Ask the patient to close his/her eyes and place a common object like coin, key in his palm and ask him to identify the object.
  - The examiner can also write a letter on the palm of the patient with his fingers or a blunt object and ask him/her to identify the letter (graphesthesia).

Q11. What are the normal range of motion (ROM) at joints of upper limb?
The functional ROM at various joints are:
- Shoulder:
  - shrugging (present/not)
  - Flexion: 0 to 180 degree.
  - Extension: 0 to 45 degree.
  - Abduction: 0 to 180 degree.
  - Adduction: 0 to 10 degree.
  - Lateral rotation (infraspinatus, Teres major [T. major]): 0 to 90 degree.
  - Medial rotation (T. major, Pec. minor): 0 to 90 degree.
- Elbow: Extension/Flexion: 0/145 degree.
- Forearm: Pronation/Supination: 70/85 degree.
- Wrist: Extension/Flexion: 70/75 degree. Radial/Ulnar deviation: 20/35 degree.
- Thumb:
  - Carpometacarpal (CMC) joint:
    - Palmar adduction/abduction: Contact/45 degree.
    - Radial adduction/abduction: Contact/60 degree.
    - Extension/Flexion: 50/50 degree.
  - MCP joint:
    - Hyperextension/Flexion: 10/55 degree.
  - Interphalangeal (IP) joint:
    - Hyperextension (H)/Flexion: 15H/80 degree.
- Fingers:
  - MCP joint:
    - Hyperextension (H)/Flexion: (0–45H)/80 degree.
  - Proximal interphalangeal (PIP) joint: Extension/Flexion: 0/100 degree.
  - Distal interphalangeal (DIP) joint: Extension/Flexion: 0/80 degree.

Q12. Do you regularly explore the plexus?
Exploration of plexus on a regular basis is not required.
- In global BPI, one can directly go for nerve transfers without exploring the plexus.
- Exploration indicated in all other cases: partial BPI, phenic as donor nerve, MRI showing rupture/stretching.

Q13. How do you perform spinal accessory nerve (SAN) transfer to suprascapular nerve (SSN) or what are the markings and landmarks in SAN to SSN transfer?
SAN to SSN transfer:
Surgical anatomy of SAN:
- The spinal accessory nerve is formed by both spinal and cranial nerve roots.
- Once it crosses the jugular foramen, it divides into cranial part which joins vagus and spinal part which supplies sterno-cleidomastoid (SCM) and trapezius.
- SAN once supplied to SCM descends down in the posterior triangle between the layers of deep cervical fascia.
- It gives two to three branches to the upper trapezius and runs on its anterior edge to provide supply to middle and lower parts of the muscles.

Approaches:
- Anterior approach: Incisions:
  - Classic supraclavicular incision starts at the angle of mandible which runs down vertically to the midpoint of clavicle. This makes the incision to be along the posterior border of the SCM. The incision then runs parallel to the lateral half of clavicle till the root of trapezius muscle (**Fig. 5.25a**).
  - Transverse cervical incision: Aesthetically more acceptable.
    - A single incision running from posterior border of SCM to the anterior edge of trapezius, parallel

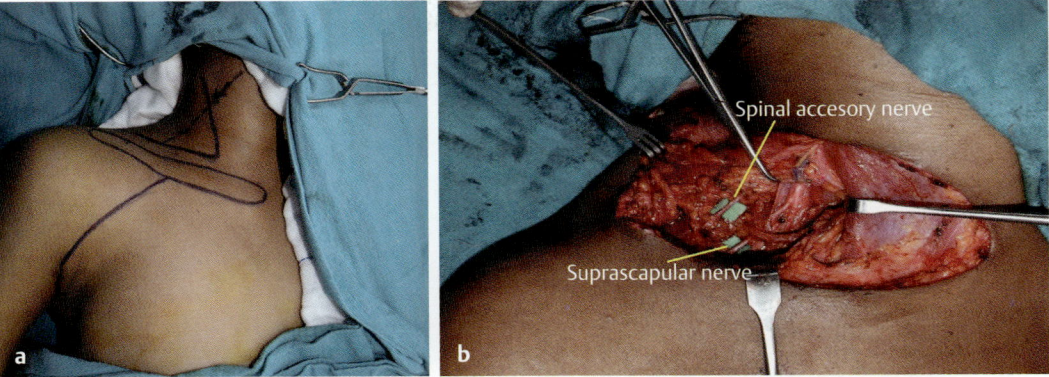

Fig. 5.25   (a, b) Anterior approach: Spinal accessory nerve to suprascapular (SAN-SSN).

and superior to the lateral half of clavicle.

- The difference between both the incisions is that in classical type, the SAN is traced from the posterior border of SCM to the anterior edge of trapezius which has the disadvantages of creating a long scar in the neck and possible damage to the nerve.
- The beginners can start with classical incision and gradually shift to the transverse incision.

- Key points in anterior approach (**Fig. 5.25b**):
  - The trapezius muscle inserted at the clavicle is exposed and the anterior fibers are detached.
  - The cut fibers are retracted posteriorly and look for the transverse cervical artery and vein which accompany the SAN.
  - Carefully look for branches of SAN in the adipose tissue around the anterior edge of the trapezius. Confirm it using a nerve stimulator. The terminal branch is dissected distally and divided at the level of the spine of scapula.
  - SAN branch is then delivered in the supraclavicular fossa for coaptation.
  - To dissect out the SSN, omohyoid muscle is dissected, cut, and retracted medially. The nerve lies deep to the omohyoid.

- It passes laterally toward the suprascapular notch, passes deep to superior transverse ligament to enter the supraspinatus fossa.
- SSN is liable to undergo crush injury while passing through the notch which may lead to unsuccessful outcome, if missed. So, one has to go posterior to the notch to dissect the part of nerve which lies distal to the notch for coaptation.
- The impact of the injury in the notch is avoidable when transfer is done through the posterior approach.

- Posterior approach:
  Markings: On the back of the patient in sitting position (**Fig. 5.26a**).
  - Mark the midline spinous process.
  - Mark the acromion process.
  - Palpate the superior border of scapula.
  - Draw a line parallel to superior border and joining the midline and acromion process.
  - Mark the SAN at the junction of medial one-third and lateral two-third on this line (literature says at a distance of 40 percent from midline).
  - Draw a line on the superior border of scapula from acromion process to the superior angle of scapula.
  - Mark the SSN at the midpoint on this line.

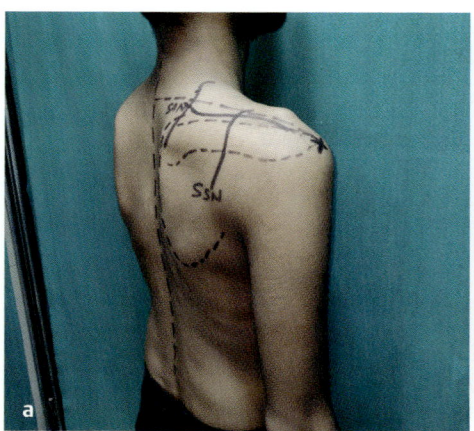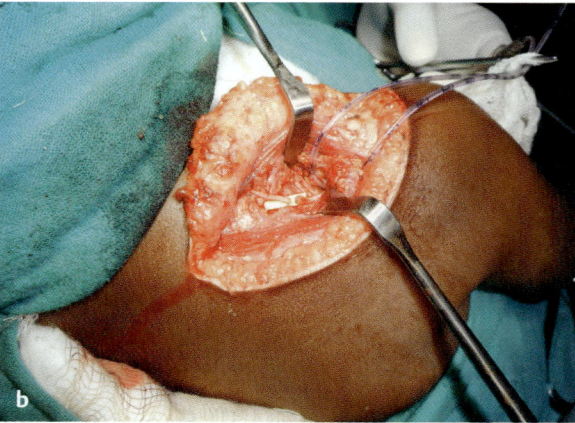

Fig. 5.26 **(a, b)** Posterior approach: Spinal accessory nerve to suprascapular (SAN-SSN).

Incision:

- A transverse incision is marked between the location of these two nerves and incision is made.
- Dissection is carried out deep into the trapezius muscle. Alternatively, the posterior fibers of trapezius muscle are dissected off their attachment at spine of scapula.
- SAN will be identified at the undersurface of trapezius muscle in the adipose tissue.
- Along the superior border of the scapula, dissection is carried out slightly deeper to the supraspinatus muscle toward the scapular notch.
- Locate the suprascapular artery which runs superior to the transverse capsular ligament that forms the roof of the notch.
- All soft tissues over the ligament are cleared, ligament is cut sharply under vision and a right-angled forceps is used to hook the suprascapular nerve.
- SSN is dissected proximally to ensure tension-free cooptation **(Fig. 5.26b).**

Advantages:

- It prevents the denervation of the upper part of trapezius muscle.
- It negates the effect of injury to SSN in the suprascapular notch.
- Nerve transfer is close to the muscle.

Q14. What are the procedures for restoration of elbow flexion?

- Nerve transfer for restoration of elbow flexion.
  - Donor nerves:
    - Intercostal nerves (ICN).
    - Ulnar nerve.
    - Median nerve.
    - Contralateral C7.
  - Indications for ICN transfer (**Fig. 5.27a, b**):
    - Global BPI or upper trunk injury.
    - Duration of injury <6 months.
    - Third, fourth, and fifth intercostal nerves are used. Second nerve is preserved as the intercostobrachial branch of second ICN is the only sensory supply to the medial arm in global BPI.
    - The more proximal part of ICN is used for cooptation as motor fiber content of ICN decreases distally.
  - Ulnar and medial nerve as donors (Oberlin's 1 and 2) (**Fig. 5.28**):
    Indications:
    - Upper trunk BPI (C5, C6).
    - In C5–C7 BPI where only ulnar nerve is used as donor.
    - Less than 6 months, sometimes up to 10 months.
    - Preferably, in younger patient.
      - In the upper half of the arm, there are 6 to 10 fascicles in ulnar

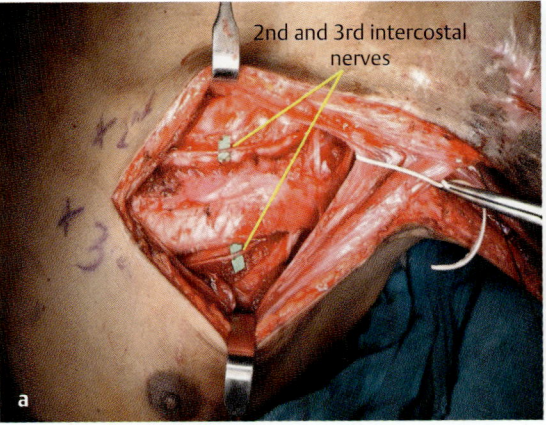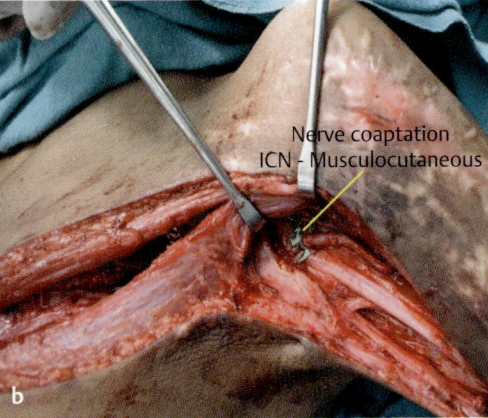

Fig. 5.27 **(a, b)** Intercostal nerve to musculocutaneous transfer (ICN-MCN).

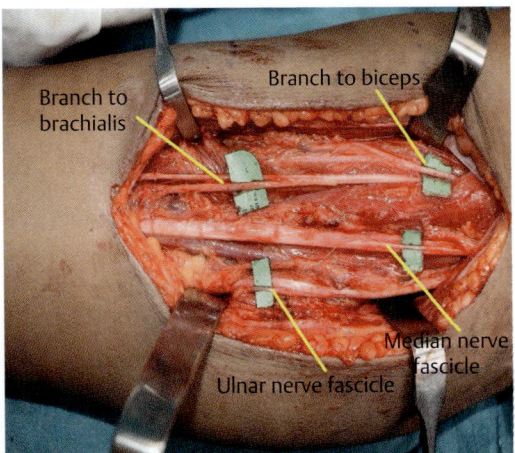

Fig. 5.28 Oberlin's procedure.

nerve containing sensory and motor fibers.

○ Posteromedial fascicles contain the motor fibers to the muscles in the forearm and anterolateral fascicles contain motor fibers to the intrinsic muscles of the hand.

○ A single fascicle of ulnar nerve is identified by epineural dissection and electrical stimulation. Few brachial plexus surgeons prefer to use one posteromedial fascicle supplying flexor carpi ulnaris (FCU) but any fascicle can be used as the level of midarm; all fascicles of ulnar nerve are mixed.

○ Ulnar nerve fascicle is transferred to musculocutaneous branch to biceps muscle (Oberlin's 1 procedure).

○ A single median nerve fascicle is transferred to the musculocutaneous branch to biceps more distally in the arm (Oberlin's 2 procedure).

– Contralateral C7 transfer:

Indications:

■ In very limited cases in global palsy or C5–C8 root ovulation in which double free functional muscle transfer is planned.

■ In children and young adults, to coapt with suprascapular nerve when ipsilateral C7 nerve root is not available.

○ Free vascularized ulnar nerve graft is used.

○ Counting of C7 nerve root is very important as there might be presence of prefixed and postfixed brachial plexus.

• Free functional muscle transfer:

Indications:

– Delayed cases of BPI >10 months of injury.

– Unsuccessful nerve repair/transfer.

– Preferably younger patients.

Donor muscles:

– Gracilis (free functional) (**Fig. 5.29a, b**).

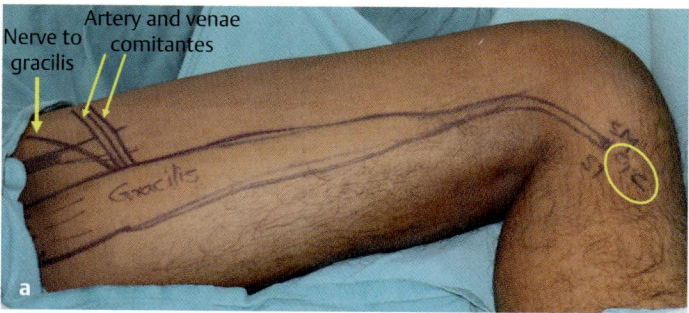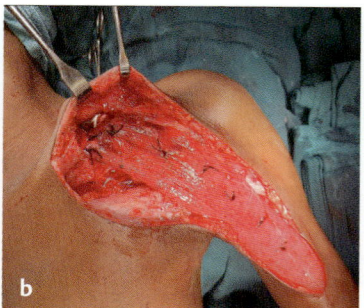

Fig. 5.29 (a, b) Free functional gracilis muscle transfer.

- Pedicled latissimus dorsi.
- Free rectus femoris.
- For elbow flexion by muscle transfer, shoulder joint stability must be restored either by nerve or muscle transfer or secondarily by arthrodesis of glenohumeral joint.
- Lateral dorsi and rectus femoris are stronger for elbow flexion as compared to gracilis which is the best choice for wrist and finger function.

Donor nerve:
- ICN in global BPI.
- Spinal accessory.
- Ulnar nerve fascicle (in C5–C6 or C5–C7 injury).
- Medial/lateral pectoral nerve.

Recipient vessels:
- Thoracoacromial artery and cephalic vein.
- Thoracodorsal artery and vein.

Q15. How will you restore movements of wrist, or what will you do for restoration of finger movements?

Double free functional gracilis muscle transfer is the technique for restoration of finger flexion and extension.

- It consists of five procedures:
  - Exploration and repair of ruptured nerves, if possible.
  - First-free functioning muscle transfer (FFMT), innervated by SAN for elbow flexion and finger extension.
  - Second FFMT, innervated by ICN 5 and 6.
  - ICN 3 and 4 transfer to nerve to triceps simultaneously with second muscle transfer.
  - ICN sensory rami coapted to the medial cord of brachial plexus for restoring the sensibility of the hand.
    - Sometimes, a sixth procedure like arthrodesis of shoulder joint or wrist joint or CMC joint is required to increase the stability of the joint.

Indications:
- Global BPI.
- Duration of injury >6 months.
- No injury to the bigger vessels or donor nerve.
- Young patient <40 years.

In patients not suitable for free functional muscle transfer, tendon transfers for only lower trunk injury involving median and ulnar nerve can be done for restoration of fingers and thumb flexion: extensor carpi radialis longus–flexor digitorum profundus (ECRL-FDP) and brachioradialis–flexor pollicis longus (BR-FPL) **(Fig. 5.30)**.

Q16. How a normal shoulder abduction is brought about, or what are the movements at shoulder joint?

Major movements at the shoulder (glenohumeral) joint:
- Abduction.
- Adduction.

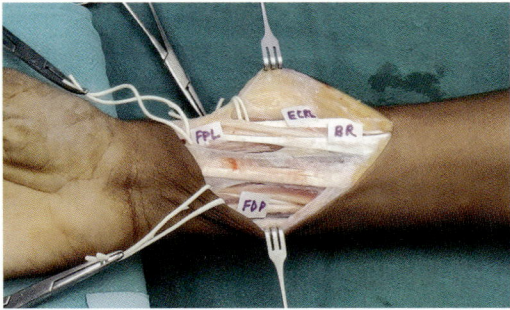

Fig. 5.30 Tendon transfer in lower trunk brachial plexus injury (BPI) (extensor carpi radialis longus–flexor digitorum profundus [ECRL-FDP], brachioradialis–flexor pollicis longus [BR-FPL]).

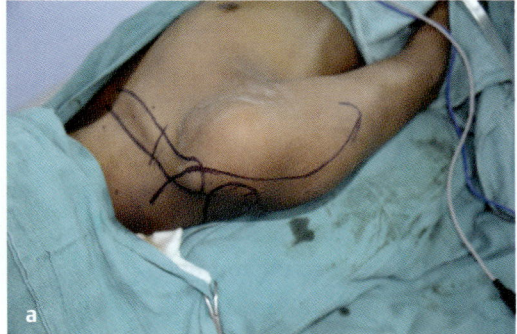

- Flexion.
- Extension.
- External rotation.
- Internal rotation.
- Abduction:
  - First 15 degrees by supraspinatus.
  - 15 to 90 degrees by primarily deltoid and assisted by supraspinatus.
  - Beyond 90 degrees and also scapular rotation by trapezius and serratus anterior.
- Adduction: By pectoralis major, latissimus dorsi, teres major, triceps, and coracobrachialis.
- Flexion: Combined actions of deltoid, pectoralis major, coracobrachialis, and biceps brachii.
- Extension: Deltoid, latissimus dorsi, teres major, and triceps.
- External rotation: Deltoid, teres minor, and infraspinatus.
- Internal rotation: Pectoralis major, latissimus dorsi, deltoid, teres major, and subscapularis.

Q17. What are the various muscle transfers done in BPI for shoulder joint?

Saha's procedure:
- Transfer of:
  - Trapezius for deltoid and clavicular head of pectoralis major (*prime movement of shoulder*) (**Fig. 5.31a, b**).

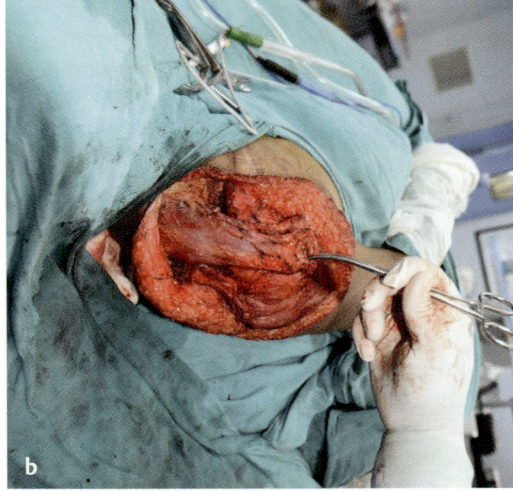

Fig. 5.31   (a, b) Trapezius transfer.

  - Levator scapulae for supraspinatus (vertical steerer).
  - Pectoralis minor or remaining pectoralis major for anterior horizontal steerers (subscapular teres minor).
- Prime movers: Deltoid, long and short head of biceps, coracobrachialis, long head of triceps and teres major.
- Steerers: Supraspinatus, infraspinatus, subscapularis, and teres minor.

Q18. What is the postoperative rehabilitation protocol in nerve transfers and muscle transfer?

- In nerve transfers:
  - After 4 to 6 weeks of surgery:
    - Passive and active ROM to be started.

- In muscle transfer:
  - Trapezius: Immobilization for 6 to 8 weeks followed by passive and active range of motion.
  - Gracilis: Passive ROM after 4 to 6 week of immobilization.

Q19. When you will do electrodiagnostic studies (NCS, electromyography [EMG]) and what are its implications? How to perform it?

Electrodiagnostic studies.

1. Nerve Conduction Studies (NCS)
   - Principle: It gives information regarding:
     - Whether nerve action potential is propagating.
     - Idea about the compound muscle action potential (CMAP) due to the activation of muscle fibers in target muscle supplied by that particular nerve.
   - Procedure: There are two electrodes placed on the skin along the course of the nerve: one electrode proximal and other distal to the site of injury.
     - Through the stimulating electrode, a mild and brief electrical stimulation is given and through the recording electrode, the response of the nerve to the stimulus is recorded on a monitor.
     - Electrodes used can be surface or needle electrodes.
   - Interpretation is done in context with:
     - The latency of the nerve.
     - Amplitude and duration of the action potential.
     - Calculate the conduction velocity and compare with normal.
     - Gradient of velocity (velocity is faster in part of the nerve closer to the central neural axis or in cephalad position as compared to the caudal and more distal nerves).
     - Size and shape of CMAP:
       - CMAP: Summated voltage response from individual muscle fiber action potentials.
       - To record CMAP during NCSs, the electrical stimulation is increased in a gradient till a point where no further increase in CMAP amplitude occurs on increasing the stimulus.
     - Sensory nerve action potential (SNAP):
       - Is received by giving electrical stimulation to the sensory fibers and recording the nerve action potential.

2. EMG
   - EMG is a neurodiagnostic procedure to assess the innervation of a muscle.
   - In EMG, a needle is directly inserted into a muscle and the electrical activity in that muscle is recorded.
   - Procedure:
     - A disposable needle electrode is used to insert into the muscle.
     - Both the appearance of muscle activity and the sound of activity amplified through a speaker can be interpreted.
   - Reading: At Rest
     - Fibrillations: Present in denervated muscles.
       - The basis for appearance of fibrillation is the super sensitivity of the muscle fibers after 7 to 10 days of nerve injury.
       - Detectable by the EMG needle and visible through skin as it is a single muscle fiber discharge.
     - Positive waves: Origin same as fibrillations and have similar importance.
     - Complex repetitive discharges:
       - May arise as jitters between the action potentials.
       - Seen in neurogenic disease.
     - Fasciculation:
       - Arises due to twitching of a part or whole of the single motor unit.
       - May be visible under the skin.
       - They are involuntary and differentiates the motor units twitching as a result of poor relaxation.

- In active movement:
  - Patient is asked to do the active movement of the target muscle.
  - Look for amplitude, duration, phasic changes, and the rate of firing of the motor unit potentials (MUPs).
  - Normal MUPs are less than 2 MV in amplitude, with a duration of 5 to 10 milliseconds in three to four phases.
  - Nascent MUPs have low voltage and shorter duration amplitude.

Suggested Reading

1. Spinner RJ, Shin AY, Elhassan BT et al. In: Green DP, eds. Green's operative hand surgery. Vol. 1. 8th ed. Elsevier; 2022:1304–1362.

6 Facial Nerve Palsy

Veena K. Singh and Saurabh K. Gupta

Learning Objectives

At the end of the chapter, the students will be able to:

1. Recognize the varied presentation of facial nerve palsy.
2. Recall the entire course of facial nerve and its supply to face.
3. Understand the assessment of a patient with facial nerve palsy.
4. Make decision on the surgical options for each region of the face.
5. Demonstrate the common surgical procedures for facial reanimation.

Introduction

Facial nerve paralysis leading to nonfunctioning of the facial muscles has many adverse effects on the patient. Vital functions like protection of eyeball, nasal airway patency, oral continence, and speech are affected. Facial expressions are worst hit by nerve palsy which harms the social integration of the patient to such an extent that few patients might suffer psychological issues. A clear understanding of the clinical examination and its correct interpretation will help in the proper planning and adequate management of the patient with better outcomes.

Chief Complaints

- Inability to close the eye on the affected side.
- Deviation of mouth on smiling.
- Watering or redness of the affected eye.
- Accumulation of food in the mouth on the affected side.
- Occasionally, patient may also complaint of drooping of eyelid or sagging of face on the affected side.

History of Present Illness

- Duration of the problems.
- Onset—Sudden/gradual.
- Progress—Slow/rapid, static/progressive.
- Any recovery over the course of time.
- Whether any history of initial recovery followed by static course.
- Any medication which he/she is taking for the current problem.
- Any history of trauma or fracture of facial bones.
- Eye symptoms: History of dryness, redness, excessive watering, incomplete closure, sand particles/foreign body sensation especially when outside and any use of eye drops or artificial tears for the eye problems. Any difficulty in reading.
- Nasal problem: History of any breathing difficulty from the nostril on affected side or dryness of nose.
- Speech problem: History of drooling of saliva due to oral incontinence or speech problem in pronouncing certain syllables.
- Eating problem: Any problem in chewing food or food particles accumulating in the

mouth or falling out of mouth. Enquire about loss of taste sensation or dryness of mouth.

- Abnormal movements: Also ask about spontaneous movement of one part of face on moving any other part of face. Any weakness in other parts of the body.
- Ear problems: History suggestive of ear infection like earache, discharge, any facial cellulitis, or other infection like herpes zoster. Any history of increased loudness of sound (hyperacusis).
- History related to the extent of their social interaction because of facial asymmetry, especially on smiling.
- Also, look for mental and emotional problems, if any in history.
- Enquire about sleep, appetite, bladder, bowel function.

Past History

- History of diabetes mellitus, hypertension, tuberculosis, or any other medical illness.
- Any surgery done in the past, around ear, eyes, or the temp-mandibular joint.

Personal History

History of addiction including alcoholism, smoking, marital status, no. of kids, employment status.

Family History

Number of family members dependent on the patient.

Treatment History

- Any medicine (like steroids) or any surgery done for the current problem.
- History of allergy to food or medications.

General Physical Examination

- Remains same as others except for specific mentioning of faces, which may be like a masked/expressionless face in cases of facial nerve palsy.
- Neck nodes—to be palpated carefully.

Systemic Examination

• Abdomen	Like others except
• CNS	of CNS which will
• CVS	be covered under
• Respiratory system	'local examination'

Local Examination of The Face

Inspection

Facies

Description will start in a sequence from above below (**Fig. 6.1**):
1. Any obvious absence of forehead wrinkles at rest on affected side.
2. Position of eyebrow, whether drooping or at a lower level compared to normal side.
3. Size of palpebral aperture if more as compared to normal side.

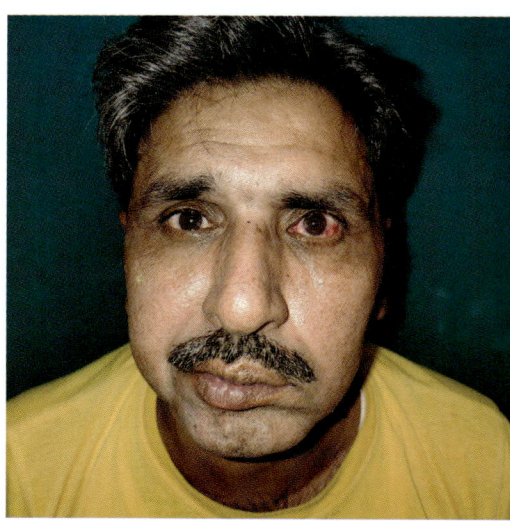

Fig. 6.1 Facies in a facial nerve palsy patient.

4. Watering/Redness of eyes, if present.
5. Ectropion of lower eyelid.
6. Sagging of cheek.
7. Obliteration of nasolabial fold.
8. Amount of philtral deviation.
9. Depression and deviation of the oral commissure/angle of mouth on the affected side.
10. Drooping of upper lip, if any.
11. Presence of vermilion inversion.

Palpation

Examination of Facial Nerve

1. Stabilize the patient head with left hand and ask him to see upward (**Fig. 6.2**).
   - Look for absence of wrinkles on the forehead on affected side.
   - This tests the frontotemporal branches of facial nerve which supplies the frontalis muscle.
2. Ask the patient to frown (**Fig. 6.3**).
   - Look for the presence/absence of vertical furrows in between the eyebrows.
     - This tests the action of corrugator supercilii.
3. Ask the patient to close his both eyes. If able to close the eye on affected side, ask him to close forcefully and try to open it (**Fig. 6.4a, b**).

- Look for patient's inability to close the eyes.
- Check for partial weakness or complete paralysis of facial nerve branch to orbicularis oculi.
4. Ask the patient to fill air in his mouth. If he is able to do so, press the affected cheek gently (**Fig. 6.5**).
   - Look for the escape of air from the affected side either on rest or on pressure from your side.
   - This tests the zygomaticobuccal branches of facial nerve supplying the buccinators and orbicularis oris.
5. Ask the patient to blow whistle (**Fig. 6.6**).
   - Look for the escape of air through the lips.
   - This tests the action of orbicularis oris.
6. Ask the patient to smile maximally (**Fig. 6.7**).
   - Look for the movement at bilateral commissure. Also, look for the extent of upper incisor shown while smiling.
   - This tests the marginal mandibular branches of facial nerve which supplies the depressors of the lip.
   - The angle of mouth is deviated to the affected side.
7. Ask the patient to stretch his neck backward (**Fig. 6.8**).

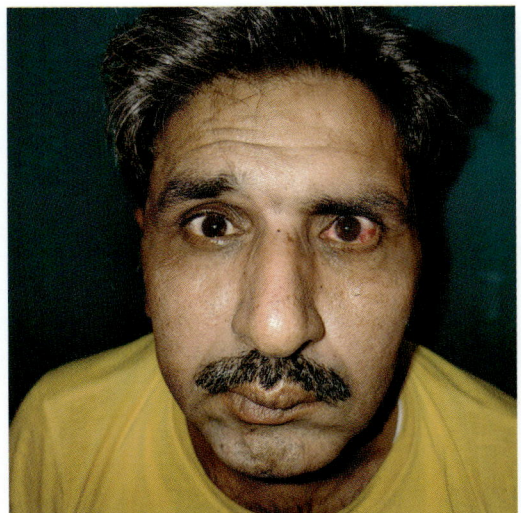

Fig. 6.2 Action of frontalis.

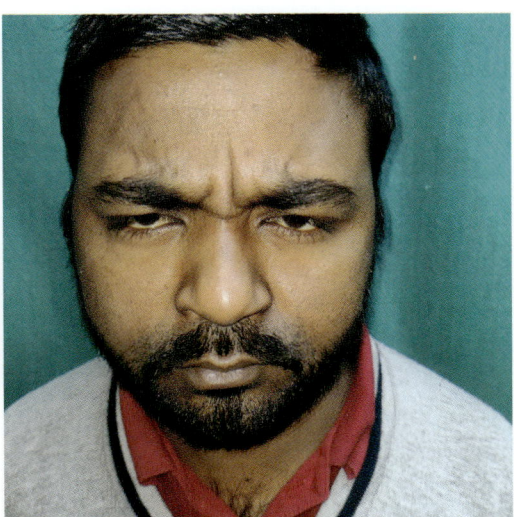

Fig. 6.3 Action of corrugator supercilia.

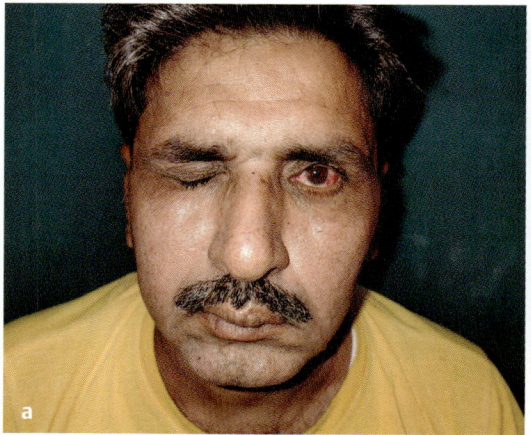

Fig. 6.4   **(a, b)** Action of orbicularis oculi.

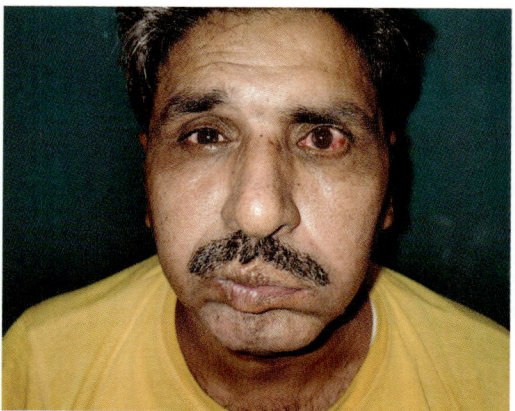

Fig. 6.5   Action of buccinator.

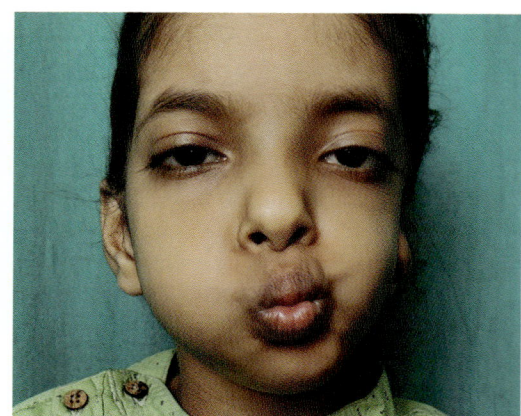

Fig. 6.6   Action of orbicularis oris.

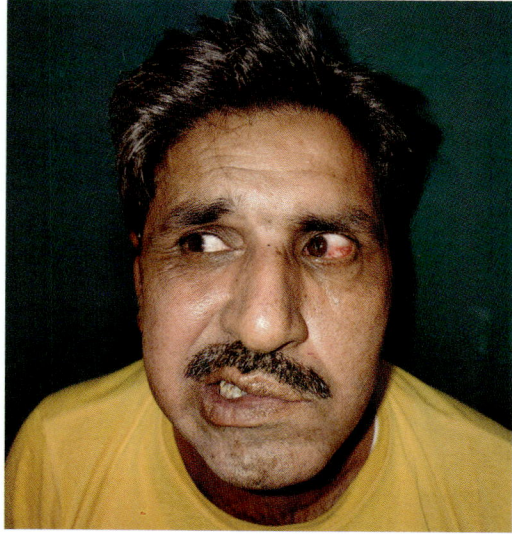

Fig. 6.7   Action of depressors of lip.

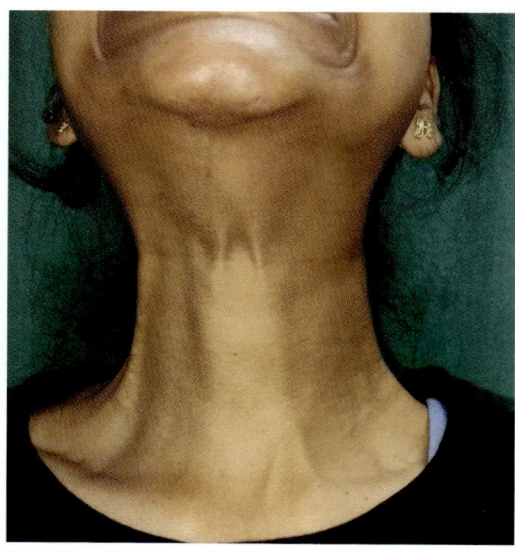

Fig. 6.8   Action of platysma.

- This tests the action of cervical divisions of facial nerve which supplied the platysma.

Examination of Nasal Airway

- Ask the patient to do forced inspiration while blocking each nostril alternately to check the patency of nasal airway.
- There might be some blockage of the nasal airway on affected side due to collapsed nostril as a result of paralyzed dilator naris and drooping of cheek.
- An intranasal examination of the nasal cavity must be done using Thudichum's speculum.

Intraoral Examination

- Look for dental hygiene.
- Look for accumulated food particles in the oral sulcus.
- Look for any evidence of cheek biting.
- Do a bimanual palpation for any thickening of parotid duct.

Assessment of Speech

- Look for pronunciation of the words producing "b" and "p" sounds (Plosives) which require lip sealing.

Examination of Eye

1. Measure the height of palpebral aperture on both affected and normal side (**Fig. 6.9a, b**).
   - Normally, when the eyes are open, the shape of the palpebral aperture is of an asymmetrical ellipse. The normal height at its widest point is 9 to 11 mm.
   - Normally, in a neutral gaze position, the upper eyelid covers 2 to 3 mm of the superior portion of corneal.
2. Look for the presence of Bell's reflex (visibility of white of eye-on-eye closure) (**Fig. 6.10**).
3. Position of lower eyelid and its tone by doing snap test.
   - Gently pinch the lower eyelid and pull it away from the eyeball.
   - Release it and check whether the eyelid immediately snaps back against the eyeball.
   - In a facial nerve palsy, this does not occur due to poor tone of eyelid.
4. Position of lower eyelid punctum: Whether applied to the globe as in normal eyelid or is it rolled away and exposed.
   - Look for redness and features of corneal ulceration, if any.

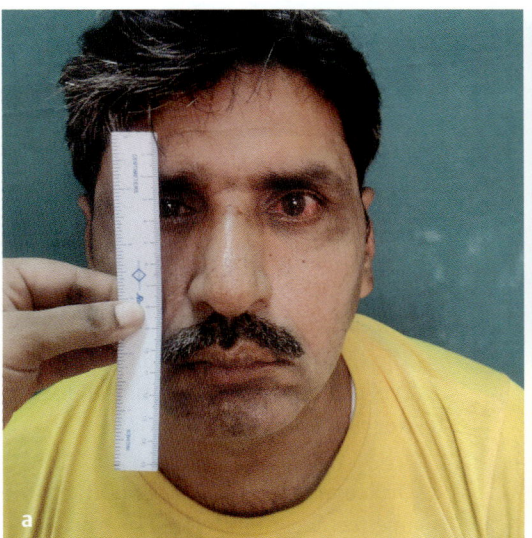
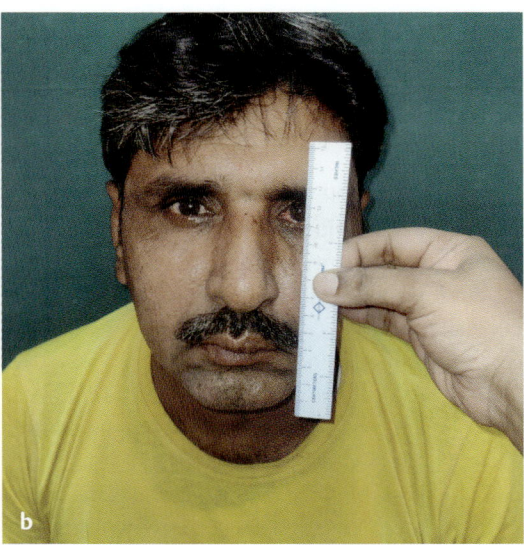

Fig. 6.9 (**a, b**) Measurement of palpebral aperture.

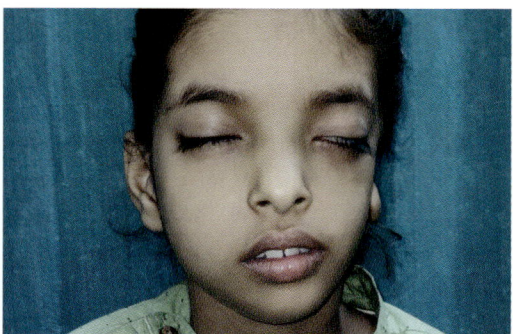

Fig. 6.10 Bell's phenomenon.

Look for Presence of Synkinesis

- Synkinesis is simultaneous contraction of two or more group of muscles that do not normally contract together.
- This happens due to misdirection of the sprouting of reinnervating axons.
  - Look whether the eye closure occurs with smiling.
  - Look whether there is wrinkling of the eyebrows when mouth is moved while speaking.
  - Look whether eye closure causes grimacing of the mouth.

Provisional Diagnosis

This is a case of a 6-month-old idiopathic left sided facial nerve palsy in a 46-year-old male of lower motor neuron type.

Questions

Q1. How will you do the clinical assessment of the level of injury?

Clinical assessment of the level of injury can be done by few tests which can be performed clinically:

- Examination of taste:
  - Ask for the loss of taste sensation over anterior two-third of the tongue on the affected side.
  - Loss of taste on ipsilateral side indicates injury to facial nerve within the

bony canal due to injury to chorda tympani nerve.

- Stapedius reflex:
  - If patient complaints of hyperacusis (increased frequency of sound) on the affected side, it indicates the level of facial nerve injury within the bony canal due to injury to nerve to stapedius.
- Secretomotor function and salivary flow test:
  - Ask for dryness of nose, mouth, or eyes which indicates decreased secretory function due to injury to facial nerve near the geniculate ganglion.
  - **Schirmer test:**
    - Place a strip in the lower fornix and ask the patient to close the eyes for 5 minutes.
    - Remove the paper strip and measure the extent to which it has become moist.
    - Less than 10 mm is a sign of insufficient tear production.

Q2. What is the functional importance of lower eyelid?

- Normally, the lower eyelid covers the inferior limbus of the cornea and there is no scleral show.
  - During majority of eye movements, the upper eyelid moves the most whereas the lower lid remains static except for 1 to 2 mm upward movement of lower eyelid during smiling or squinting.
- The main functions of the lower lid is in drainage of tears.
  - Due to repetitive blinking, the tear film spreads in a lateral-to-medial inferior fornix.

    ↓

  - The tear then migrates along the lower eyelid margin to the inferior and superior puncta.

    ↓

  - Orbicularis oculi has an important role in effective drainage of tears by causing a pumplike effect on the lacrimal sac to facilitate the effective clearance of tears.

Q3. Why do dryness and watering occur in the facial nerve palsy?

The secretory functions of facial nerve are compromised in cases of paralysis.

↓

Dryness and corneal exposure

↓

Reflex production of excessive tears

↓

Ineffective drainage due to paralyzed lower eyelid

↓

Excessive watering (epiphora)

↓

Can be increased by the downward inclination of face while reading or doing some near work.

Q4. How will you assess taste sensation in a patient with facial nerve palsy?

- Tongue has taste sensations in the sensory endings of the papillae which are of four types (**Fig. 6.11**):
  - Surface of tongue → Fungiform ⎤
  - Lateral sides → Foliate ⎟ Papillae
  - Form an inverted "V" at the ⎟ containing taste buds
    base of tongue → Circumvallate ⎟
  - Filiform → transmits ⎟
    touch, temp- ⎟
    erature, and ⎟
    nociception. ⎦
- Four basic taste sensations have been described:
  - Sweet and salty: at the tip of tongue.
  - Sour: at the sides.
  - Bitter: at the posterior surface/base of tongue.
- Taste from anterior two-third of the tongue is carried by chorda tympani, a branch of facial nerve, and other sensations by lingual nerve, a branch of trigeminal nerve.

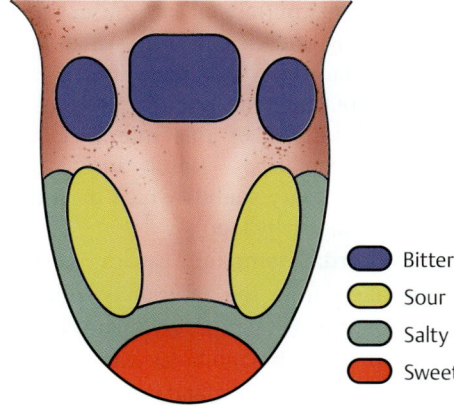

Bitter
Sour
Salty
Sweet

Fig. 6.11 Distribution of taste zones on tongue.

- Taste from posterior one-third of the tongue is carried by glossopharyngeal nerve.

Q5. What is the intracranial course of facial nerve?

The part of the facial nerve which lies within the cranium is its intracranial part.

- It originates from pons as two roots—a large motor and a small sensory.

↓

- The two roots travel through the petrous part of the temporal bone in the internal acoustic meatus (~1 cm long).

↓

- It then leaves the meatus to enter the facial canal where the two roots join to from the facial nerve and the geniculate ganglion.

↓

- Within the canal, facial nerve gives three branches:
  - **Greater petrosal nerve**, which carries parasympathetic fibers to the lacrimal gland.
  - **Nerve to stapedius**, which supplies the stapedius muscle in middle ear.
    - Stapedius is the smallest skeletal muscle in the human body.

- On contraction, it causes stiffening of ossicular chain which in turn dampens the intensity of sound reaching the inner ear.
- Paralysis of this muscle leads to hyperacusis (intolerance toward ordinary sounds which may appear unusually loud).
  - **Chorda tympani** carries gustatory fibers from the anterior two-thirds of the tongue and parasympathetic fibers to the submandibular and sublingual glands (parotid gland is supplied by the glossopharyngeal nerve).

    ↓

  - The nerve then leaves the cranium by exiting through the stylomastoid foramen located deep to the styloid process of temporal bone.

Q6. What is the extracranial course of facial nerve?

- Facial nerve exits at the stylomastoid foramen and lies in a deep plane below the earlobe (**Fig. 6.12**).

  ↓

- Three branches arise from facial nerve immediately after coming out from the foramen.
  - Posterior auricular nerve:
    - Supplies muscles of external ear.
  - Nerve to posterior belly of digastric (anterior belly of digastric receives its supply from mylohyoid nerve, a branch of inferior alveolar nerve arising from mandibular branch of trigeminal nerve).
  - Nerve to stylohyoid muscle.

    ↓

- It becomes superficial to pass between the superficial and deep portions of the parotid gland where it divides into two main trunks which further divides within the gland.

  ↓

- It then exits from the parotid gland to lie approximately 10 mm deep to the surface of the skin and gradually becomes superficial.

  ↓

- It then divides into 8 to 10 branches which makes a total of five divisions.

  ↓

The branches further divide and connect with each other leading to much functional overlap between the branches.

Q7. What are the major divisions of the facial nerve?

There are five major divisions of facial nerve:

- **Frontotemporal branches:**
  - They are three to four in number.
  - They run under the temporoparietal fascia and cross the zygomatic arch 3 to 5 cm lateral to the lateral orbital wall.
  - The upper two branches enter the frontalis muscle at the level of supraorbital ridge and lies 3 cm above the level of lateral canthus in the subcutaneous plane.
  - Its relation to the frontal branch of superficial temporal artery is that nerve lies approx. 1.5 to 2 cm inferior to the artery.
  - Approx. 1 cm above the line joining the tragus and lateral canthus, dissection above this like must be deep to temporoparietal fascia.
  - It supplies the frontalis, orbicularis oculi, corrugator supercilii.
- **Zygomatic branch:** Supplies the muscles of middle face.
- **Buccal branch:** Muscles of cheek including buccinators.
  - Both are combined as zygomaticobuccal division which consists of three to eight branches with much of overlapping and interconnections so that one or more branches may be divided without causing weakness.
  - These branches supply the lower orbicularis oculi, buccinator, orbicularis oris, and lip elevators.

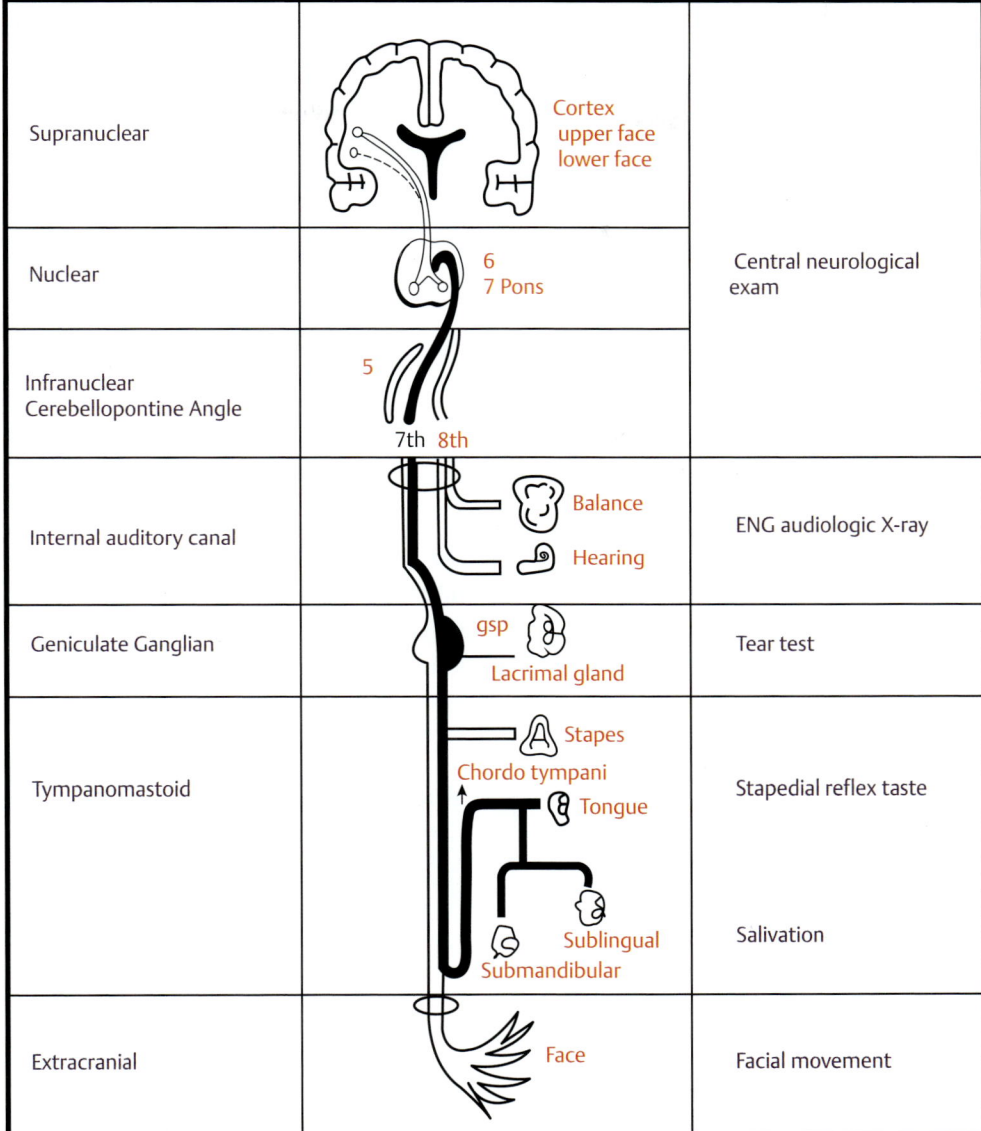

Supranuclear		Cortex upper face lower face
Nuclear	6 7 Pons	Central neurological exam
Infranuclear Cerebellopontine Angle	5 7th 8th	
Internal auditory canal	Balance Hearing	ENG audiologic X-ray
Geniculate Ganglian	gsp Lacrimal gland	Tear test
Tympanomastoid	Stapes Chordo tympani Tongue Sublingual Submandibular	Stapedial reflex taste Salivation
Extracranial	Face	Facial movement

Fig. 6.12 Course of facial nerve.

- The plane of these nerves is same as that of parotid duct.
- **Marginal mandibular branch:**
  - Consists of one to three branches.
  - Runs 2 cm below the ramus of the mandible and courses upward, crossing at the middle of the mandibular body to supply lower orbicularis oris, depressors of lip, and platysma.

- These branches run deep to platysma and pass superficial to facial vessels.
- **Cervical branch:**
  - This is mostly a single branch which passes below the angle of mandible to run on the undersurface of platysma.
  - It enters the platysma at the junction of upper and middle thirds.

Q8. What are the muscles of facial expression?

They are divided into various groups:

- Orbital group:
  - Corrugator supercilii: Pulls the eyebrows median and downward.
  - Orbicularis oculi: Closes the eyelids.
  - Efferent limb of corneal/blind reflex.
- Nasal group:
  - Nasalis: Pulls the nasal cartilage laterally to open the nostrils.
  - Procerus: Pulls the medial end of eyebrows downward to produce a transverse wrinkle at the bridge of nose.
  - Depressor septi: Pulls the tip of nose downward.
- Oral group:
  - Depressor anguli oris.
  - Depressor labii inferioris.
  - Levator labii superioris.
  - Levator labii superioris alaeque nasi.
  - Zygomaticus major and minor.
  - Orbicularis oris.
  - Buccinator.
  - Risorius.
  - Mentalis.
- Other muscles:
  - Anterior, posterior, and superior auricular muscles: Elevate the ear.
  - Occipitofrontalis:
    - Frontalis: Raises the eyebrows.
    - Occipital: Pulls the scalp backward.

Q9. How do you classify facial nerve injuries?

- Multiple classification of facial nerve injuries are found in the literature.
- Most commonly used is House-Brackmann scale (**Table 6.1**).

House and Brackmann also staged from grade 1-6 with different chances of recovery:

- **Grade I**
  - Neuropraxia (spontaneous recovery most likely).
- **Grade II–III**
  - Axonotemesis (longer compression of nerve).
  - Temporary interruption.
- Subsequent Wallerian degeneration (partial facial weakness often remains).
- **Grade IV**
  - Neurotomesis (permanent loss of axons).
  - Demyelination leading to moderate to severe facial musculature dysfunction.
  - Regeneration impaired → Facial synkinetic movements, mass movements or contracture.
- **Grade V–VI**
  - Partial and complete transection of facial nerve.
  - Retainment of minimal facial musculature movements or complete loss of function.

Q10. What are the investigations which you will perform in a case of facial nerve palsy and why?

Electrophysiologic studies are conducted to assess:

Electrophysiology		
Extent of nerve disruption	Possible outcome	Treatment options

- Electrodiagnostic tests including electromyography (EMG) and nerve conduction study (NCS).
- Electroneuronography (ENoG) is an objective test to record the evoked compound muscle action potential to quantify the degeneration of nerve fibers. Tests are performed with percutaneous stimulation of facial nerve.
- Electroneuronography (ENoG) determines the timing and necessity of surgical intervention.
  - ENoG records CAP (compound action potential) as well as latency after nerve stimulation.
  - Defunction of 90% means poor prognosis without surgical intervention.
- Multisliced computed tomography (CT) scan and magnetic resonance imaging (MRI) of brain in case any intracranial or

Table 6.1 House-Brackmann scale for clinical classification of the facial nerve injuries

Grade	Characteristics
1. No dysfunction	Normal facial function in all areas
2. Mild dysfunction	**Gross** • Slight weakness noticeable on close inspection • Slight synkinesis may be present • At rest, normal symmetry and tone **Motion** • Forehead: Moderate to good function • Eye: Complete closure with minimal effort • Mouth: Slight asymmetry
3. Moderate dysfunction	**Gross** • Obvious but not disfiguring difference between sides • Noticeable (but not severe) synkinesis, contracture or hemifacial spasm • At rest, normal symmetry and tone **Motion** • Forehead: Slight to moderate movement • Eye: Complete closure with effort • Mouth: Slightly weak with maximum effort
4. Moderately Severe dysfunction	**Gross** • Obvious weakness and/or disfiguring asymmetry • At rest, normal symmetry **Motion** • Forehead: None • Eye: Incomplete closure • Mouth: Asymmetrical with maximum effort
5. Severe dysfunction	**Gross** • Only barely perceptible motion • At rest symmetry **Motion** • Forehead: None • Eye: Incomplete closure • Mouth: Slight movement
6. Total paralysis	**No movement**

intratemporal cause of facial nerve palsy is suspected.

- To determine the anatomical site of the lesion, tests like salivary flow test, Schirmer's test, stapedius reflex, and taste examination can be done.

Q11. What are the goals of treatment?

In general, the goals are to protect the eye, to provide symmetry at rest, and to provide movement.

- **Goals of treatment for eye:**
  - To protect and maintain the vision.
  - To maintain the eyelids function.
  - To enable the eye to express emotion.
- **Goals of treatment for mouth:**
  - To achieve symmetry.
  - To achieve oral continence.
  - To achieve good coherent speech.
  - To provide a balanced smile which the patient can use socially.

Q12. What are the nonsurgical measures for immediate protection of eyes?

- Artificial tears containing hydroxypropyl methyl cellulose, three to four times/d.
- Eye ointment during night hours, at sleep.
- Lid taping while sleeping.
- Eye patches/shields while sleeping.
- Forced blinking exercises in patients with weak eye closure.
- Temporary tarsorrhaphy.

Nonsurgical methods can protect the eyes while surgery is being planned.

Q13. What are the surgical options for immediate/early nerve injury?

- **Direct end-to-end repair (Fig. 6.13):**
  - In cases of sharp transaction of the nerve, (e.g., parotid surgery), surgery over temporomandibular joint.
  - End-to-end coaptation with epineurial sutures is the best method.
- **Nerve grafting (Fig. 6.14):**
  - Sural nerve grafts can be used for managing a wide neural gap.
  - Synkinesis may occur if done in the intraosseous part of the facial nerve.
- **Cross-facial nerve graft (Fig. 6.15):**
  - Indications:
    - Unavailability of proximal stump.
    - Loss of distal stump/muscles required for facial expression.
  - Recipient is contralateral unaffected facial nerve by selecting a specific branch and is connected to the affected side via a nerve graft that crosses the face.
  - It is a two-stage procedure in which the first stage is laying over of the cross facial nerve graft and the second stage which is 9 to 12 months later in which the nerve graft is coapted to the branches of the affected facial nerve or direct neurotization of the target facial muscle (if distal neural stump is not available).
  - **"Baby sitter" concept:**
    - Cross facial nerve transfers are required when the facial nerve trunk of the affected side is nonusable.
    - Sural nerve grafts are taken and coapted to the upper and lower trunks of normal facial nerve of contralateral side. In this surgery the ends of sural grafts are marked and banked at the suitable site.
    - In the same sitting, a donor motor nerve either hypoglossal or masseter nerve is used and attached to the facial nerve of affected side so that the tone of paralyzed side muscles is regained.
    - At the second surgery the banked sural graft from the C/L facial nerve

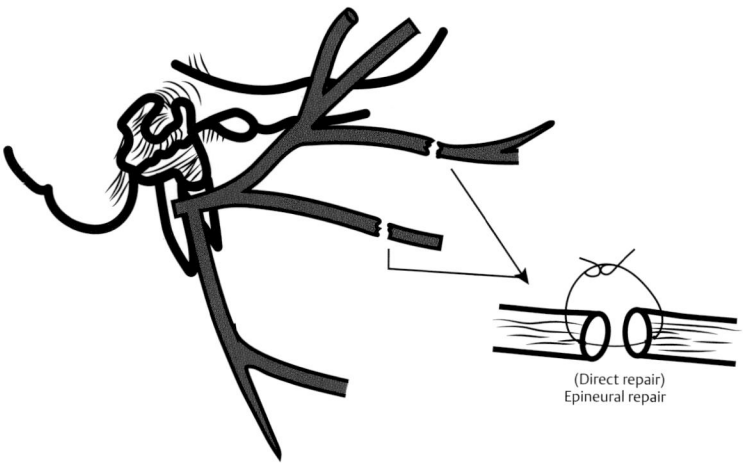

Fig. 6.13 End-to-end direct repair.

(Direct repair)
Epineural repair

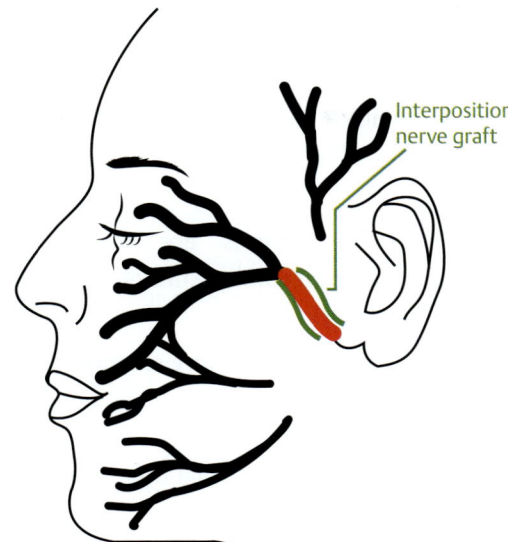

Interposition nerve graft

Fig. 6.14 Sural nerve grafting.

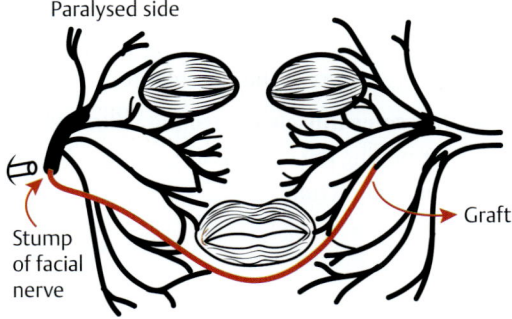

Paralysed side

Stump of facial nerve

Graft

Fig. 6.15 Cross facial nerve grafting.

are coupled distally to the previous anastomosis.

- **Nerve transfers:**
  - Other cranial nerves as donors with end-to-side coaptation.
  - Indications:
    - Unavailability of proximal stump.
    - Intact distal nerve.
    - Intact motor end plates of facial muscles.

- Contraindication in using the contralateral facial nerve as donor (in moebius syndrome).
- **Direct neurotization** of the target muscle in case no distal nerve stump is present.

Q13. What are the surgical options for the specific region of face?

- **Brow:**
  - Direct brow lift (brow excision).
  - Coronal brow lift with static suspension.
  - Endoscopic brow lift.
- **Upper eyelid (lagophthalmos):**
  - Gold weight.
  - Temporalis muscle transfer.
  - Spring.
  - Tarsorrhaphy.
- **Lower eyelid (ectropion):**
  - Tendon sling (a better option).
  - Lateral canthoplasty.
  - Horizontal lid shortening.
  - Temporalis muscle transfer.
- **Nasal airway:**
  - Static sling.
  - Alar base elevation.
  - Septoplasty.
- **Commissure and upper lip:**
  - Microneurovascular muscle transfer with ipsilateral seventh nerve or cross facial nerve graft.
  - Temporalis muscle transfer and masseter transfer.
  - Static slings.
  - Soft tissue balancing procedures (rhytidectomy, mucosal excision or advancement).
- **Lower lip:**
  - Selective myectomy of depressor labii inferioris of normal side.
  - Muscle transfer (platysma, digastric).
  - Wedge excision of the paralyzed side of the lower lip.

Q15. How do you perform a temporalis muscle transplantation/transfer for eyelid reanimation?

Antegrade temporalis muscle transplantation: This procedure was initially described by Gillies.

- A zig-zag incision is given along the parietal branch of superficial temporal artery starting from the anterior edge of sideburn up to the superior temporal line.

  ↓

- After elevating the skin flaps in subfollicular plane, the superficial temporal fascia is incised and deep temporal fascia is exposed.

  ↓

- 1.5 to 2 cm wide flap of temporalis muscle based inferiorly is raised along with the overlying deep temporal fascia.

  ↓

- The blood supply of temporalis muscle and deep temporal fascia is by deep temporal artery which enters the muscle from below in the deeper plane.

  ↓

- The fascia is then separated from the underlying muscle in a proximal to distal direction and the superior most ends of both muscle and fascia are enforced with two to three sutures.

  ↓

- The fascia is split at distal end for few centimeters and passed subcutaneously through the lateral canthus and tunneled along the upper and lower eyelid margins as much as closed to the margins.

  ↓

- Both the fascial strips are sutured to the medial canthal ligament.

  ↓

- When the patient clenches his teeth to contract the temporalis muscle, the fascial strips are pulled tight leading to eyelid closure.

The disadvantages of this procedure are:

- The shape of the palpebral aperture changes from oval to slit-like.
- Bunching of skin and muscle bulge over lateral canthal region.
- Movement of eyelids during chewing.

Q16. What procedures are there for reanimation of oral commissure or dynamic smile reconstruction?

Procedures for oral commissure reanimation:

- **Retrograde temporalis muscle transfer:**
  - First described by Gillies.
  - The muscle is detached from its origin at temporal fossa and turned over the zygomatic arch and extended to the oral commissure.
  - A fascial graft may be required to achieve the length to reach the mouth (**Fig. 6.16**).
  - It produces an oblique lift to the angle of mouth.
- **Masseter muscle transplantation** is done for pulling the commissure in a more horizontal direction.

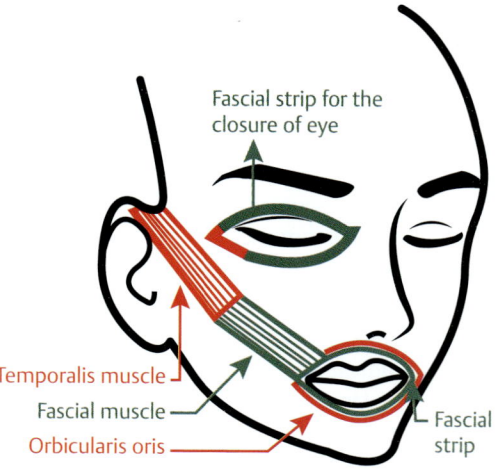

Fig. 6.16 Temporalis transfer for eyelid reanimation and retrograde temporalis transplantation for oral commissure reanimation.

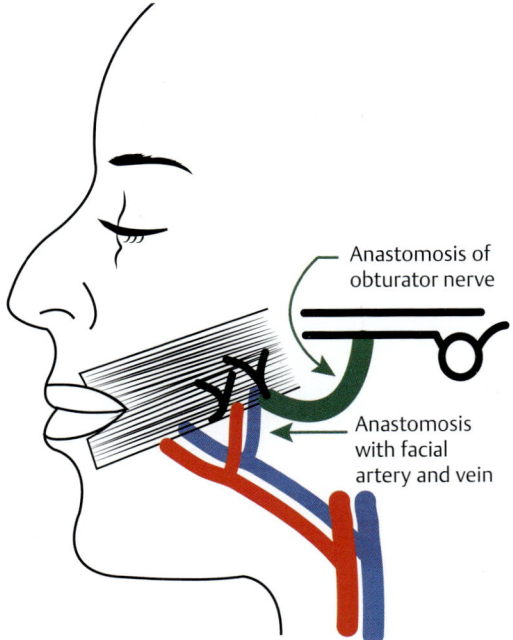

Anastomosis of obturator nerve

Anastomosis with facial artery and vein

Fig. 6.17 Free functional gracilis transfer for smile reconstruction.

- **Microneurovascular muscle transplantation (Fig. 6.17):**
  - Free functioning muscle transfers can be done for restoring the smile of the patient.
  - Generally, gracilis is used.
  - Patient factors play a major role as it is assessed whether patient can sustain such long duration of procedure and anesthesia as well.

Suggested Readings

1. Zuker RM, Hussain G, Gur E, Manktelow RT. In: Neligan PC, ed. Plastic surgery: craniofacial, head and neck surgery, and pediatric plastic surgery. Vol. 3. 4th ed. Canada: Elsevier; 2018:329–357
2. Zuker RM, Manktelow RT, Hussain G, Mathes SJ, eds. Plastic surgery: the head and neck. Part 2. Vol. 3. 2nd ed. Canada: Elsevier; 2006:883–916
3. House JW, Brackmann DE. Facial nerve grading system. Otolaryngol Head Neck Surg 1985;93(2):146–147

7 Ulnar Nerve Palsy

Veena K. Singh and Anupama Kumari

Learning Objectives

At the end of this chapter, the student will be able to:
1. Describe the clinical presentation of a patient with ulnar nerve palsy.
2. Recall the course and supply of ulnar nerve.
3. Demonstrate the motor and sensory examination of ulnar nerve.
4. Make a decision on the right surgical intervention in context to timeline.
5. Understand the various tendon transfers in ulnar nerve palsy.

Introduction

Ulnar nerve palsy may be due to trauma, Hansen's disease, or compression neuropathies. There is loss of all extrinsic and intrinsic muscles supplied by the ulnar nerve if involvement is at the proximal level and of only intrinsic muscles if distally affected. The choice of surgical interventions depends upon the level of injury and the specific functional disability of the patient. Ulnar nerve palsy leads to many functional problems of the hand. There is no universal method of reconstruction, and the treatment is highly individualized.

Chief Complaints

- Inability to straighten the ring and little fingers.
- Deformity of the ring and little fingers.
- Weakness/Loss of power in hand.
- Loss of/decreased sensation over the ring and little fingers.
- Patch over forearm/arm/anywhere else in the body (in cases of leprosy).
- Ulceration/Blisters.

History of Present Illness

- **Duration of complaints:** The duration of the deformity, the severity of the weakness, the daily activities which are affected, history of disabilities due to loss of sensation.
- **Mode of trauma:** Whether sharp cut injury or blunt trauma, which part of the limb is affected. In cases of road traffic accidents, ask if there is history suggestive of crush injury or associated fracture.
- **Duration of injury:** To guide what surgical options are available: end-to-end repair, nerve graft, or tendon transfer.
- **In case of associated fracture:** History of splintage, any surgical intervention for fracture fixation, presence of any implant in the wound.

Past History

Same as in other cases. History of any surgical intervention, (e.g., any suturing or attempt at repair of the nerve if done previously).

Personal History

History of addiction including alcoholism, smoking, marital status, no. of kids, employment status.

Family History

No. of family members dependent on the patient.

Treatment History

Any physiotherapy since the injury or any use of splintage.

History of Allergy

To food or medications.

General Physical Examination

Same as in other cases.

Local Examination of the Hand

After proper exposure of bilateral hands up to forearm in adequate light with informed consent.

Inspection

Inspection of outstretched hands with palm facing upward and rested on the top of a table.

1. **Attitude:**
   - Claw deformity (benediction hand) needs to be described in detail—hyperextension at metacarpophalangeal (MCP) joints and flexion at interphalangeal (IP) joints of the ring and little fingers.
   - Claw deformity is more pronounced in low ulnar nerve palsy (**Fig. 7.1**).
   - The deformity is less obvious in high ulnar nerve palsy.
2. **Atrophy:**
   - Flattening of the palm with flattening of hypothenar eminence (**Fig. 7.2**).
   - Longitudinal furrowing between the long flexors of the hand is visible in slender hands (due to wasting of lumbricals).
   - The appearance of the hand is that of an isosceles triangle with distal base (the normal configuration of the hand is rectangular). This is due to atrophy of the hypothenar eminence leading to loss of bulge medial to the fifth metacarpal which in combination with loss of fullness of the first web space (due to atrophy of the adductor pollicis [AP] and the first dorsal interosseous muscles) give triangular shape to the hand.
3. **Ulcers/Blisters/Healed scars:**
   - These may be present in the areas of loss of sensation due to ulnar nerve palsy.

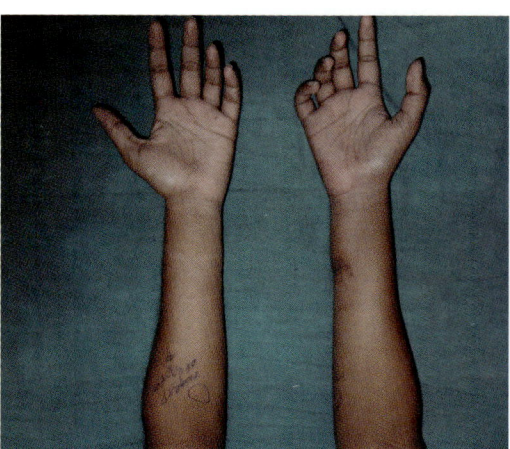

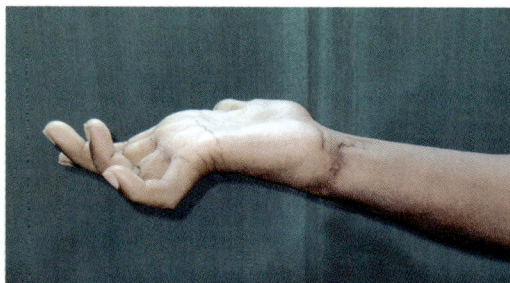

Fig. 7.1 Claw deformity in low ulnar nerve palsy.

Fig. 7.2 Atrophy of hypothenar eminence.

4. Condition of the skin/signs of atrophic changes in the skin.
5. Details of the scar in terms of length, width, pigmentation, hypertrophy, etc.

Palpation

1. Feel of the hand.
2. Details of ulcer/scar, if any.
3. Palpate ulnar nerve in nontraumatic cases (see details later).
4. Palpate the ulnar and radial artery and perform Allen's test to confirm the injury, if any.
5. Tinel's sign must be seen and documented (refer to the chapter on "brachial plexus injury").

Movements

Movements and tests for motor dysfunction in ulnar nerve palsy:

1. **Duchenne's sign** (**Fig. 7.3**):
   - It indicates the claw deformity or "intrinsic minus deformity," i.e., the attitude of the hand with hyperextension at MCP joints and flexion at proximal interphalangeal (PIP) joints and distal interphalangeal (DIP) joints of the ring and little fingers.
     – **Reason:** Due to paralysis of the two ulnar lumbricals muscles and interossei muscles (which brings flexion at MCP joints and extension of IP joints).

2. **Bouvier's maneuver** (**Fig. 7.4**):
   - Passive flexion at MCP joints and straightening of the IP joints on applying dorsal pressure on the proximal phalanx leading to temporary correction of claw hand indicates positive Bouvier's sign.
   - A positive sign is pathognomonic of claw finger caused by intrinsic muscle paralysis.
     – **Reason:** When proximal phalanx is stabilized, the extensor digitorum tendon can cause extension at PIP and DIP joints, leading to temporary correction of claw deformity.

3. **Andre-Thomas sign** (**Fig. 7.5**):
   - When the patient unconsciously tries to extend the fingers by palmar flexing the wrist, there is an increase in the claw deformity. This is called Andre-Thomas sign.

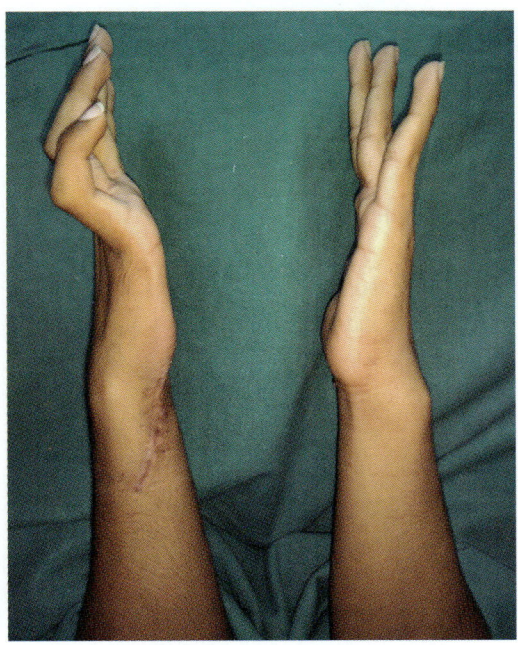

Fig. 7.3 Duchenne's sign.

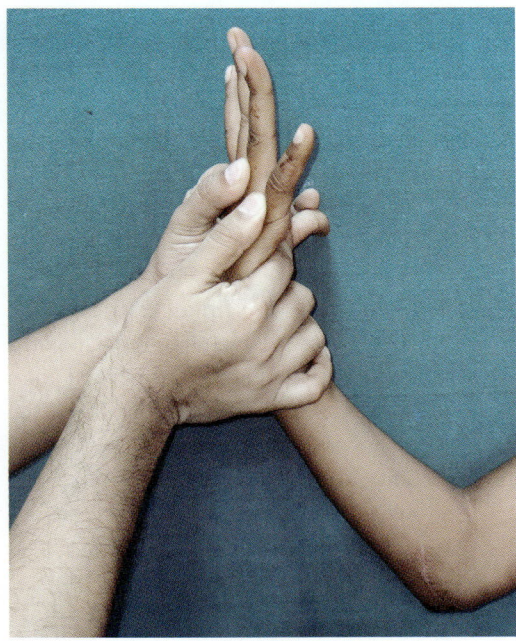

Fig. 7.4 Bouvier's maneuver.

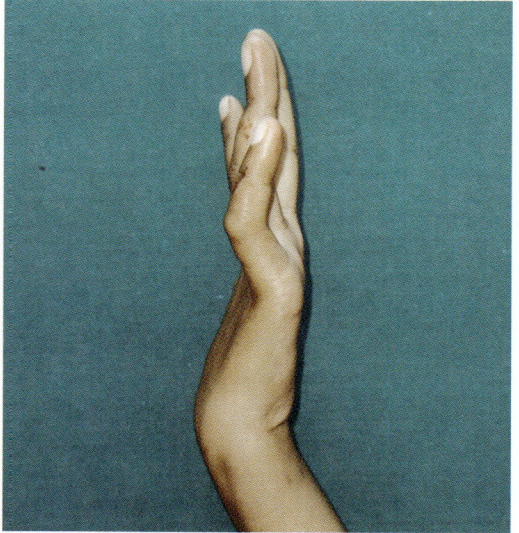

Fig. 7.5 Andre-Thomas sign.

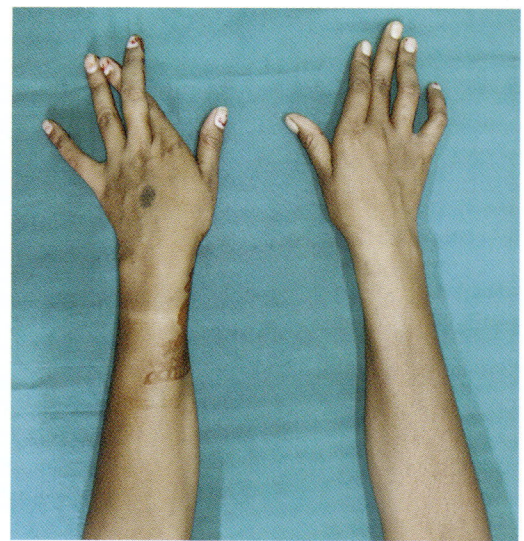

Fig. 7.6 Earle's sign.

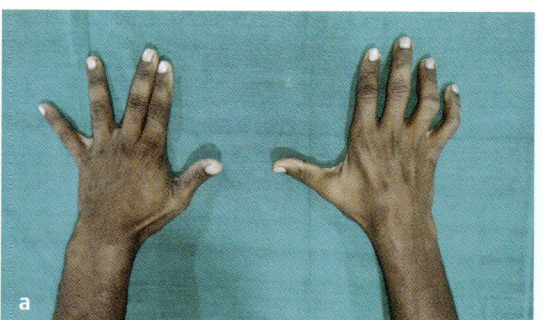

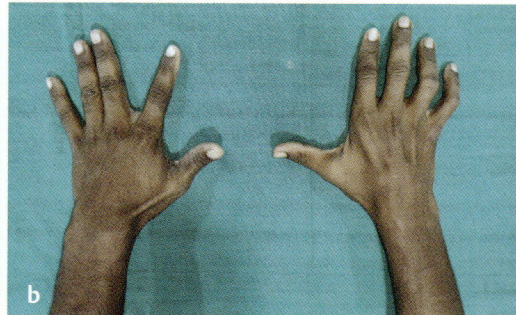

Fig. 7.7 **(a, b)** Pitres Testut sign.

- **Reason:** Due to the tenodesis effect of the long extensor tendons, flexing the wrist leads to exaggeration of the hyperextension deformity at MCP joints.

4. **Earle's sign (cross your finger test)** (**Fig. 7.6**):
   - The patient is asked to place the hand on a table top with palm facing down and cross the middle finger over the dorsum of the index finger and vice versa.
   - Inability to do so indicates Earle's sign.
     - **Reason:** It tests the paralysis of the first palmar interosseous and second dorsal interosseous muscles.

5. **Pitres Testut sign** (**Fig. 7.7a, b**):
   - The patient is asked to place his hand on the top of a table with palm facing down

and move the middle finger in radial and ulnar direction.
   - Inability to do so indicates Pitres Testut sign.
     - **Reason:** It tests the paralysis of the second and third dorsal interosseous muscles.

6. **Flatt's sign/Brand's sign:**
   - Ask the patient to grasp an object like glass/bottle. Look carefully at the sequence of flexion at MCP and IP joints.
   - In ulnar nerve palsy, there is loss of integration of flexion at MCP and IP joints as a result of which the fingers curl up into the palm pushing the object away on trying to grasp it.

– **Reason:** This loss of integration of MCP and IP flexion is due to paralysis of the ulnar lumbrical muscles. Normally, while trying to grasp an object, the flexion is first at MCP joints followed by flexion at IP joints.

7. **Jeanne's sign (loss of key pinch of thumb)** (**Fig. 7.8**):

   • The patient is asked to hold a key between thumb and index finger (in a proper key holding fashion). While trying to do this, there is hyperextension at the MCP joint of thumb, indicating the loss of key pinch/lateral pinch of the thumb.

   – **Reason:** Loss of key pinch of thumb is due to the paralysis of AP. (Normally, there is adduction at first metacarpal, flexion at MCP joint, and extension at IP joint of the thumb.)

8. **Masse's sign** (**Fig. 7.9**):

   • Ask the patient to place his hand on a table top.

   • Look for the flattening of metacarpal arch and loss of hypothenar eminence (always compare it with the contralateral normal hand).

   – **Reason:** Masse's sign indicates the loss of opponens digiti minimi (ODM).

9. **Smith's sign** (**Fig. 7.10**):

   • Ask the patient to do the abduction and adduction movement of the individual finger in extension.

   – **Reason:** This indicates paralysis of interossei and hypothenar muscles.

10. **Wartenberg's sign** (**Fig. 7.11**):

    • Ask the patient to place his hand on a table top with dorsum facing upward. Then ask him to adduct his extended little finger toward the extended ring finger. Patient will be unable to do so.

    – **Reason:** This indicates paralysis of palmar interosseous of the little finger (third palmar interosseous). It also indicates the isolated palsy of deep motor branch of ulnar nerve in

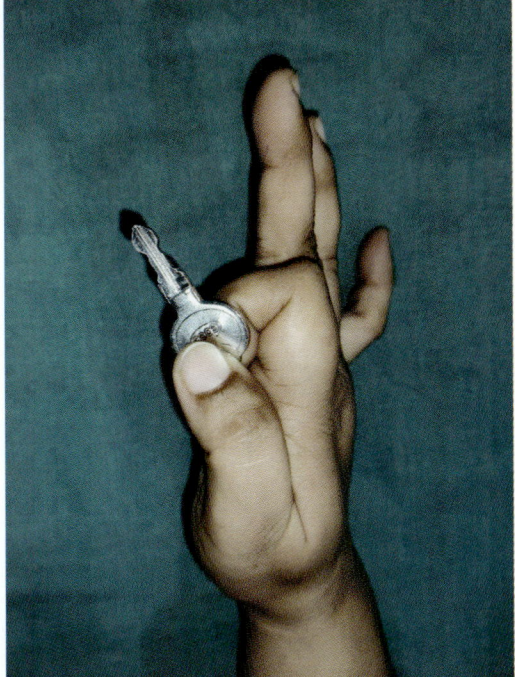

Fig. 7.8 Jeanne's sign.

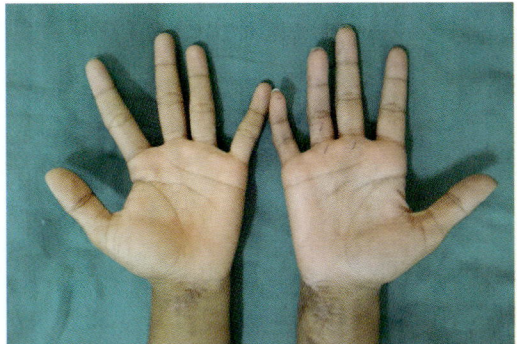

Fig. 7.9 Masse's sign.

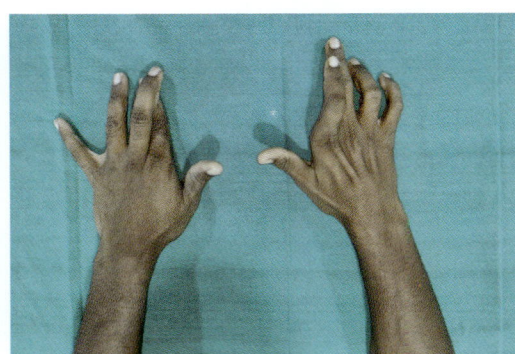

Fig. 7.10 Smith's sign.

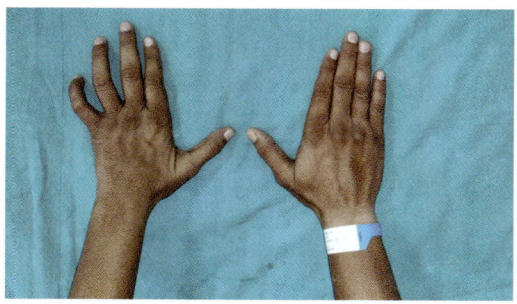

Fig. 7.11 Wartenberg's sign.

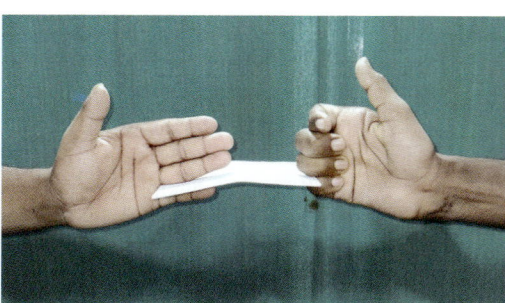

Fig. 7.12 Card test.

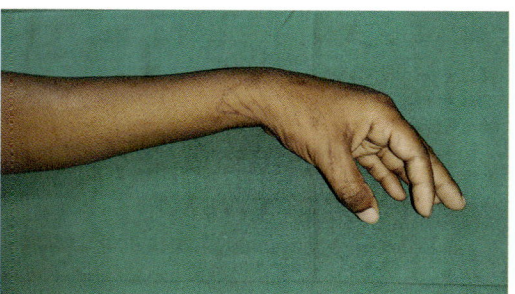

Fig. 7.13 Pitres Testut sign.

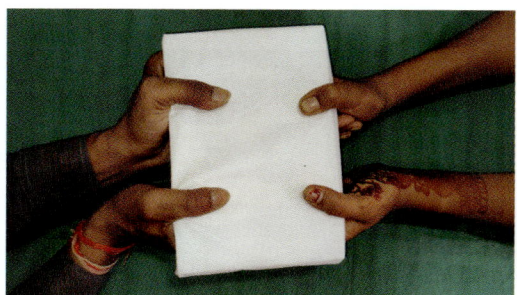

Fig. 7.14 Froment's sign.

which abductor digiti minimi (ADM) is spared and opposes the third palmar interosseous.

11. **Card test** (**Fig. 7.12**):
    - Ask the patient to hold a small card between the fingers of the affected hand. The examiner also holds this card in the same fashion. The examiner will pull the card while the patient will try to resist it. If the card is easily pulled out from the patient's fingers, card test is said to be positive.

12. **Pitres Testut sign** (**Fig. 7.13**):
    - Patient is asked to make a cone with the tips of all extended fingers and thumb.
       – **Reason:** Inability to do so is due to the paralysis of AP muscle.

13. **Froment's sign/Book sign** (**Fig. 7.14**):
    - The patient is asked to hold a book in between thumb and index finger of both hands.
    - The examiner will also hold the book in the same fashion and try to pull the book while the patient will try to hold it back.

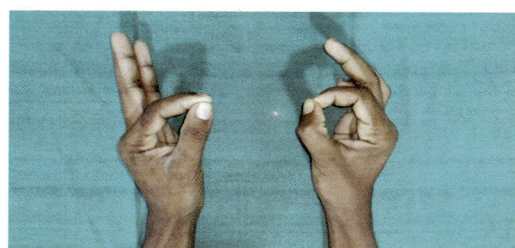

Fig. 7.15 Bunnell's O sign.

- Carefully observe for hyperflexion at the IP joint of the affected hand's thumb while resisting the pulling back of the book by the examiner. This indicates positive Froment's sign.
   – **Reason:** Due to the paralysis of AP and loss of lateral pinch, the force is applied by flexor pollicis longus (supplied by median nerve) which leads to flexion at IP joint of the thumb.

14. **Bunnell's O sign** (**Fig. 7.15**):
    - Ask the patient to hold an object (like thread or a cotton piece) between the tips of thumb and index finger.

- The replacement of the normal spindle-shaped configuration with a circular one in ulnar nerve palsy indicates positive Bunnell's sign.
  - **Reason:** This is due to hyperextension at MCP joint and hyperflexion at IP joint of the thumb.

15. **Pollock's sign (Fig. 7.16)**
- Ask the patient to clench the fist and note the little finger from medial side.
- If it remains extended and the normal "X" configuration formed by folded creases of the little finger is replaced by "Y" configuration, then Pollock's sign is said to be positive.
  - **Reason:** This is due to weakness of ulnar-innervated position of flexor digitorum profundus (FDP) which results in the inability to flex the DIP joints of the ring and little fingers. Loss of DIP flexion at little finger leads to "Y" configuration of its creases in a clenched fist.

16. **Bowden and Napier's sign:**
- Ask the patient to do power grip by clenching the fist with wrist in neutral position.

- Bring the wrist gradually in dorsiflexion and feel the loss of power grip.
  - **Reason:** There is partial loss of wrist flexion due to paralyzed flexor carpi ulnaris (FCU).

Note: Jeanne's sign (loss of key pinch of thumb), Pitres Testut sign, and Froment's sign/Book sign are for thumb; Pollock's sign and Bowden and Napier's sign for extrinsic muscles, and the rest for finger intrinsic muscles.

Measurement

1. **Atrophy of forearm.**
   Measure the girth of the forearm at the same distance from a fixed landmark on both normaml and affected side
2. **Angle measurements:** Must be done during preoperative assessment using a goniometer. All angles are measured at PIP joint.
   a. **Unassisted angle** (Fig. 7.17):
   - With the elbow rested on a table, the patient is asked to keep the hand in an "intrinsic plus" or "lumbrical plus" position (which actually brings the MCP joints of fingers in flexion and IP joints in extension).

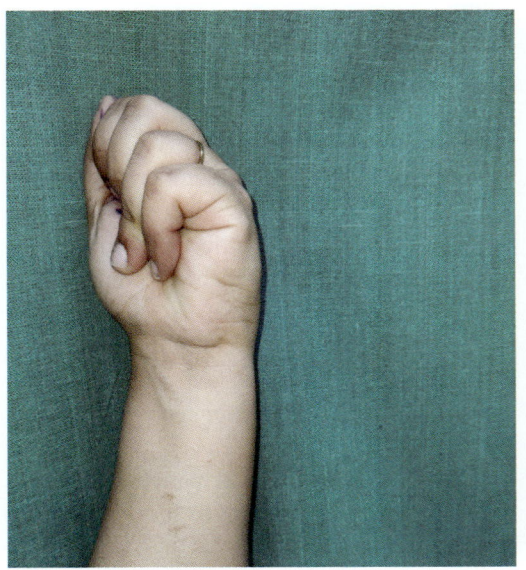

Fig. 7.16 Pollock's sign.

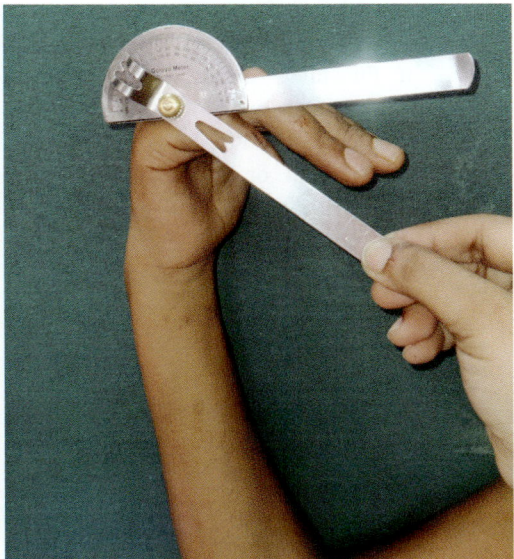

Fig. 7.17 Unassisted angle.

- Measure the lag in extension (extension deficit) at PIP joint.
- This checks the ability of intrinsic mechanism to bring active extension at IP joints of fingers.
- The more is the extension lag, the less are the chances of complete recovery after corrective surgery.

b. **Assisted angle:**
- In the same "lumbrical plus" or "intrinsic plus" position, stabilize the proximal phalanx by putting dorsal pressure on it (Bouvier's maneuver).
- Ideally, the IP joints should get completely extended and there should not be any extension lag at PIP joint. This is because of the active action of long extensors of hand.
- A finger with incomplete extension at PIP joint is not ideal for claw corrective surgery because even with restoration of MP joint flexion, the long extensors would not be able to extend the IP joints.
- So, only when assisted angle is "zero," claw corrective surgery targeted at the prevention of MP joint extension should be performed.

c. **Contracture angle:**
- In cases of fixed flexion contracture at PIP joint, measure the angle of contracture.
- This may be due to contracture of palmar skin or contracture of volar plate with/without PIP joint capsule. The underlying cause needs to be addressed first before attempting for a claw correction surgery.

d. **Adaptive shortening angle of extrinsic/ long flexors:**
- Ask the patient to rest the elbow on a table top and gradually extend the wrist.
- If there is an increase in angulation of PIP joint flexion with wrist extension, it indicates shortening of extrinsic flexors due to habitual positioning of wrist in flexion to minimize the claw deformity.
- Measure the change in angle of PIP joint flexion in fully extended wrist from flexed posture.

e. **Hypermobile angle:**
- Measure the extension angle during hyperextension at PIP joint in patients with hypermobile joints due to laxity of ligaments.
- In a patient with hypermobile angle more than 20 degrees, the tension of the transferred tendons during corrective surgery needs to be adjusted accordingly; otherwise the patient might develop intrinsic plus deformity in the finger.

Note: X-ray must be seen if available to look for any underlying bony injury.

Provisional Diagnosis

This is a case of a 3-months old posttraumatic low ulnar nerve palsy at 2 cm proximal to wrist joint with ulnar artery injury in a 45-year-old male patient without any underlying bony injury.

Questions

Q1. How will you proceed?
- We will plan for exploration and nerve repair for which we will go for baseline investigations to get the anesthetic fitness.
- Photographic and video recording of the deformity.
- Patient's counseling and consent regarding requirement of nerve graft and loss of sensation in the area supplied by the donor nerve.
- We will also start the patient on preoperative physiotherapy to make the joints supple.

Q2. Would you like to go for any other investigation?

We will also go for a nerve conduction study to confirm the type of injury and whether there is any neural regeneration. (Refer 'Nerve conduction studies in chapter on 'Brachial plexus injury')

Q3. What is the mechanism of claw hand development?

Keeping in mind the intrinsic mechanism of hand, it has been made clear by Landsmeer that the movements at MCP and IP joints are independent, but there is coordination between the two IP joints as flexion at DIP joint brings flexion at PIP joint. Therefore, it appears that it is a biarticular system of MCP and PIP joints with proximal phalanx as the intercalated bone.

- In a normal finger, when the patient extends the finger, the tension placed on the extensor tendon at MCP joint is transmitted distally to extend the IP joints.
- In a claw hand, this tension is diverted to the sagittal band leading to hyperextension at MCP joint which blocks the extensor mechanism to extend the IP joint. Hence, without intrinsic function, the middle and distal phalanx collapse into flexion. This leads to disruption of normal cascade of finger extension.
- The normal sequence of finger closure is also reversed, i.e., IP joint flexion precedes the MP joint flexion.
- So, intrinsic paralysis of the hand leads to claw deformity and loss of independence

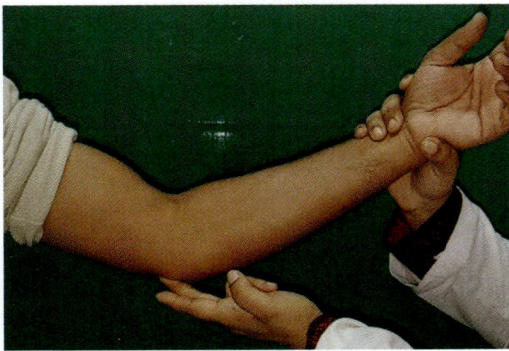

Fig. 7.18 Palpation of ulnar nerve.

of the movement at MCP joint, and PIP joint becomes the principal disability.

Q4. How will you palpate ulnar nerve? (Fig. 7.18)

Sit in front of the patient and rest his/her forearm with flexed elbow on your forearm/hand.

- Place the index, middle, and ring finger tips of the other hand behind the medial epicondyle and roll the fingers backward and forward to palpate the ulnar nerve in the olecranon groove along the long axis of the nerve.
- Nerve is only palpable if enlarged to more than 5 mm in diameter.

Q5. What is the course of ulnar nerve? (Fig. 7.19)

Ulnar nerve originates from the medial cord of brachial plexus (root value: C_8 and T_1 with sometimes contribution from C_7 also).

- **In the arm:** It descends from the axilla to the arm lying medial to the axillary artery. In the arm, it runs on the medial aspect of the arm, lying medially to the brachial artery and biceps muscle.
  - **At mid-arm level**, it enters the posterior compartment of the arm by piercing the medial intramuscular septum and lies anteriorly to the medial head of triceps muscle.
  - **At elbow**, it passes behind the medial epicondyle in the olecranon groove where it lies in a subcutaneous plane and is easily palpable, especially if thickened.
  - Ulnar nerve gives no branches in arm.
- **At forearm level**, it passes through the cubital tunnel (superficial to the posterior and oblique fibers of the ulnar collateral ligament.
  - Cubital tunnel is formed by the olecranon process, medial epicondyle of ulna, and the arcuate ligament which connects the two heads of FCU.
  - Through the ulnar and the humeral heads of FCU, it then enters into the anterior compartment of the

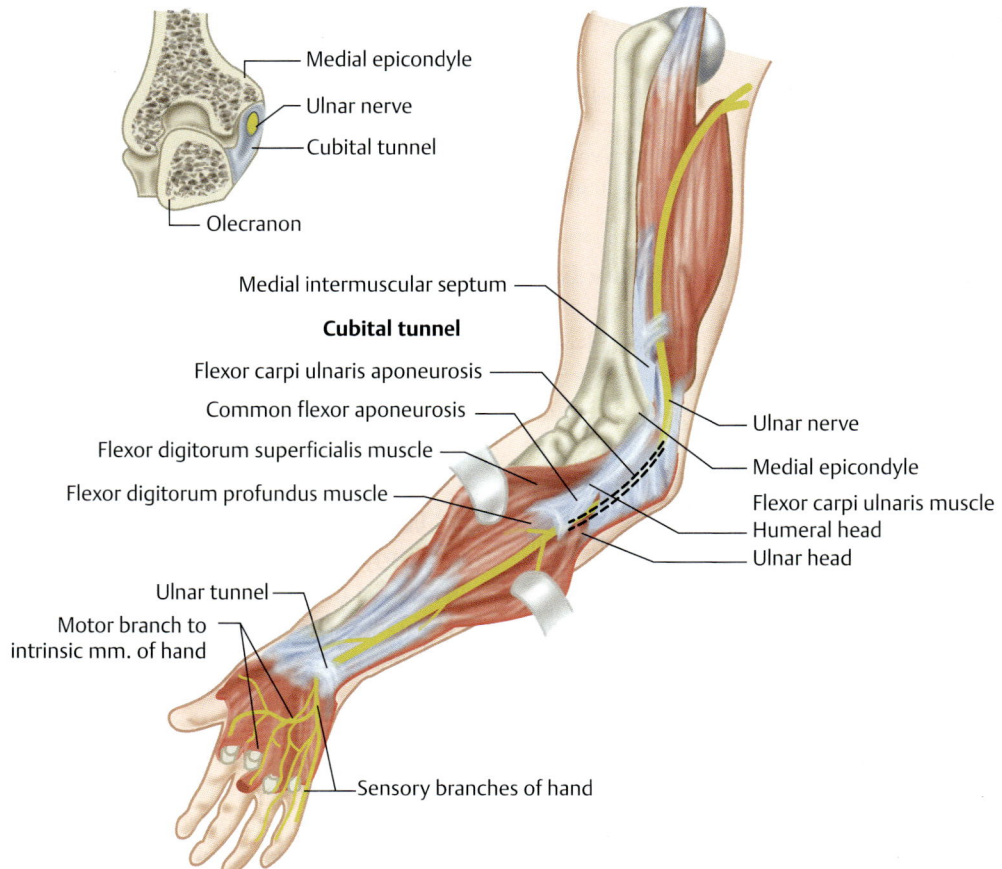

Fig. 7.19 Course of ulnar nerve.

forearm and runs in the medial forearm between FCU (superficially) and flexor digitorum superficialis (FDS) (beneath)

- **At wrist,** it emerges lateral to FCU and runs lateral to the ulnar artery. Both ulnar nerve and artery runs superficial to carpal tunnel and lateral to pisiform bone through the Guyon's canal and enter the hand.
- **Guyon's canal** is a groove formed between pisiform and hook of hamate bone and is covered by the palmar carpal ligament.
  - The ulnar nerve then enters the hand and divides into two branches: superficial and deep.
  - The **superficial branch** provides sensory supply to the palmar aspect of little finger and ulnar half of ring finger and also to ulnar half of the palm.

It also provides motor supply to palmaris brevis (PB) muscle.

- The **deep branch** of ulnar nerve courses in the hand between the hypothenar muscles and provides motor supply to hypothenar muscle, all interossei, two ulnar lumbricals, deep head of flexor pollicis brevis (FPB), and AP.

Q6. What is the sensory distribution of ulnar nerve? (Fig. 7.20 a, b)

The sensory supply from ulnar nerve distributes through three branches:

- **Palmar cutaneous branch:**
  - Originates from ulnar nerve at the level of mid-forearm.
  - It descends along with the ulnar artery, and in the distal forearm, it pierces the

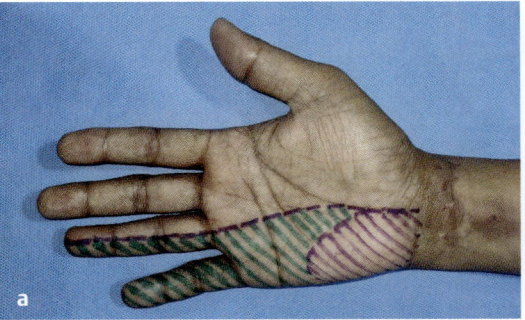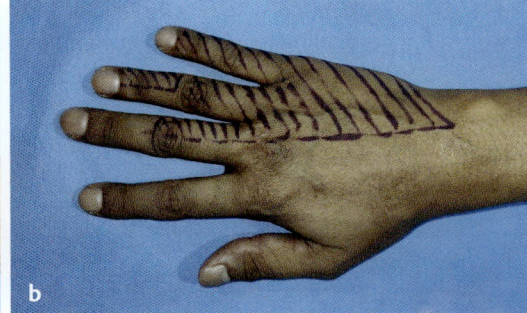

Fig. 7.20   (a, b) Sensory mapping of ulnar nerve in hand.

deep fascia to provide sensations to the skin over the base of the palm.

- **Dorsal cutaneous branch:**
  - Emerges from the ulnar nerve at the distal aspect of forearm, just proximal to wrist joint.
  - It lies deep to the FCU and passes posteriorly to pierce the deep fascia and lie on the dorsomedial aspect of the palm.
  - It divides into two to three dorsal digital nerves and provides sensory supply to the dorsomedial skin of hand and proximal aspect of medial one-and-half digits.
- **Superficial branch of ulnar nerve:**
  - It originates from ulnar nerve at the distal aspect of pisiform bone and divides into two palmar digital branches.
  - It provides sensory supply to the palmar aspect of medial one-and-half fingers.
  - It also provides motor supply to PB in the hypothenar region.

Q7. What are the basic functions of the hand?

There are three basic functions of the hand—grip, grasp, and precision movements. Thumb is responsible for 40 to 50% of the overall function of the hand.

Q8. What is intrinsic mechanism?

The intrinsic mechanism of the hand consists of muscles which are divided into four groups:

- **Thenar muscles:**
  - Abductor pollicis brevis (APB), FPB, opponens pollicis (OP), AP.
  - APB, superficial head of FPB, and opponens pollicis (OP) are innervated by median nerve.
  - Deep head of FPB and AP are supplied by ulnar nerve.
- **Hypothenar muscles:**
  - PB, ADM, ODM.
  - All are supplied by ulnar nerve.
- **Lumbricals:**
  - Unique muscle with no bony attachment.
  - Arises from the radial side of FDP and inserts on the radial aspect of extensor apparatus via lateral bands.
  - Lumbricals are the major flexors at MCP joint.
  - In combination with interossei, it flexes the MCP joint and extends the IP joints.
  - **Mechanism:** FDP contracts → Lumbricals move proximally → Flexion at MCP joint → Simultaneously lumbrical insertion moves distally → It tends to pull the profundus distally → Shortening of lateral bands → Extension at IP joints.
- **Interossei:**
  - Three palmar interossei and four dorsal interossei.
  - All are innervated by ulnar nerve.
  - They originate from metacarpals and along with lumbricals form the lateral bands.

– Action is ulnar and radial deviators of fingers leading to adduction and abduction. Along with lumbricals these cause MCP joint flexion and IP joint extension leading to intrinsic plus position of hand.

Q9. How do you classify the claw hands?

The classification of paralytic claw hands is based on etiology and chronicity of the claw deformity and also on the presence of hypermobility of joints:

- Type I—Claw hands with supple joints.
  - No hypermobility of joints.
  - No contracture of IP joints.
- Type II—Claw hand with supple joints.
  - Hypermobility at PIP joints of ≥20 degree of painless passive hyperextension.
- Type III—Claw hand with supple joints.
  - Adaptive shortening of long flexors (commonly FDS).
  - No contracture of IP joints.
- Type IV—Contracted claw hands.
  - PIP joint flexion contracture of ≥15 degrees (cause may include contracture of palmar skin, volar plate or joint capsule).
  - ±Adaptive shortening of long flexors.
- Type V—Contracted claw hands.
  - "Hooding deformity" due to attrition of extensor apparatus at PIP joint.
  - PIP joint ankylosis, may be fibrous or bony.
  - MP joint in extension contracture.

The type of claw hand helps to choose the appropriate corrective surgery.

Q10. What is "Z" thumb deformity?

- The **"Claw"** thumb in ulnar nerve palsy is also known as "Z" thumb deformity (**Fig. 7.21**).
- The thumb has sequential movements at three joints: the carpometacarpal (CMC) joint, MCP joint, and IP joint.
- The CMC joint is affected by the paralysis of AP, FPB, and the first dorsal interosseous.

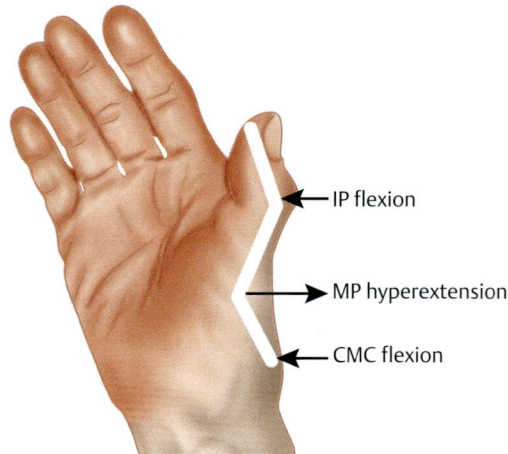

Fig. 7.21   Z-thumb deformity

In case of intrinsic paralysis, on applying the Landsmeer's model of biarticular system, the two distal joints—MCP joint and IP joint—get controlled by the extrinsic flexors and extensors with proximal phalanx forming the intercalated bone.

- Therefore, the MP joint goes into hyperextension and IP joint into flexion leading to a "Z" thumb deformity.
- For correcting this "Z" thumb deformity reconstruction of thumb adductor is required which is done by the transfer of one extrinsic tendon to any of the three sites: adductor tubercle, APB insertion, or proximal phalanx.

Q11. What is ulnar paradox?

In all nerve injuries, the more proximal the site of injury is, the more severe the deformity is.

- But in ulnar nerve injury, as we move distally, the deformity is more pronounced. This is because in low ulnar nerve injury, the medial half of FDP is intact and causes flexion at PIP and DIP joints leading to more obvious appearance of claw hand.
- In proximal injuries where even FDP is paralyzed, there is absent flexion at IP joints and hence clawing is less visible.
- This is called ulnar paradox.

Q12. What are the prerequisites for reconstructive surgery in post-Hansen's ulnar claw hand?

Prerequisites for reconstructive surgery in ulnar nerve palsy due to leprosy are:

- The patient's medical treatment should be completed.
- Skin smears for the bacillus are negative.
- The bacteriological index is negative on two successive tests.
- The disease has been inactive for at least a year before embarking upon the reconstructive surgery.
- The patient should also be off steroids treatment for several months before surgery.

The aim of surgical reconstruction in leprosy is to make the paralyzed hand functional so the patient can integrate well in the society both at occupational and societal level.

Q13. What are static and dynamic procedures of claw hand correction?

- **Static procedures:**
  - These are the surgical procedures intended to bring some degree of flexion at MCP joint or to prevent (MCP) joint hyperextension.
  - By preventing the hyperextension at MCP joint, the long extensors are able to extend the IP joints.
    - Flexor pulley advancement (Bunnell).
    - Fasciodermodesis (Zancolli).
    - Volar capsulodesis (Zancolli).
    - Static Tenodesis techniques.
      - Without tendon grafts (Riordan).
      - With tendon grafts (Parkes).
    - Wrist tenodesis techniques (Fowler).

The disadvantage of the static procedures is that it does not provide additional movements, and recurrence is a rule.

- **Dynamic procedures:**
  - Transfer of a functional motor to a specific insertion site in the finger so as to correct the deformity and also allowing additional motor power to carry out some lost functions.

- The basis of all dynamic procedures is to replace the lost function of lumbricals.
  - Superficialis tendon transfer (Stiles-Bunnell).
  - EIP and EDM transfer (Flower, Riordan).
  - Wrist motors transfer.
    - Extensor carpi radialis brevis (ECRB).
    - Flexor carpi radialis (FCR).
    - Extensor carpi radialis longus (ECRL).
    - PL transfer (Fritschi).

Q14. What are the key points in few common static procedures for claw hand?

- **Flexor pulley advancement (Bunnell):**
  - The proximal pulleys are split 1.5 to 2.5 cm up to the middle phalanx.
  - Leads to "bowstringing" of flexor tendon so as to bring flexion at MCP joint.
- **Fasciodermodesis (Zancolli):**
  - Excision of 2 cm of volar skin at the level of MCP joint along with shortening of pretendinous band of the palmar aponeurosis.
  - This procedure is done in claw hands with weak extensors.
  - Recurrence of clawing is high.
- **Volar capsulodesis (Zancolli):**
  - Consists of release of A1 pulley with advancement of volar plate at MCP joint.
  - Through a transverse incision at distal palmar crease, A1 pulley is split longitudinally, and after tendons are retracted, volar plate at MCP joint is incised along its length to create two distally based volar plate flaps. A hole is then drilled in the metacarpal neck and the volar plate flaps are anchored into the neck via a monofilament wire in 5 degrees of flexion at MCP joint.
- **Static tenodesis techniques:**
  - **Riordan (without tendon grafts):**
    - One half of ECRL and ECU are used as pedicled "grafts" based distally on

their insertions at dorsal base of the metacarpals.

- These two halves are further divided into four slips and passed on the radial side of metacarpals to be sutured to the radial lateral band of each finger.
- This tenodesis is sutured with wrist in 30 degrees of dorsiflexion and MCP joints in 80 degrees of flexion.
  - **Parkes (with free tendon grafts):**
    - Two free grafts from plantaris or palmaris longus or toe extensors are taken.
- **Wrist tenodesis techniques (Fowler):**
  - Free tendon grafts are sutured to the extensor retinaculum of the wrist and passed in dorsal to palmar direction through the intermetacarpal spaces and lumbrical canals and sutured to the lateral bands.
  - With wrist in 30 degrees of dorsiflexion, MCP joints in 80 degrees of flexion, and IP joints in full extension.

Q15. What is modified Stiles-Bunnell procedure?

Superficialis tendon transfer techniques (Stiles-Bunnell) (Fig. 7.22):

- Sir Harold Stiles transferred one slip of each FDS tendon to the extensor digitorum over the proximal phalanx.
- Bunnell modified by transferring both slips of all FDS through the lumbrical canals and anchored to both sides of the lateral bands (**Stiles-Bunnell procedure**).
- Littler modified by using FDS of only middle finger and splitting into four slips

for each finger (**modified Stiles-Bunnell procedure**).

- Tension maintained at wrist in 30 degrees of palmar flexion, MCP joints in 80 to 90 degrees of flexion, and IP joints in full extension.
- Not done in high ulnar nerve injury.
- The four primary insertion sites for FDS slips are:
  - Lateral band insertion.
  - Phalangeal insertion.
  - Pulley insertion.
  - Interosseous insertion.

Important to know: Brand recommended that any reconstructive surgery in claw hand must be done in all fingers as ulnar nerve injury results in weakness in all four fingers. The clawing deformity may not be obvious in index and middle fingers but becomes apparent only during power pinch.

Q16. What is Lasso technique?

Lasso technique (Zancolli) (Fig. 7.23):

- The FDS tendon slip is passed through the entire A1 pulley and sutured upon itself to create a loop.
- The FDS of middle or ring finger is made free till the proximal palmar aspect so that all four slips can be easily looped through the A1 pulley.

Q17. What is the position of joints in splint after tendon transfer/Lasso technique?

The below-elbow splint is maintained in a position of wrist in 45 degrees of palmar flexion, MCP joints in 90 degrees of flexion and IP joints in full extension.

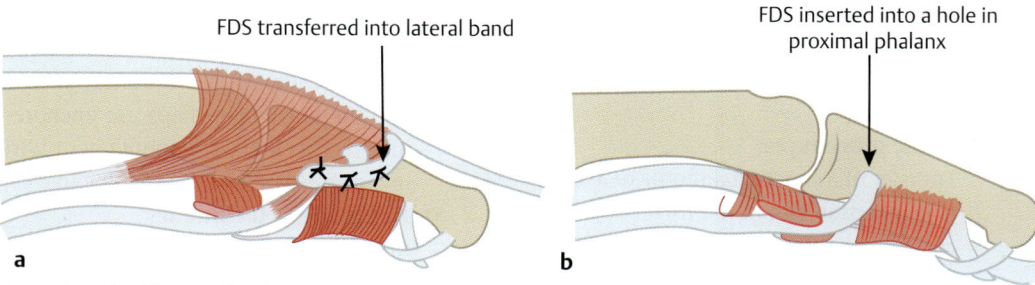

FDS transferred into lateral band

FDS inserted into a hole in proximal phalanx

a   b

Fig. 7.22 **(a, b)** Superficialis tendon transfer technique (Stiles-Bunnell).

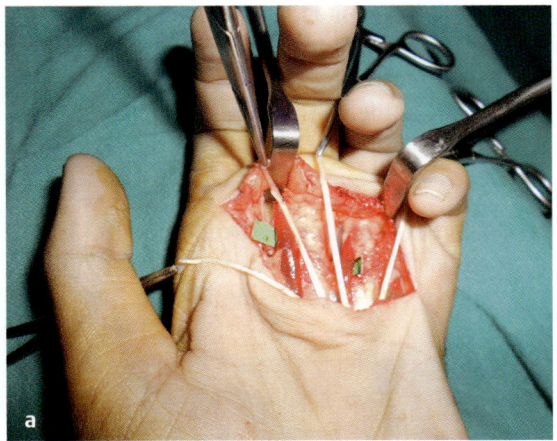

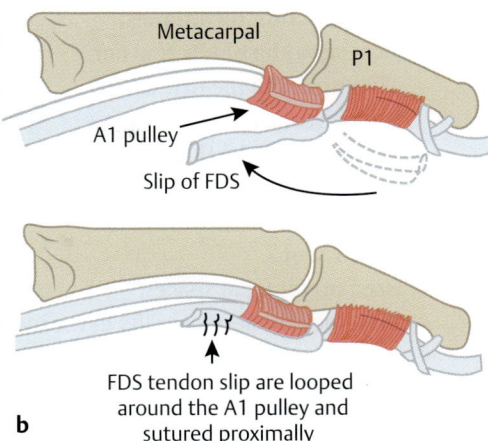

Metacarpal

P1

A1 pulley

Slip of FDS

FDS tendon slip are looped around the A1 pulley and sutured proximally

Fig. 7.23 (a, b) Lasso technique.

Q18. What is the postoperative physiotherapy protocol after a tendon transfer?

- **Post-operative week 3-4:**
  - Immobilization in the cast for 3 to 4 weeks.
  - Gentle active range of motion (AROM) and passive range of motion (PROM) within the restraints of the dorsal blocking splint (DBS).
- **Week 4:**
  - AROM out of splint, avoiding composite extension.
- **Week 6:**
  - Discard DBS and begin using hand-based MCP block splint.
  - Complete unrestricted AROM/PROM, avoiding composite digital extension.
  - May introduce light resistance.
  - Closely monitor MCP joint flexion; a slight flexion contracture is the goal of intrinsic rebalancing procedures, to provide an internal splint.
- **Week 8:**
  - Preferably frequent low-resistance exercise session rather than occasional high-resistance exercises.
  - It is important not to fatigue the transfer.
- **Week 12:**
  - The hand-based splint may be needed until this time.
  - Resume unrestricted activities; continue to avoid composite digital extension with resistance.

Q19. What is the role of pre-operative physiotherapy in claw hand?

The prerequisite for dynamic corrective surgery in claw hand is that the preoperative assisted angle should be 0 degree.

- If the assisted angles are between 30 and 60 degrees, preoperative physiotherapy may be done to correct it.
- Wax bath, oil massage, exercises, and splints are various modalities.
- In PIP joint contracture of ≥45 degrees, serial static plaster splinting can be done.
- In associated Boutonniere deformity, a dynamic splint and preoperative exercise program may be required for 6 to 8 weeks to reduce the assisted angle.

Q20. What are the procedures to restore thumb-index key pinch and tip pinch (restoration of thumb adduction)?

- **Thumb adduction techniques use various motors:**
  - ECRB (Smith).
  - Brachioradialis (Boyes).
  - FDS: transferred to AP (Littler).
  - Transferred to adductor tubercle (Edgerton Brand).
  - EIP (Brown).

- **Index abduction techniques:**
  - Accessory slip of APL transfer.
  - EIP transfer to the first dorsal interosseous.
  - PL transfer to the first dorsal interosseous.
  - EPB transfer to the first dorsal interosseous.
- **Wasted metacarpal spaces:**
  - Placement of dermal grafts in the inter-metacarpal space between thumb and index finger.
  - This is only an aesthetic procedure.

Q21. Which are the procedures in claw hand that are named after Indian leprologists?

- Brand.
- Fritschi.

Common Questions Related to Hansen's Disease:

Q1. What are the types of facies in leprosy?

Facies can be of different types: masked, leonine, sagging.

Q2. What are the cardinal signs of leprosy?

The cardinal signs are:

- Hypopigmented patches.
- Anesthesia.
- Thickened nerves.
- Acid fast bacilli (AFB).

Q3. What are the different classifications used in leprosy?

Classifications in leprosy:

- Madrid:
  - Tuberculoid.
  - Borderline.
  - Lepromatous.
- WHO classification:
  - Paucibacillary, single skin lesion.
  - Paucibacillary, two to five skin lesions.
  - Multibacillary, more than five skin lesions.

- Ridley-Jopling:
  - Tuberculoid leprosy (TT).
  - Borderline tuberculoid (BT).
  - Borderline borderline (BB).
  - Borderline lepromatous (BL).
  - Lepromatous leprosy (LL).

Q4. What is Bacteriological Index (B.I.)?

Bacteriological index denotes the load of lepra bacilli in the sputum smear (both, living and dead).

According to Ridley's scale, B.I. can be:

- 6+ >1000 bacilli in each oil immersion field.
- 5+ 100–1000 bacilli in each oil immersion field.
- 4+ 10–100 bacilli in each oil immersion field.
- 3+ 1–10 bacilli in each oil immersion field.
- 2+ 1–10 bacilli in 10 oil immersion field.
- 1+ 1–10 bacilli in 100 oil immersion field.
- 0 No bacilli in 100 oil immersion field.

Another index is Morphological Index (M.I.) which denotes the presence of viable bacilli as solid-stained ones in the smear.

Q5. What are the treatment protocols in leprosy?

In paucibacillary:

- Dapsone 100 mg for 6 months.
- Rifampicin 600 mg once monthly.

In multibacillary:

- Dapsone 100 mg for 6 months.
- Rifampicin 600 mg once monthly for 24 months.
- Clofazimine 50 mg OD.

Suggested Readings

1. Davis TRC. In: Green DP, eds. Green's operative hand surgery. Vol. 1. 8th ed. Elsevier; 2022: 1189–1242
2. Jones NF, Khiabini KT. In: Mathes SJ, eds. Plastic surgery: the hand and upper limb. Part 2. Vol. 8. 2nd ed. Canada: Elsevier; 2006:453–488

8 Median Nerve Palsy

Veena K. Singh

Learning Objectives

At the end of this chapter, the student will be able to:
1. Describe the clinical presentation of a patient with median nerve palsy.
2. Recall the course and supply of median nerve.
3. Demonstrate the motor and sensory examination of median nerve.
4. Make a decision on the right surgical intervention in context to timeline.
5. Understand the various tendon transfers in median nerve palsy.

Introduction

The median nerve palsy affects the laborers most and functions lost are opposition and abduction of thumb, and flexion of thumb and radial two fingers as it innervates the flexor-pronator group of muscles and the intrinsic muscles on the radial aspect of hand. The injury can be classified as high or low based on the site of injury, (i.e., whether proximal or distal to the origin of anterior interosseous nerve). The goal of reconstruction in a median nerve palsy is according to the target restoration of lost functions.

Chief Complaints

- Inability to bend the thumb, index, and middle fingers.
- Inability to touch the thumb tip to the tip of other fingers.
- Loss of grip/power in the affected hand.
- Loss of sensation over palmar aspect.

History of Present Illness (As in Cases of Other Nerve Injuries)

- **Duration of complaints**: The duration of the deformity, the severity of the weakness, the daily activities which are affected, history of disabilities due to loss of sensation.
- **Mode of trauma**: Whether sharp cut injury or blunt trauma, which part of the limb is affected. In cases of road traffic accidents, ask if there is history suggestive of crush injury or associated fracture.
- **Duration of injury**: To guide what surgical options are available: end-to-end repair, nerve graft, or tendon transfer.
- **In case of associated fracture**: History of splintage, any surgical intervention for fracture fixation, presence of any implant in the wound.

Past History

- History of diabetes mellitus, hypertension, tuberculosis, or any other medical illness.
- Any surgery done in the past for nerve injury or intervention for fracture.

Personal History

History of addiction including alcoholism, smoking, marital status, no. of kids, employment status.

Family History

Number of family members dependent on the patient.

Treatment History

Any physiotherapy since the injury or any use of splintage.

History of Allergy

To food or medications.

General Physical Examination

Same as in other cases.

Local Examination of the Hand

After proper exposure of B/L hands up to forearm in adequate light with informed consent.

Inspection

Inspection of outstretched hands with palm facing upward and rested on the top of a table.
1. Attitude of the hand:
   - Look carefully for pointing index (straight index finger)—it is the most pathognomonic sign of median nerve palsy (**Fig. 8.1**).
   - Claw deformity of the involved fingers (index and middle fingers), if any, needs to be described in detail.

2. Atrophy:
   - Prominent on the thenar eminence and radial aspect of the palm.
   - Also visible in the forearm in cases of high median nerve palsy.
3. Scar:
   - From trauma or from previous surgical intervention. It needs to be mentioned in detail.
4. Condition of the skin:
   - Whether dry, rough, coarse.
   - Any blisters due to sensory loss in median nerve territory.

Palpation

1. Inspection findings need to be corroborated.
2. Feel of the hand—whether warm/cold, rough skin.
3. Details of the scar, if any.

Movement

Motor Examination

1. **Flexor pollicis longus (FPL)** (**Fig. 8.2**)
   Place the hand on the table with palm facing upward and hold the proximal phalanx of the thumb steady. Ask the patient to flex the interphalangeal joint (IP joint). If he is able to do so, apply resistance to flexion by applying pressure over distal phalanx and check the power against resistance.
2. **Abductor pollicis brevis (APB)** (**Fig. 8.3**)
   Place the hand on the table with palm facing upward. A pen is held by the examiner above

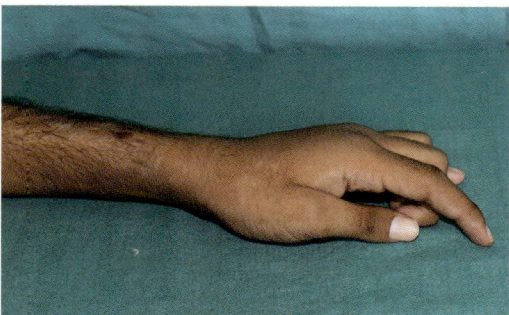

Fig. 8.1 Pointing index in median nerve palsy.

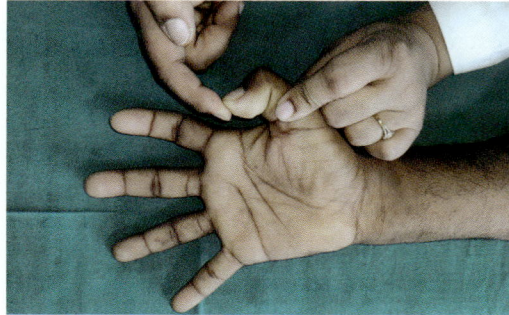

Fig. 8.2 Examination of flexor pollicis longus (FPL).

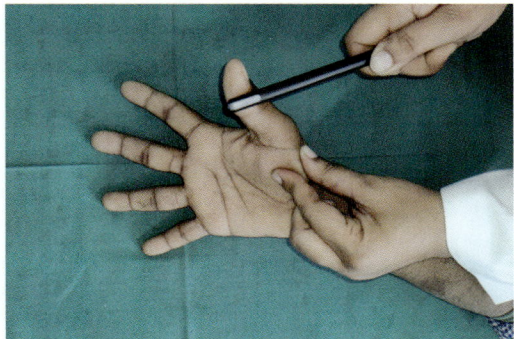

Fig. 8.3 Examination of abductor pollicis brevis (APB).

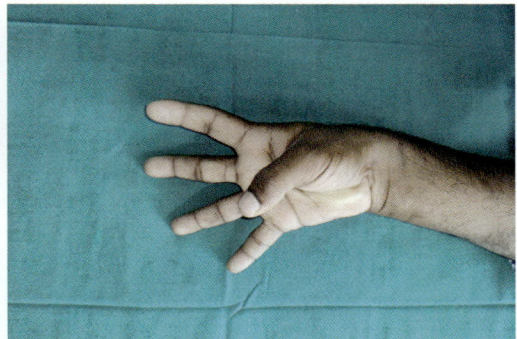

Fig. 8.4 Examination of flexor pollicis brevis (FPB).

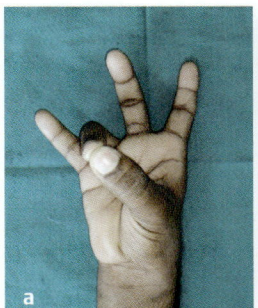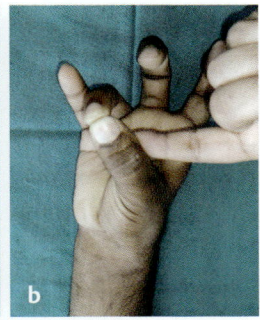

Fig. 8.5 **(a, b)** Examination of opponens pollicis.

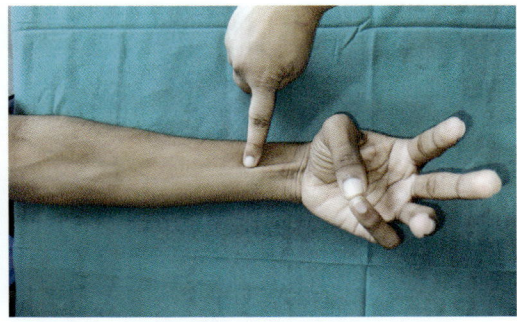

Fig. 8.6 Examination of palmaris longus (PL).

the thumb at some distance and the patient is asked to touch the pen by moving the thumb at 90 degrees to the palm. This abduction movement of thumb is brought by APB. If he is able to do so, apply resistance to the perpendicular movement of thumb to check the power against resistance.

3. **Flexor pollicis brevis (FPB)** (**Fig. 8.4**)
   Ask the patient to rest his hand on a table top. Ask him to flex the thumb at metacarpophalangeal (MCP) joint. If he is able to do so, check against resistance by putting pressure to the proximal phalanx. Flexion at MCP joint is brought by FPB.

4. **Opponens pollicis** (**Fig. 8.5**)
   Place the hand on the table with palm facing upward. Ask the patient to touch the tip of all fingers one by one with the tip of thumb (opposition). If the patient is able to do so, resistance can be applied to the tip of thumb

to check the power against resistance. Take care that the thumb tip should touch the other finger tips and not pulp-to-pulp.

5. **Palmaris longus (PL)** (**Fig. 8.6**)
   The patient is asked to place his hand on the top of a table and asked to touch the thumb tip to the tip of little finger with wrist in flexed position. You will be able to see and feel the taut tendon of PL in distal wrist (Schaeffer's test).

6. **Flexor digitorum superficialis (FDS)** (**Fig. 8.7**)
   Ask the patient to rest his/her hand on the table top. The examiner must stabilize the proximal phalanx either by his left hand or with the help of a pen and the patient is asked to flex the proximal interphalangeal (PIP) joint. Check the power against resistance by putting pressure on the middle phalanx. All fingers are examined separately.

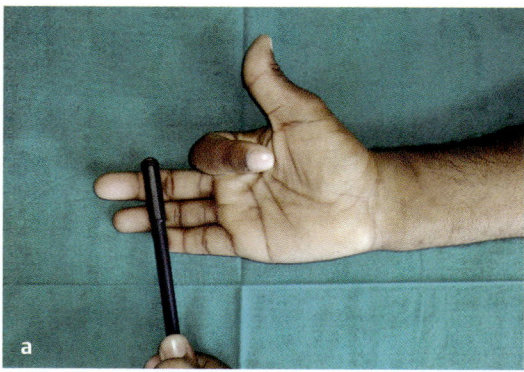
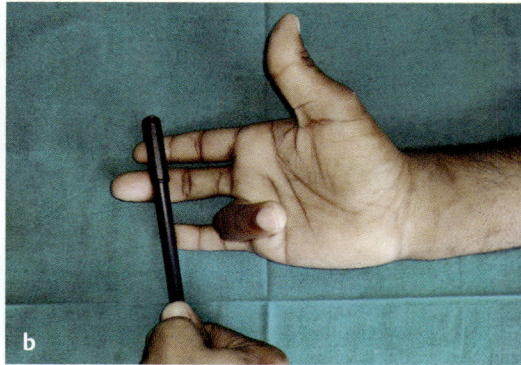

Fig. 8.7 **(a, b)** Examination of flexor digitorum superficialis (FDS).

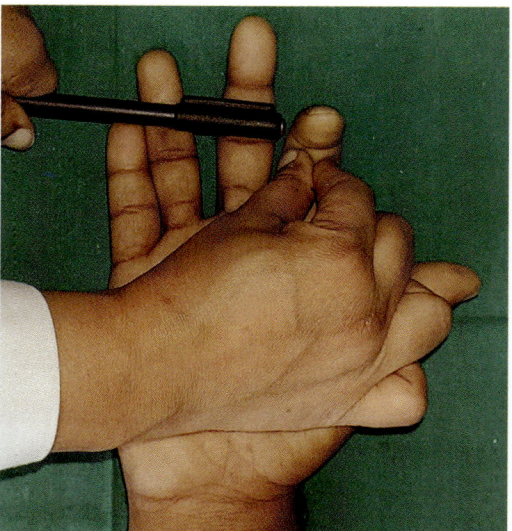

Fig. 8.8 Examination of lateral half of flexor digitorum profundus.

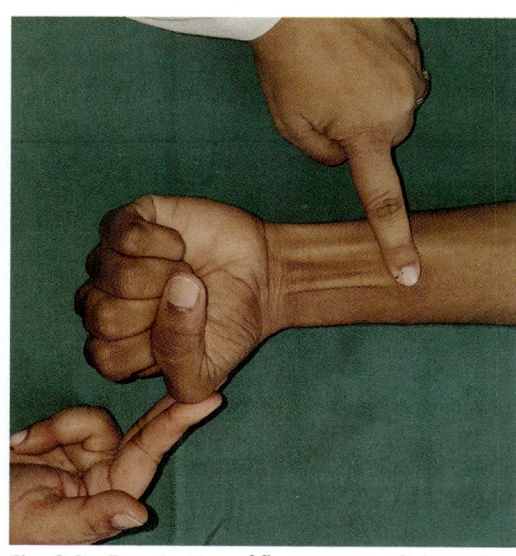

Fig. 8.9 Examination of flexor carpi radialis (FCR).

7. **Flexor digitorum profundus (FDP) of index and middle fingers (lateral half)** (**Fig. 8.8**)
   Ask the patient to rest his/her hand on the table top. Stabilize the PIP joint or middle phalanx with your left hand. Also, press the distal phalanx of other fingers except the finger under examination. Then ask the patient to flex the distal interphalangeal (DIP) joint and check against resistance also. This test must be done separately for each finger.

8. **Flexor carpi radialis (FCR)** (**Fig. 8.9**)
   Ask the patient to rest the forearm on a table and flex the wrist in a fist position. Both FCR and flexor carpi ulnaris (FCU) will become taut on either side of PL. FCR may again be felt when patient is asked to do the radial deviation of wrist in flexed position. If he is able to do so, some resistance can be applied to the closed fist to check the power against resistance.

9. **Pronator teres (PT)** (**Fig. 8.10**)
   In high median nerve palsy, PT is paralyzed which leads to the supine position of the forearm. Place the patient's forearm and hand on a table top. Ask the patient to pronate the forearm from supine position. If the patient is able to do so, some resistance can be applied to check the power against resistance.

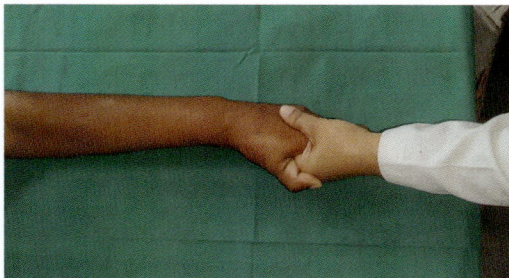

Fig. 8.10 Examination of pronator teres (PT).

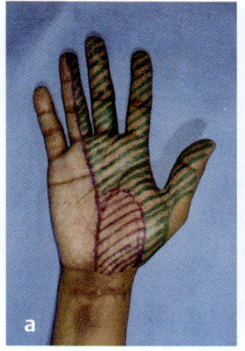 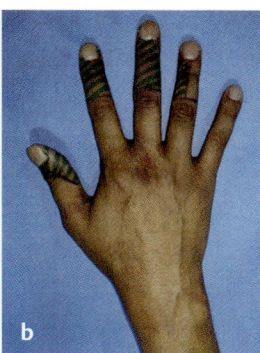

a   b

Fig. 8.11 (a, b) Sensory mapping of median nerve.

Sensory Examination

The sensory supply of median nerve in the hand is radial half of the palm and palmar and dorsal aspect of radial three-and-half fingers (**Fig. 8.11a, b**). So, a detailed sensory examination in the territory of median nerve supply needs to be checked. (Refer to the chapter on brachial plexus injury.) (refer chapter 5 on Brachial plexus injury)

Measurement

a. **Girth of forearm**: The circumference of the arm and forearm at a fixed distance from a bony landmark need to be measured in the affected limb and compare with the normal side to rule out atrophy, if any.
b. **Range of movements at joints**: The functional range of movements at elbow, wrist, MCP, PIP, and DIP joints must be measured to rule out any stiffness.

Tinel's Sign

Gentle tapping with examiner's fingertip is done along the course of median nerve from distal to proximal.

- Ask the patient if he/she feels pins and needles sensation or an electric shock sensation at the fingertips.
- If the patient feels tingling sensation, Tinel's sign is said to be positive.
- Mark the point where tapping elicits maximum tingling sensation and note the distance from a fixed landmark.
- Interpretation

- Progressive Tinel's sign indicates nerve regeneration.
- Nonprogressive Tinel's sign indicates no regeneration or a neuroma formation at the site of injury.

Provisional Diagnosis

This is a case of 2 months old glass cut injury just proximal to left wrist joint with low median nerve palsy in a 17 year old male patient without any bony abnormality.

Questions

Q1. What are the goals of surgery in median nerve injury?

- Restoration of lost motor functions viz. opposition and flexion of thumb (FPL function) and flexion of index finger.
- Restoration of sensations over thumb tip, may be with neurovascular island skin flaps.

Q2. When do you say a "high" or "low" median nerve palsy?

When the injuries in median nerve are proximal to anterior interosseous nerve (AIN), it is termed as "high" palsy and injuries distal to it are "low" median nerve palsy.

Q3. How do you plan to proceed?

Since the injury is only 2 months old, I will go for exploration and end-to-end repair of median nerve via nerve graft.

Q4. For your plan, what is the workup you would require?

Following investigations would be carried out for the patient:

- Nerve conduction studies
  - to see the status of injured nerves and
  - documentation purpose
- Baseline investigations for preanesthetic fitness
- Informed and written consent for sural nerve to be used as nerve graft and loss of sensation over the lateral aspect of the donor foot as a result of sural nerve harvest.

Q5. How do you manage a nerve gap?

- Nerve gap up to 1 cm
  - The standard procedure of choice is tension-free monofascicular repair with "end-to-end neurorrhaphy" and proper fascicular alignment.
  - Direct coaptation is achieved by various maneuvers.
    - fascial release,
    - release of adventitial attachment,
    - dissecting tethering bands,
    - mobilization and transposition of nerve,
    - adjusting the position of joint, or
    - some shortening of bone.
  - Stretching of the peripheral nerve for over 10% of the resting length has been shown to decrease the blood flow by 50%.
  - Polyfascicular repair raises the accuracy of fascicular apposition and a straightforward technique is to use superficial landmarks, like tiny arteries in vasa nervorum to match geographics arrangement of the fascicles.
- Nerve gap from 1 to 5 cm
  - Monofascicular nerve gaps from 1 to 5 cm with available proximal stump are managed with techniques like
    - nerve autografts
    - cellular and acellular nerve grafts
    - nerve conduits

- For polyfascicular larger nerves (diameter > 7 mm), cable nerve grafts (autografts or allografts) are the ideal choice.
- Nerve gap >5 cm
  - In nerve gaps over 5 cm, the options are
    - vascularized nerve grafts (VNGs)
    - nerve transfers

Q6. What are the factors affecting the choice of nerve autografts?

- The size of the nerve gap
- The caliber of the involved nerves
- The locations of the nerve repair
- Considerations to the donor site morbidity

Q7. What are the donor options available for nerve autografts?

- Sural nerve
- Medial and lateral cutaneous nerves of the forearm
- Dorsal cutaneous branch of the ulnar nerve
- Superficial peroneal nerve
- Intercostal nerves
- Posterior and lateral cutaneous nerves of the thigh

Q8. Why free nerve grafts cannot be used in longer gaps?

- Two types of revascularization occur after neural coaptation:
  - Centripetal revascularization from the surrounding tissue bed
  - Inosculation or longitudinal neovascularization from the donor nerve anastomosis.
- Free nerve grafts do not have their own blood supply and the survival depends upon their revascularization in the recipient area. More important one is centripetal mode.
- Several studies have found that on third postoperative day, only 42% of grafts undergo the process of inosculation and the nerve graft is dependent upon centripetal revascularization for its survival.

- For the same reason, whenever a long nerve graft is used for bridging the gap, there is central necrosis and fibrosis which affects the final outcome.
- This initial ischemia period leading to intraneural fibrosis is avoided using VNGs which in turn improves the axonal regeneration.

Q9. How will you manage a neuroma in continuity?

- Complete neuroma in continuity
  - No transmission on nerve stimulation and no functional component
  - Treatment is resection and neural repair via grafting
- Incomplete neuroma in continuity
  - See in mixed (sixth degree) type of nerve injuries
  - A portion of the nerve is functional
  - Nerve stimulator and microneurolysis technique is used to separate the functional fascicles from the neuroma.
  - Sometimes, separating the functional fascicles within the neuroma is more damaging, so, nonfunctioning fascicles are cut at proximal and distal ends and then repaired via nerve graft.

Q10. What topographical landmarks you will keep in mind while repairing median nerve?

- The internal topography of median nerve is complex as compared to ulnar nerve as it contains more number of fascicles.
- In the proximal forearm, the anterior interosseus nerve is situated on the radial or posterior aspect of the median nerve.
- Distally, the motor fascicles to the thenar muscles are located on the radial side and sensory fibers to the third webspace are located on the ulnar side.

Q11. What is neurotropism and neurotrophism?

- Neurotropism: The tendency of regenerating nerve fibers to show tissue and

end-organ specificity and grow distally towards another nerve.
- The affinity of a nerve fiber to respond to the influences of the distal nerve and grow towards a nerve rather than any other tissue is affected by the critical gap which a nerve fiber has to cross.
- Neurotrophism: effect of nutritive factors on the survival of neurons

Q12. Which muscles are supplied by median nerve?

- **In the arm**: NIL.
- **In the forearm:** Both pronator quadratus (PQ) and teres (PT), FCR, PL, FDS of all fingers, FDP of middle and index fingers, and FPL.
- **In the hand:** Hypothenar muscles viz. APB, opponens pollicis, and superficial head of FPB.

Q13. What is the course of median nerve?

Median nerve is constituted by combining two roots—lateral root from the lateral cord and medial root from the medial cord of brachial plexus (C5–T1) (**Fig. 8.12**).

- After the two roots are combined to form median nerve, it lies lateral to the axillary artery in the axilla.
  - It enters the arm at the inferior border of teres major between the tendons of biceps and triceps.
- **In the proximal arm**, it lies on the coracobrachialis muscles lateral to the brachial artery. It then crosses the brachial artery from lateral to medial position in the arm and lies on the muscles of brachialis.
  - Median nerve lies medial to the brachial artery and the tendon of biceps brachii in region of cubital fossa (MBBR). MBBR indicates arrangement of structure in cubital fossa from medial to lateral - median nerve, brachial artery, biceps tendon and radial nerve.
- **Just above the elbow**, it supplies the muscle of PT, and enters the forearm between the two heads of PT giving origin to AIN.

MEDIAN NERVE

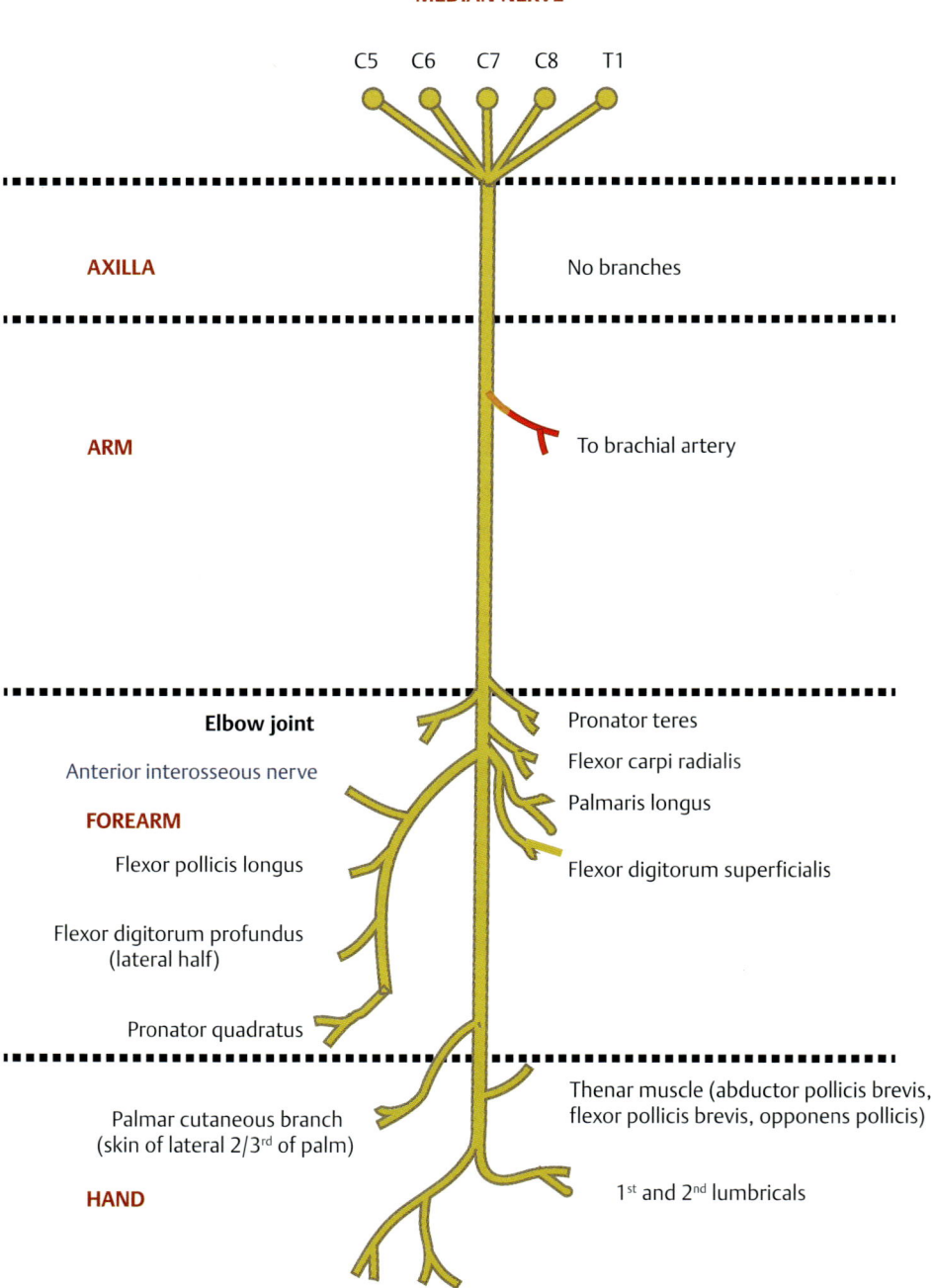

C5   C6   C7   C8   T1

AXILLA

No branches

ARM

To brachial artery

Elbow joint

Pronator teres

Flexor carpi radialis

Anterior interosseous nerve

Palmaris longus

FOREARM

Flexor pollicis longus

Flexor digitorum superficialis

Flexor digitorum profundus
(lateral half)

Pronator quadratus

Thenar muscle (abductor pollicis brevis,
flexor pollicis brevis, opponens pollicis)

Palmar cutaneous branch
(skin of lateral 2/3rd of palm)

HAND

1st and 2nd lumbricals

Palmar digital branches to supply skin of
lateral 3½ digits

Fig. 8.12 Course of median nerve.

- AIN supplies FPL, PQ, and radial half of FDP and courses further down in the forearm between the FDS and FDP.
- **Below elbow**, it gives branches to FCR, PL, and FDS.
- **About 5 cm proximal to the wrist**, median nerve becomes lateral to FDS and gives the palmar cutaneous branch at this level which passes superficial to the flexor retinaculum between PL and FCR and supplies the skin over thenar eminence lateral half of the palm.
  - The main trunk of the median nerve then passes deep to the flexor retinaculum in the carpal tunnel and enters the palm.
- **In the palm**, it gives sensory and motor branches.
  - The motor recurrent branch of median nerve supplies the thenar muscles viz. APB, superficial head of FPB (deep head of FPB is innervated by ulnar nerve), opponens pollicis, and the radial two lumbricals.
  - The sensory branches of median nerve in palm supplies the palmar and dorsal aspects of thumb index, middle and radial half of the ring fingers including the nail beds.
- Median nerve also gives articular branches to the joints of elbow, wrist, and fingers.

Q14. What are the variations in median nerve anatomy?

There are few anomalous connections between the median and ulnar nerve (**Fig. 8.13**). It may be evident on either clinical examination or electromyographic studies.

- **Martin-Gruber anastomosis**: Between the main trunk of median nerve or its anterior interosseous branch and ulnar nerve at the level of proximal aspect of the forearm (5–40%, avg. 17%).
- **Reverse Martin-Gruber or Marinacci anastomosis**: When the anastomotic branch arises from ulnar nerve and joins the median nerve. (In Martin-Gruber, the anastomotic branch arises from median nerve.)
- **Riche-Cannieu anastomosis**: At the level of wrist or hand between the recurrent branch of median nerve and the deep branch of ulnar nerve (77–83%).
- **Berrettini anastomosis**: At the level of digits between the digital sensory branches of median and ulnar nerve (4–94%).

Q15. What is pointing index and its cause?

The FDS and FDP tendon to index finger are supplied by the median nerve so in case of palsy, there is loss of extension both at proximal and distal IP joints.

Q16. What is ape thumb deformity?

Injuries of median nerve leading to complete paralysis of the intrinsic muscles of thumb may develop a supinated and adducted position representing an "ape thumb" deformity (**Fig. 8.14**).

Q17. How is opposition done?

Opposition is a hand movement in which the tip of thumb touches the tips of other fingers.

- The prime muscle responsible for bringing thumb opposition is APB with assistance from opponens pollicis and FPB.
- It consists of a sequence of movements: abduction, flexion, and pronation. This movement takes place at the first carpometacarpal joint, also known as trapeziometacarpal joint.
- Due to diverse pattern of innervation of the thenar muscles by both median and deep branch of ulnar nerve, thumb abduction and opposition are frequently preserved in isolated median nerve injury as a result of preserved lunar nerve function.

Q18. What are the types of opponensplasty?

There are four widely used standard opponensplasties:

- FDS: Royle Thompson and Bunnell technique.
- Extensor indicis proprius (EIP) opponensplasty (Burkhalter's technique).

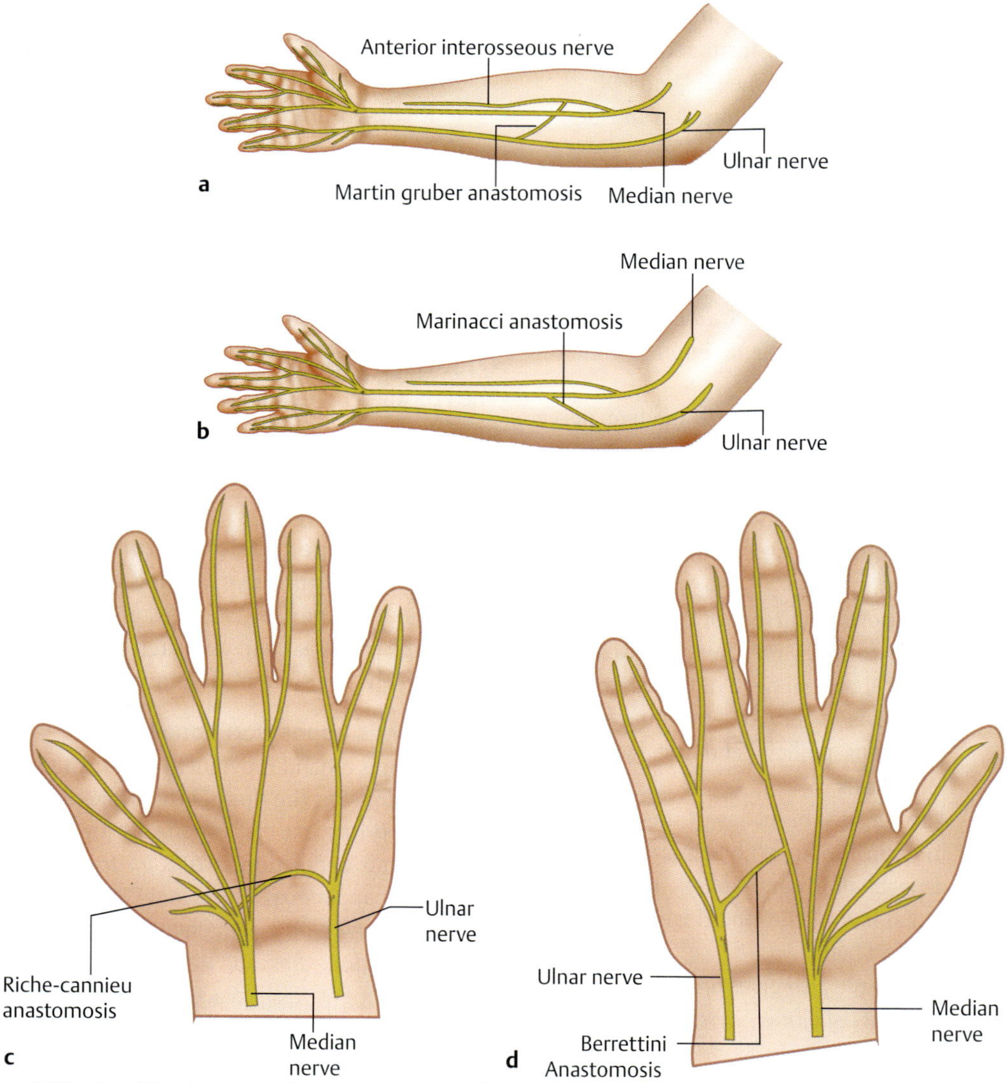

Anterior interosseous nerve

Ulnar nerve

a

Martin gruber anastomosis   Median nerve

Median nerve

Marinacci anastomosis

b

Ulnar nerve

Ulnar nerve

Riche-cannieu anastomosis

c

Median nerve

Ulnar nerve

Berrettini Anastomosis

d

Median nerve

Fig. 8.13 **(a–d)** Variations in the anatomy of median nerve.

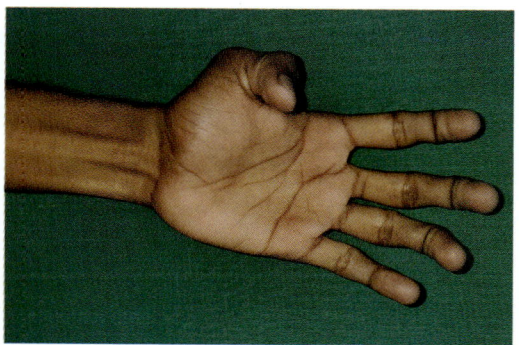

Fig. 8.14 Ape thumb deformity.

- Huber transfer (abductor digiti minimi [ADM]).
- Camitz procedure (PL).

Q19. What are the guidelines for opponensplasty?

Guidelines for opponensplasty

- Procedure is only indicated when an actual deficit in the function occurs due to loss of opposition.
- General principles of tendon transfer must be followed.

- Any contracture of the skin or surrounding tissues must be addressed before embarking upon opponensplasty.
- The ideal motor for opponensplasty must have a tension fraction of around 3.0 and muscle fiber length at least same as that of APB.
  - **Tension fraction**: The strength of a muscle is proportional to its cross-sectional area. This strength is expressed in terms of tension fraction.
  - **Potential excursion**: The range of movement of a muscle is determined by the fiber length of that muscle.
  - Tension fraction of an ideal opponensplasty motor = combined tension fraction of APB and opponens pollicis tendon, i.e., (1.1+1.9 = 3.0).
  - And length of muscle fiber should be at least as long as that of APB.
- Tendon graft should not be used.
- Rehabilitation may become simpler if the selected donor has action synergistic with APB.
- A single insertion site is preferred.

Q20. How is Bunnell's opponensplasty done?

Use of FDS as donor tendon is also known as Bunnell's opponensplasty

- **Donor**: FDS of ring finger is commonly used. Some may prefer middle finger superficialis also.
- **Tendon harvest:** Either through a single incision at distal palmar crease or separate incision at the base of donor finger. Palmar incision is preferred.
- Just proximal to the chiasma, FDS tendon is divided through a window in the flexor sheath between A1 and A2 pulley.
- This prevents injury to the flexor tendon sheath at the level of PIP joint and a 3 cm free length of FDS tendon is left behind to glide freely inside the sheath. This leads to the prevention of swan neck deformity.
- **Pulley:**
  - The transferred tendon is passed through a subcutaneous tunnel in the hypothenar eminence and the fibrous raphe between the deep fascia and the overlying skin is used as the pulley.
  - Another technique for creating a pulley is to make a loop using a strip of FCU tendon graft attached to pisiform and pass it around the FCU tendon where it passes between the pisiform and the base of the fifth metacarpal.
  - Other structures used as pulley can be created by making a hole in the flexor retinaculum or Guyon's canal.

Q21. What is Burkhalter opponensplasty?

EIP opponensplasty: It is also known as Burkhalter opponensplasty.

- Commonly done in high median nerve injury where FDS tendons are not available as donors.
  - **Donor**: EIP is the donor tendon.
  - **Tendon harvest:**
    - A dorsal incision is given on the MCP joint of index finger and proximal to extensor hood and EIP is divided.
    - Another incision is given over the dorsoulnar aspect of the forearm distally and through this incision, EIP tendon is delivered into the forearm proximal to the extensor retinaculum.
  - **Pulley:**
    - Small incision is made in the area of pisiform and another incision is made on the dorsoradial side of the thumb MCP joint.
    - A tunnel is made subcutaneously from extensor aspect of the forearm up to the incision over the thumb while passing the EIP tendon around the ulnar border of the wrist and across the palm.
    - Through this tunnel, EIP tendon is passed superficial to the FCU tendon.
  - **Insertion:**
    - In isolated injuries of median nerve, the tendon is inserted at APB tendon with:
      - Wrist in 30-degree flexion.
      - Thumb in maximum opposition.

- In combined injuries of median and ulnar nerve with intrinsic minus thumb, the transfer is attached in sequence to the APB tendon, MPJ capsule, and extensor pollicis longus (EPL) tendon over the proximal phalanx of thumb with:
  - ○ Wrist in flexion.
  - ○ Thumb in maximum opposition.

Q22. What is Huber opponensplasty?

ADM (Huber) opponensplasty

This transfer improves the appearance of the hand by increasing the thenar eminence bulk.

- **Donor**: The donor tendon in Huber opponensplasty is ADM.
- **Tendon harvest:**
  - A midlateral incision is placed on the proximal phalanx of little finger on ulnar side. It is then extended proximally and radially to the distal palmar crease.
  - The same incision continues along the radial aspect of the hypothenar bulge and extends ulnarly to reach the distal palmar crease.
  - ADM has two insertions at the base of the proximal phalanx and extensor apparatus. The insertions are cut and muscle is mobilized.
- **Pulley**: Near pisiform.
- **Insertion:**
  - Second incision is placed at the base of thenar eminence and third incision at the dorsoradial aspect of MPJ.
  - The subcutaneous tunnel is prepared joining the third incision up to proximal to the pisiform.

Q23. What is Camitz opponensplasty?

When PL tendon is used, it is also known as Camitz opponensplasty.

- Usually performed for loss of abduction and opposition occurring as a complication of severe carpal tunnel syndrome.
- Restores more of palmar abduction rather than opposition.

  - Not recommended in traumatic median nerve injuries as PL lies over the median nerve and gets damaged and scarred simultaneously.

Technique:

- First, confirm the presence of PL by asking the patient to oppose his thumb to the little finger with wrist in flexion.
- A long skin incision extending from the distal crease of wrist to the proximal crease of the palm is made in line with the ring finger.
- A wide strip of palmar aponeurosis of approximately 1 cm is cut out in continuity with the tendon.
- A second incision on dorsoradial aspect of thumb MCP joint is made and a wide subcutaneous tunnel is developed.
- PL tendon is passed through this tunnel and attached to APB insertion.
  - **Thumb**: In full opposition.
  - **MPJ**: In extension.
  - **Wrist**: In neutral.
- Cast holding the wrist in neutral and thumb opposed is applied for 4 weeks followed by night splintage for another 1 week.

Q24. What are the other donor muscles for opponensplasty?

Other opponensplasties include:

- ECU, extensor carpi ulnaris.
- ECRL, extensor carpi radialis longus.
- EDM, extensor digiti minimi.

Q25. What is the difference between single insertion and dual insertion?

Duel-insertion technique:

- Aims for insertion of donor tendon to allow dual functions: opposition of thumb along with stabilization of metacarpophalangeal (MCP) joint passively or to restrict the flexion at the IP joint, beneficial in combined injuries of ulnar and median nerve.
- The disadvantage of duel insertion is that the efficiency of tendon transfers increases

when it does only one function actively (whenever a transferred tendon is inserted at two sites to do two different functions, the tighter insertion will act in a dominant fashion).

- The sites for insertion can be: duel insertions into the APB insertion and either the dorsal MPJ capsule or the extensor expansion of the thumb.

Single-insertion technique:

- Tendon transfers with insertion at APB site are commonly used in isolated median nerve palsy.
- The transferred opponensplasty tendon is attached to the APB insertion on the radial aspect of the MCP joint.

Q26. Why pulleys are required and how are they reconstructed?

In the tendon transfers to restore opponensplasty, the donor tendon has to pass subcutaneously across the palm to lie parallel to the APB muscle.

- To lie parallel to APB, all the true extrinsic opponensplasties must pass around a stout fixed pulley in the region of the pisiform on the ulnar border of the wrist.
- The advantage is that it makes the line of the tendon transfer lie in a straight line. If it is not followed, there will be constant friction with the soft tissues and to overcome this friction, tendon would apply extra force and will migrate so as to lie in a straight line.

Q27. What are the various tendon transfers done in high median nerve injuries?

The goals of tendon transfer in high median nerve injury are:

- To restore the index finger flexion and thumb flexion.
- To restore the opposition.
  - The available donors are brachioradialis, ECRL, and ECU for transfer to extrinsic flexors.
  - ECU may also be used for opponensplasty.

ECRL → Index profundus transfer
BR → FPL transfer

- As the excursion of BR, ECRL, and ECU is less, so in order to achieve the full flexion and extension of thumb and fingers, the patient needs to use the tenodesis effect of wrist extensions and flexion, respectively.
- Tendon transfers are done in end-to-side fashion if motor recovery after nerve repair or graft is anticipated. In all cases when there is no hope of recovery, end-to-end tendon transfer is performed.

Complications after tendon transfers in high median nerve paralysis:

- These are predominantly common in patients with hypermobile joints and therefore transfers may be modified in these patients:
  - ECRL—for FDS of index and middle fingers.
    - In these two fingers, the profundus tendons are used to tenodese their DIP joints in 30 degrees of flexion.
  - ECRL—for FDP of index and middle fingers.
    - In these fingers, the profundus tendons are then sutured to A4 pulleys to maintain the DIP joint in 30 degrees of flexion so as to create the tenodesis effect. The transferred tendon will then primarily cause flexion of the PIP joints.
  - Transfer may be accompanied with DIP joint arthrodesis.
- The most critical part in high injuries of median nerve is least likelihood of sensory recovery and therefore opponensplasty is not at all beneficial.

Q28. What is post-operative rehabilitation protocol after opponensplasty?

The postoperative management guidelines of opponensplasty are as follows:

- The thumb is immobilized in opposition for 3 weeks after most opponensplasties.

- Wrist should also be immobilized if the tendon transfer crosses the flexor surface of this joint.
- When muscles with short excursions like EIP are used for transfers, then the wrist is immobilized in 30-degree flexion and thumb in full opposition.
- However, after transfer of muscles with larger excursions, such as FDS, the wrist is immobilized in neutral with thumb in full opposition.
- If transfer is attached either to extensor mechanism or APB insertion, the IP joint of the thumb should also be immobilized in full extension.

Q29. What is the physiotherapy protocol?

Physiotherapy protocol in both high and low median nerve palsy differs:

Low median nerve injury

Opponensplasty:

Week 0–3

- FDS of ring finger (RF) or PL to APB (Camitz): Long opponens splint with:
  - Wrist in 20° flexion.
  - Thumb in maximum palmar abduction with index finger.
- **EIP to APB**: Long opponens splint with:
  - Wrist in neutral to flexion/extension (depending on the route of transfer).
  - Thumb in maximum palmar abduction.
- **ADM to APB (Huber)**: Hand-based long opponens with:
  - Wrist position neutral.
  - Thumb in maximum palmar abduction.

Week 3

Begin AROM of thumb in splint to activate transfer, six to eight times per day.

Week 4

Begin AROM of thumb and other joints out of splint. Focus on activation of transfer; may use light grasp.

Week 6

- Discontinue splint and begin unrestricted A/PROM.

- May introduce light resistance.

Week 8

- Preferably the patient should complete frequent low-resistance exercise sessions rather than occasional high-resistive exercises.
- *It is important not to fatigue the transfer.*

Week 12

- Resume unrestricted activities.

High median nerve palsy

BR/FDS to FPL

Week 0–3

- DBS (possibly long arm splint with elbow in 90-degree flexion for BR).
- Wrist in 20-degree flexion.
- Thumb MCPI in 20-degree flexion, IPJ in 20-degree flexion, and CMC in full palmar abduction.

AROM of MCP/IP within splint to activate transfer six to eight times per day.

Week 4

AROM out of splint for transfer activation and light prehension.

Week 6

Discontinue splint, PROM, and splintage to decrease tightness if present.

Week 8

Progressive Resistive Exercises (PRE).

Suggested Readings

1. Davis TRC. In; Green DP, editors. Green's Operative Hand Surgery. Vol.1. 8th ed, Elsevier; 2022.
2. Jones NF, Khiabini KT. In; Mathes SJ, editors. Plastic Surgery: The Hand and Upper Limb Part 2. Vol. 8. 2nd ed. Canada: Elsevier; 2006. P. 453-488.
3. Klein MA. Tendon transfers for median nerve palsy. In: Saunders RJ, Astifidis RP, Burke SL, Higgins JP, Mcclinton MA, eds. Hand and upper extremity rehabilitation: a practical guide. St. Louis, MO: Elsevier; 2006:167–171

9 Radial Nerve Palsy

Veena K. Singh

Learning Objectives

At the end of this chapter, the student will be able to:
1. Recall the course and supply of radial nerve.
2. Describe the clinical presentation of a patient with radial nerve palsy.
3. Demonstrate the motor and sensory examination of radial nerve.
4. Understand the timeline and choose the right surgical intervention.
5. Perform the tendon transfers for radial nerve palsy.

Introduction

Radial nerve palsy leads to significant functional disability in the hand. There is loss of grasp and power grip due to loss of thumb and finger extension and wrist extension. Nerve repair and various tendon transfers are the options available with predictable results but low margin of errors. In a case of radial nerve palsy, it is equally important to differentiate between complete radial nerve palsy and posterior interosseous nerve (PIN) palsy.

Chief Complaints

- Inability to straighten/lift the wrist.
- Inability to straighten the base of the finger's and thumb.
- Inability to grasp an object.
- Weakness in the grip of the hand.

History of Present Illness

- History of trauma in details.
- History of operative intervention, (e.g., fracture fixation, nerve repair).

- Any physiotherapy followed by the patient and for how long.
- Splintage use (static/dynamic).
- Loss of sensation, pain, tingling sensation over specific points.

Past History

- History of diabetes mellitus, hypertension, tuberculosis, or any other medical illness.
- Any surgery done in the past for nerve injury or intervention for fracture.

Personal History

- History of addiction including alcoholism, smoking, marital status, no. of kids, employment status.

Family History

- Number of family members dependent on the patient.

Treatment History

Any physiotherapy since the injury or any use of splintage.

History of Allergy

To food or medications.

General Physical Examination

Like other cases.

Systemic Examination

- Abdomen.
- Central nervous system.
- Cardiovascular system.
- Respiratory system.

Local Examination

After proper consent, with adequate exposure and light.

Adequate Exposure

Exposure of affected limb from shoulder level up to the finger tips. The affected limb has to be rested on a table with forearm slightly raised and rested on elbow.

Inspection

1. Attitude of the affected limb (**Fig. 9.1**): Carefully watch the posture of the affected limb from shoulder to the fingertips. In the radial nerve palsy, the wrist is in flexed

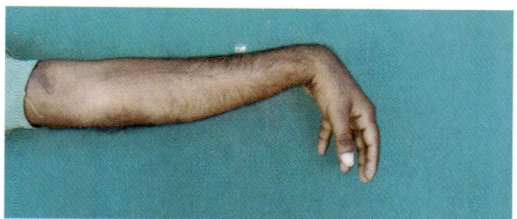

Fig. 9.1   Attitude of hand in radial nerve palsy.

posture, and in the fingers, metacarpophalangeal (MCP) joints are in flexion along with the extension of interphalangeal (IP) joints.
2. Generalized muscle wasting of the arm, forearm, and hand. Always compare with normal limb.
3. Scars, tattoos: There may be presence of scars from previous injuries or any previous surgery.
4. Look for soft tissue loss and joint contracture, if any.
5. Bony abnormalities: Humerus, elbow joint, forearm bones.
6. Presence of external fixator, if any.

Palpation

Motor Examination

1. Remember MRC grading.
2. If any muscle is weak, then again check the muscle by eliminating the effect of gravity.
3. Few things to be remembered while testing the muscle:
    - Look for the contraction of the muscles.
    - Feel for the bulk during contraction.
    - Move against resistance.
    - Normal side first followed by affected side.
    - Passive range of movements to be checked at all the joints.

Sequence of examination must be targeted to localize the lesion.

1. Elbow:
   Triceps: The triceps muscle is responsible for the extension of elbow. Ask the patient to extend his elbow from flexed posture. If the patient is able to extend his elbow, then check against resistance by applying force on the forearm and patient will continue extending the elbow. With the other hand, palpate the triceps muscle bulk at the back of the arm (**Fig. 9.2**).
   Brachioradialis (BR): The BR muscle brings flexion of the elbow in midprone position. The forearm is rested on the table at elbow in midprone position and ask the patient to

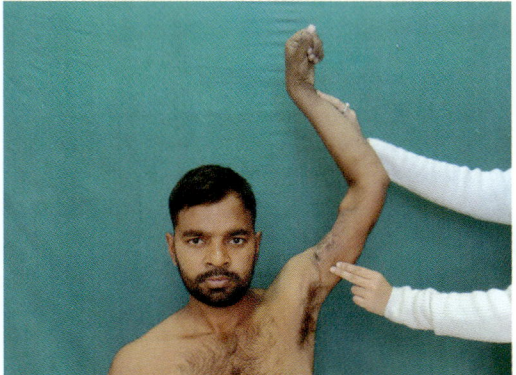

Fig. 9.2 Examination of triceps muscle.

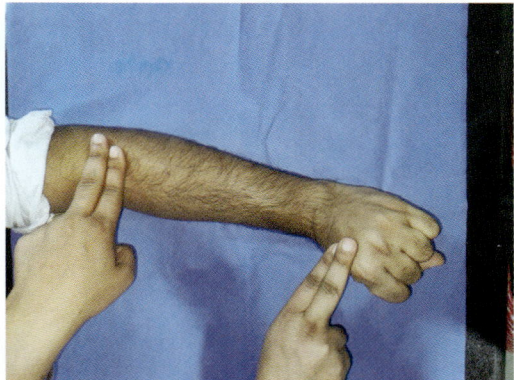

Fig. 9.3 Examination of brachioradialis.

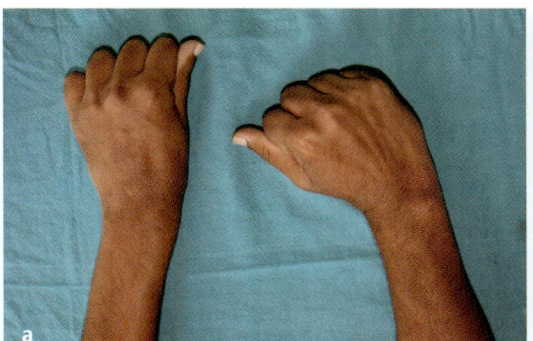

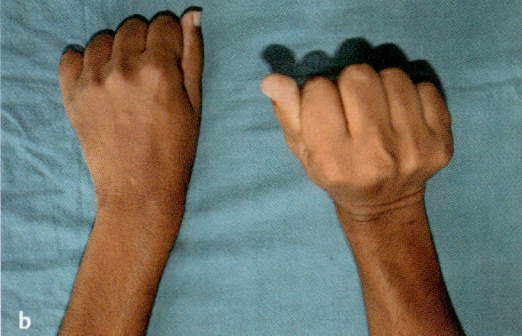

Fig. 9.4 **(a, b)** Difference between the action of extensor carpi radialis longus (ECRL) and extensor carpi radialis brevis (ECRB).

flex his elbow. Check against resistance by applying force at the wrist while the patient continues flexing the elbow in midprone position. Palpate the muscle bulk in the proximal forearm just beneath the elbow joint crease (**Fig. 9.3**).

2. **Wrist:**

   Extensor carpi radialis longus (ECRL) and extensor carpi radialis brevis (ECRB): They are wrist extensors. With the patient forearm slightly raised from the table with elbow at rest, ask the patient to straighten his wrist. Check whether he is able to do so and if straightening is possible, then ask him to fully extend the wrist (**Fig. 9.4**).

   Extensor carpi ulnaris (ECU): ECU is an ulnar deviator of the wrist in extension. Ask the patient to make a fist and extend his wrist. If the patient is able to extend the wrist, then

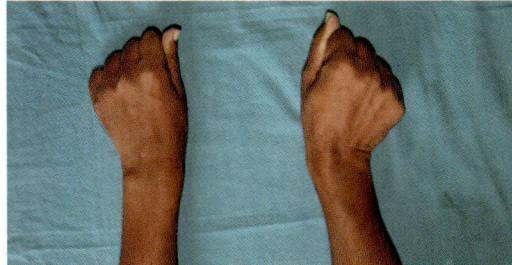

Fig. 9.5 Examination of extensor carpi ulnaris (ECU).

ask him to do the ulnar deviation. If he is able to do so, also check the power against resistance (**Fig. 9.5**).

3. **MCP joint:** Once extension at wrist is examined, then check the extension at MCP joints by asking the patient to straighten his fingers. Loss of MCP extension with intact wrist extension indicates PIN palsy (**Fig. 9.6**).

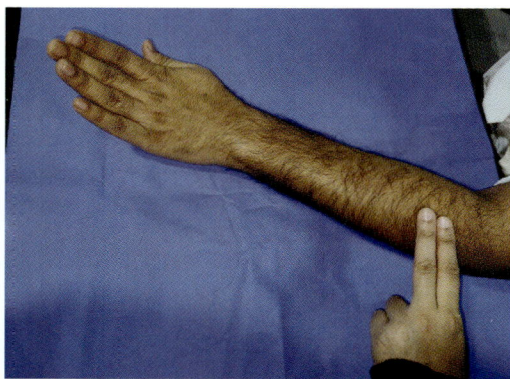

Fig. 9.6 Demonstration of extension at metacarpophalangeal (MCP) joints.

4. **IP joint:** Look for the position of IP joints in all fingers while the patient is trying to extend his MCP joints. Note that the patient is able to completely extend his fingers but not his MCP joint.

Sensory Examination

The sensory supply of radial nerve in the hand is in the area of anatomical snuff box and first web space. So, a detailed sensory examination in the territory of radial nerve supply needs to be checked. (Refer to chapter 5 on "Brachial plexus injury.")

Measurements

1. **Girth of forearm:** The circumference of the arm and forearm at a fixed distance from a bony landmark need to be measured in the affected limb and compared with the normal side to rule out atrophy, if any.
2. **Range of movements at joints:** The functional range of movements at elbow, wrist, MCP, and IP joints must be measured to rule out any stiffness.

Provisional Diagnosis

This is a case of 3 months old posttraumatic right-sided radial nerve palsy with underlying fracture shaft of humerus in a 35-year-old male patient.

Questions

Q1. How will you proceed?

I would like to go for surgical exploration and nerve repair via nerve graft along with internal splintage.

- Before surgery, I would like to do some assessments:
  - X-ray arm—anteroposterior (AP) and lateral views to confirm the fracture union.
  - High-resolution ultrasonography to have a rough idea about the nerve gap (magnetic resonance imaging [MRI] cannot be done as metal implants are in situ).
  - Nerve conduction study.
- Baseline investigation required to assess the anesthetic fitness of the patient for surgery:
  - Complete blood count, erythrocyte sedimentation rate (ESR), prothrombin time/international normalized ratio (PT/INR).
  - Renal function tests: Serum creatinine, blood urea.
  - Liver function tests.
  - Viral markers: HbsAg, HCV, HIV1 and 2.
  - Chest X-ray: Posteroanterior (PA) view. ⎤
  - Electrocardiography: In all 12 leads ⎦ in patients >30 years of age
- The standard protocol is:
  - <4 months: Nerve repair wherever indicated.
  - >4 months: Tendon transfer.

Q2. How will you differentiate complete radial nerve palsy from posterior interosseous nerve (PIN) palsy?

Wrist extension will be preserved in PIN palsy as radial nerve innervates the muscles of BR and ECRL after emerging from the spiral groove and before dividing into its two terminal branches: superficial radial nerve (the sensory branch) and PIN (the motor branch) (**Fig. 9.7**).

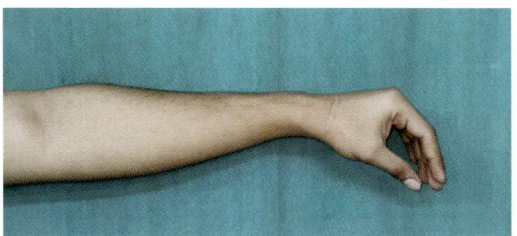

Fig. 9.7 Wrist extension preserved in posterior interosseous nerve (PIN) palsy.

Q3. Describe the anatomy of radial nerve.

Radial nerve (root value: C5–T1) is a branch arising from the posterior cord of the brachial plexus and lies posterior to the axillary artery (**Fig. 9.8**). It emerges from axilla and enters the posterior aspect of arm through the triangular space and then enters the spiral groove. Before entering the spiral groove, it supplies long and lateral heads of the triceps muscle.

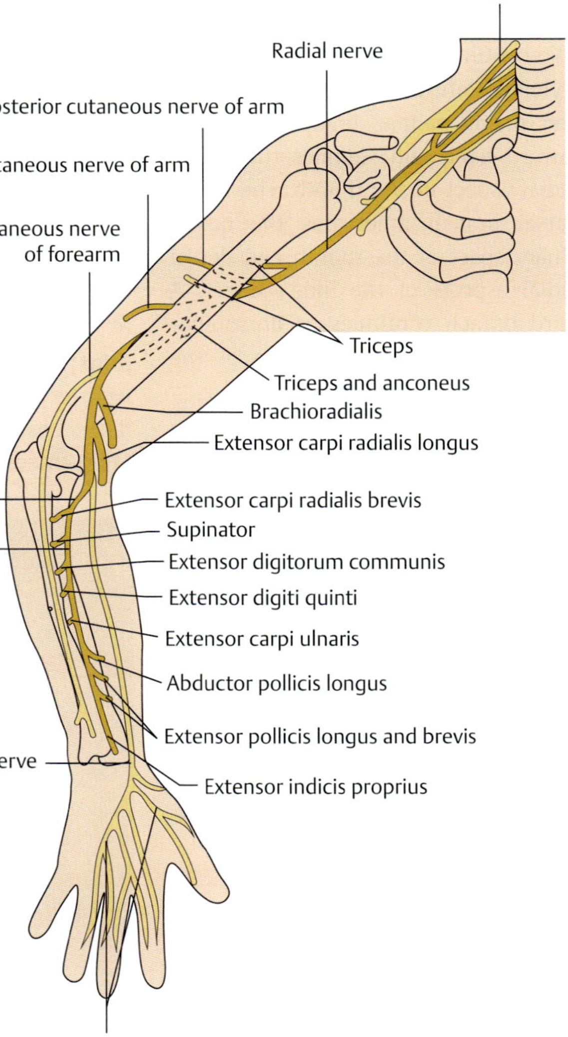

C5

Radial nerve

Posterior cutaneous nerve of arm

Lower lateral cutaneous nerve of arm

Posterior cutaneous nerve of forearm

Triceps

Triceps and anconeus

Brachioradialis

Extensor carpi radialis longus

Deep radial motor nerve

Posterior interosseous nerve

Extensor carpi radialis brevis

Supinator

Extensor digitorum communis

Extensor digiti quinti

Extensor carpi ulnaris

Abductor pollicis longus

Extensor pollicis longus and brevis

Superficial radial- sensory nerve

Extensor indicis proprius

Dorsal digital nerves

Fig. 9.8 Illustrations showing course of radial nerve.

From the spiral groove, it gives branch to the medial head of the triceps. In the spiral groove, it is accompanied by profunda brachii, the deep branch of the brachial artery.

After emerging from the spiral groove, it gives branches to BR, ECRL, ECRB. It enters the forearm by emerging from the cubital fossa and divides into two terminal branches.

- **Superficial sensory branch**: It courses below the BR and enters the subcutaneous tissue between the tendons of the BR and ECRL.
    - Five centimeter proximal to the radial styloid, it bifurcates into two branches. The major palmar branch continues toward hand and supplies the dorsal radial aspect of the thumb. The major dorsal branch innervates the dorsal ulnar aspect of the thumb and dorsal radial aspects of the index finger. A third branch continues as dorsoulnar and dorsoradial digital nerve of the index and the middle fingers.
- **Posterior interosseous nerve**: It originates at the radioulnar joint and emerges from the supinator under arcade of Frosche (supinator arch) about 8 cm distal to the elbow joint.
    - The nerve then runs in a fascial plane between the superficial and deep extensor muscles and eventually reaches interosseous membrane.
    - It supplies the four superficial extensor and five deep extensors in forearm.

Q4. What is the order in which radial nerve innervates the muscles of forearm?

- Brachioradialis (BR).
- Extensor carpi radialis longus (ECRL).
- Extensor carpi radialis brevis (ECRB).
- Supinator.
- Extensor digitorum communis (EDC).
- Extensor carpi ulnaris (ECU).
- Extensor digiti minimi (EDM).
- Abductor pollicis longus (APL).
- Extensor Pollicis Longus (EPL).

Q5. What is the pattern of sensory loss in radial nerve palsy?

The sensory loss in radial nerve palsy is not substantial and can be ignored. Only when there is a painful neuroma, it is bothersome to the patient. Sensory loss on the radial side of the dorsum of the hand may be the only positive finding in clinical examination of superficial branch of the radial nerve (**Fig. 9.9**). In long standing cases, its function is overlapped by the lateral antebrachial cutaneous nerve.

Q6. How to differentiate between the actions of ECRL and ECRB?

ECRL extends the wrist in radial axis, that is, extension of wrist in radial deviation is caused by ECRL (**Fig. 9.4a, b**).

ECRB causes extension of wrist in central axis or neutral position.

Q7. How will you test the loss of extension at the metacarpophalangeal joint (MCP joint)?

Ask the patient to straighten the MCP joint from flexed position. Inability to do so indicates loss of MCPJ extension.

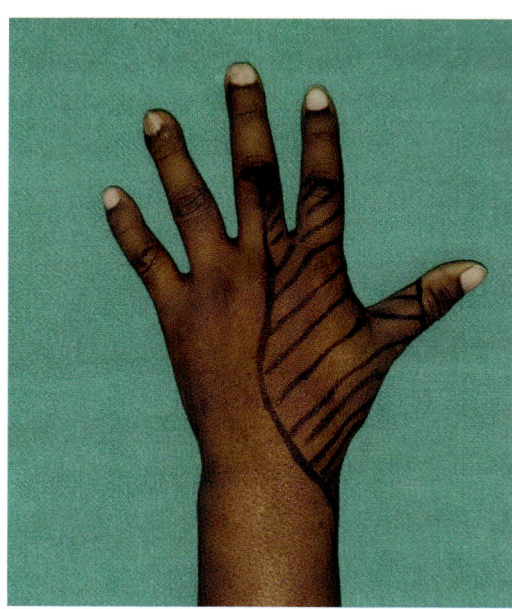

Fig. 9.9 Mapping of sensory loss in radial nerve palsy.

Q8. How will you test the action of triceps?

Ask the patient to extend his elbow from flexed posture. If the patient is able to extend his elbow, then check the extension of elbow against resistance by applying force on the forearm. With the other hand, palpate the triceps muscle bulk at the back of the arm (**Fig. 9.2**).

Q9. How will you test the action of EPL, APL, and extensor pollicis brevis (EPB)?

EPL: Place the hand on the table and hold the distal phalanx of the thumb to keep the IP joint in flexed position. Ask the patient to extend his thumb while applying force to maintain the flexion at IP joint (**Fig. 9.10**).

APL: Place the hand on the table and stabilize the proximal phalanx of thumb. Ask the patient to abduct the thumb away from the palm at right angle. Once the patient starts abducting the

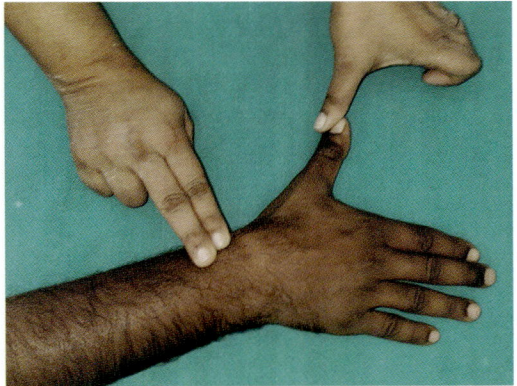

Fig. 9.10 Examination of extensor pollicis longus (EPL).

thumb, apply force to check against resistance (**Fig. 9.11**).

EPB: Place the hand on the table and hold the proximal phalanx of the thumb to keep MCP joint in flexed position. Ask the patient to extend the thumb while applying force to maintain the flexion at MCP joint (**Fig. 9.12**).

Q10. How to decide whether to go for nerve grafting or tendon transfer?

In acute injuries, repair of radial nerve should always be attempted, either end-to-end or via a nerve graft. Even late repair in radial nerve palsy has good results because the nerve is almost entirely motor and the branches are close to the site of injury.

When there is any doubt in the outcome of nerve repair, it is strongly recommended to go for tendon transfer at an early stage.

Conditions to go for early tendon transfer:
- Nerve gap >4 cm.
- Crush injury leading to massive scarring.
- Loss of skin over the site of nerve injury.

In all other cases:
- Go for nerve repair whenever possible.

Q11. What is internal splint and when is it recommended?

The concept was given by Burkhalter. Internal splint is early tendon transfer of pronator teres (PT) to ECRB. It provides a temporary splint and therefore obviates the need for an external splint.

The advantage is restoration of significant amount of power grip to the patient's hand.

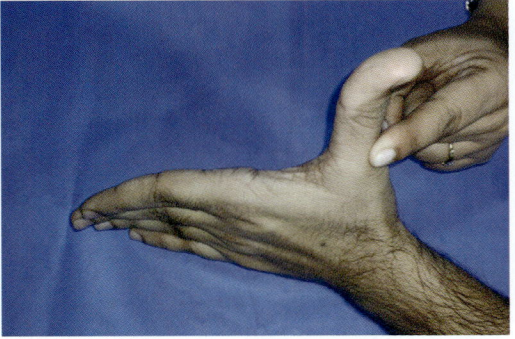

Fig. 9.11 Examination of abductor pollicis longus (APL).

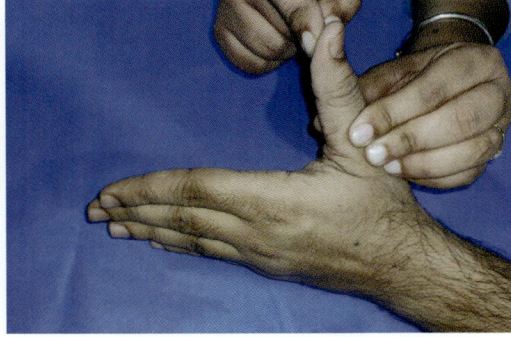

Fig. 9.12 Examination of extensor pollicis brevis (EPB).

Indications of internal splint are:

- During waiting time of nerve regeneration to exclude the requirement of external splint.
- Reinforces the power of the reinnervated muscle.
- Acts as a substitute where the expected outcome of nerve repair is poor.

In the light of above-mentioned advantages it should be done simultaneously with an end-to-side radial nerve repair. Tendon weaving is done in an end-to-side fashion and continuity of ECRB is maintained.

Q12. What are the principles of tendon transfer?

OR

What factors will you take into account before proceeding for tendon transfer?

The principles of tendon transfers are:

- **Joints should be supple:** The essential principle is to have maximum passive range of motion (PROM) at all joints before a tendon transfer is done as no tendon transfers can cause movement on a stiff joint.
- **Adequate motor strength of the donor tendon:** Preferred strength of the donor tendon is MRC grading power of 5 as any muscle loses one grade of strength after transfer.
- **Amplitude of motion:** The amplitude of the donor tendon must be taken into consideration while performing a tendon transfer as a wrist flexor would not be able to provide the range of motion (ROM) for a finger extensor.
  - Wrist flexors and extensors: 33 mm.
  - Finger extensors and EPL: 50 mm.
  - Finger flexors: 70 mm.

Two maneuvers can be done to increase the amplitude of motion:

  - A muscle can be converted from mono-articular to biarticular or polyarticular (e.g., opponensplasty).
  - Extensive dissection of fascial attachments of the donor muscle (e.g., in case of BR).

- **Line of pull must be in a straight path:**
  - It should be followed for most efficient transfer.
  - Important in FCU to EDC transfer.
- **One tendon—one function:**
  - One tendon must perform only one action for maximum efficiency.
  - If a muscle is inserted into two tendons having separate functions, the force and amplitude of the donor tendon will be divided and less efficient as compared to insertion in one tendon.
- **Synergism/synergistic action:**
  - Synergistic muscles are used for transfer whenever possible, (e.g., finger flexors acting in synergism with wrist extensors and vice versa).
  - The advantage is that it is easier to retrain muscle function after synergistic muscle transfers.
- **Donor muscles/tendon should be expendable:** Sacrifice of the donor tendon must not compromise the function normally done by that tendon.
- **Tissue equilibrium:** For a successful outcome after tendon transfer, it is crucial that the local tissues must be in optimal condition at the time of transfer. No inflammation or immature scar, adequate soft tissue cover.

Q13. What tendon transfers are available and how do you choose?

Sir Robert Jones advocated transferring both FCU and FCR in radial nerve palsy.

Brand transfer	Boyes	FCU transfer
PT to ECRB	PT to ECRL and ECRB	PT to ECRB
Flexor carpi radialis (FCR) to EDC	Flexor digitorum superficialis (FDS) III to extensor digitorum superficialis (EDS)	Flexor carpi ulnaris (FCU) to EDC
Palmaris longus (PL) to EPL (rerouted)	FDS IV to EIP and EPL	PL to EPL (rerouted)
	FCR to APL and EPB	

- In cases of isolated PIN palsy, FCR transfer is indicated because if FCU is used, static radial deviation postural deformity may occur. This happens because FCU is the prime ulnar stabilizer of the wrist.
- The advantage of Boyes transfer is because of their greater excursion (70 mm), FDS tendon is ideal for replacing finger extensors.

Q14. What incisions are given and what technical points are kept in focus?

- **Exposure of PT, ECRL, and ECRB:**
  - A long curvilinear incision with ulnar concavity extending from radial aspect of the mid-forearm up to the radial styloid process is given (**Fig. 9.13a–c**).
  - Insertion of PT from radius removed with 2 to 3 cm of strip of periosteum.
  - PT passed over radial border of forearm superficial to BR and ECRL.
  - Weaved into the tendon of ECRB and ECRL just distal to musculotendinous junction with tension adjusted to wrist in 45 degrees of extension and PT under maximum tension.
- **Exposure of FDS III and IV:**
  - A single incision over distal palmar crease or two separate incisions over the base of middle and ring fingers given (**Fig. 9.14a, b**).

- Tendons are divided proximal to the chiasma and delivered through a separate incision over distal forearm, proximal to pronator quadratus.
- Two small openings are made in the interosseous membrane on either side of the anterior interosseous artery and tendons are delivered on the dorsal aspect of forearm through the same incision used for PT and ECRB.
- The tendon transfers FDS III to EDC and FDS IV to EPL and extensor indicis proprius (EIP) are interwoven with tension:
  - Wrist in 20 degrees of extension.
  - Fingers and thumb held in a fist.
  - FDS under maximal tension.
- **Exposure of FCR and PL:**
  - A straight long incision is given over the distal half of the volar radial aspect of the forearm between FCR and PL (**Fig. 9.15a, b**).
  - FCR and PL are divided near their insertion and freed up to mid-forearm. FCR is passed around the radial border of forearm in a subcutaneous plane and delivered through a separate incision on the dorsal aspect from extensor retinaculum to mid-forearm.

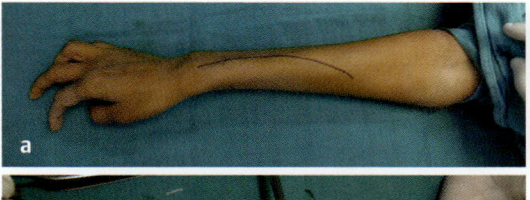
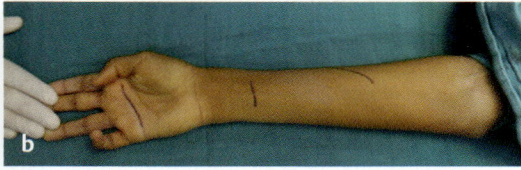
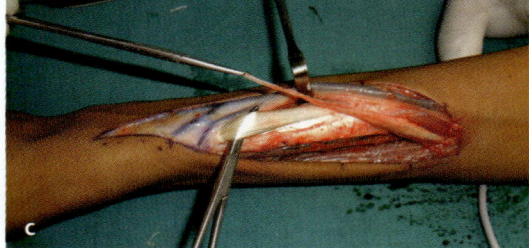

Fig. 9.13 (a–c) Incision marking for the exposure of pronator teres (PT), extensor carpi radialis longus (ECRL), and extensor carpi radialis brevis (ECRB).

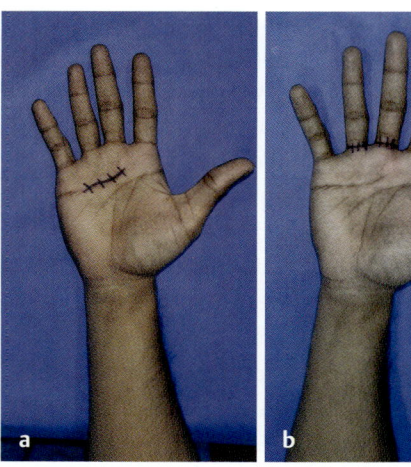

Fig. 9.14 (a, b) Incision marking for exposure of flexor digitorum superficialis (FDS) tendons.

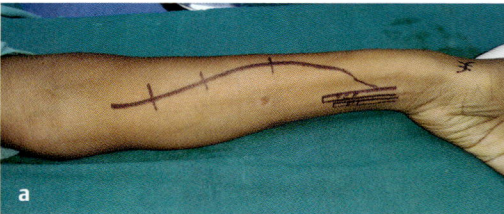

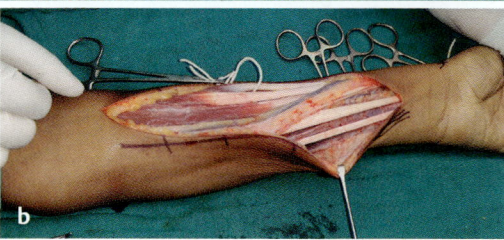

Fig. 9.15 (a, b) Incision marking for exposure of flexor carpi radialis (FCR) and palmaris longus (PL).

– EDC tendons are divided proximal to retinaculum and repositioned superficial to it.
– EDC tendons are interwoven into FCR tendon at wrist in neutral position, MCP joint also in neutral position, and FCR under maximum tension.
– PL is identified and divided at the wrist and muscle-tendon unit is made free. It is then interwoven with EPL which has already been divided at musculotendinous junction and rerouted out of Lister's canal toward the anatomical snuff box.

• **Exposure of FCU:**
– A J-shaped incision over volar aspect of distal forearm with longitudinal part over the FCU and transverse part over the PL tendon.
– FCU tendon is exposed and transected just proximal to the pisiform and freed up proximal as far as possible.
– Another incision is given approximately 5 cm below the medial epicondyle and FCU tendon is delivered into this wound. (Take care that the nerve to FCU enters at this point.)

– The third incision is same as for exposure of PT and ECRL and ECRB.
– The line of pull from medial epicondyle to EDC must be a straight one and tendon juncture is weaved.
– FCU–EDC at 0-degree wrist extension (neutral).
– MPJ in neutral (0 degree).
– FCU in maximal tension.

Q15. How do you apply a postoperative splint?
The tension of the transferred tendons is always checked on table after weaving is completed in the prescribed tension (according to the method of tendon transfer) (**Fig. 9.16**).
• A long-arm splint (**Fig. 9.17**) is applied with:
– 15 to 30 degrees of forearm pronation.
– 45 degrees of wrist extension.
– 10 to 15 degrees of MPJ flexion.
– Maximum extension and abduction of thumb.
– Proximal interphalangeal (PIP) joints are left free.
• Splint is applied for 4 weeks followed by short-arm splint for another 2 weeks.

Q16. What is the physiotherapy protocol in tendon transfers for radial nerve palsy?

The physiotherapy protocol followed in tendon transfers for radial nerve palsy is as follows:

Pre-operative Therapy

Precaution: Do not over stretch donor muscle.

- Minimize edema by limb elevation, encourage active range of motion (AROM), compression fluid flushing massage, and electrical muscle stimulation (EMS).
- Maximize AROM and PROM.
- Strengthening of uninvolved muscles of upper extremity.
- Strengthening of donor muscle as indicated.

Post-operative Therapy

Week 0 to 3–4

- Immobilization as mentioned previously in Q.15.
- Maintain ROM of uninvolved joints: AROM of distal interphalangeal (DIP), shoulder, and neck joints.

Week 3–4

- Protective ROM of individual joint: Extend all other joints while flexing one joint at a time:
  - Wrist, PIP, and DIP joints are fully extended while flexing MCP joint.
  - With full forearm pronation and digit extension, protective ROM to the MCP and IP joint permitted.
  - Limited ROM to the wrist at 10 to 30 degrees.

- Avoid composite wrist and digit flexion.
- Edema management: Elevation, EMS (electrical muscle stimulation), fluid flushing massage.
- Desensitization techniques: Gentle stroking, touching, and tapping to tolerance and application of TENS (transcutaneous electrical nerve stimulation).

Week 5–6

- **Muscle re-education**: Brief session of in contraction (place, hold technique to gentle active contraction, palpation of tendon, biofeedback exercise) and education of transferred muscle.
- Progress to full ROM during light pick up-release activities for digit and twisting activities of thumb (e.g., nut and bolt assembly).

Week 7

- Dynamic flexion splinting if extrinsic extensors tendon tightness present.

Week 8

- Discontinue protective daytime splinting, begin restrictive exercise, passive wrist flexion to gain maximum PT length.

Week 12

- Resume unrestricted activities.

Q17. What is Tubiana's method of rerouting the ECRL?

- To reduce the excessive radial deviation of the wrist in cases where FCU transfer for radial nerve palsy has been planned,

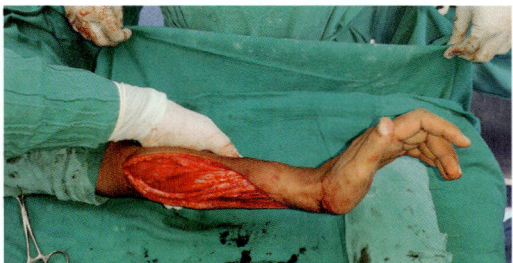

Fig. 9.16 Position of hand after tendon transfer.

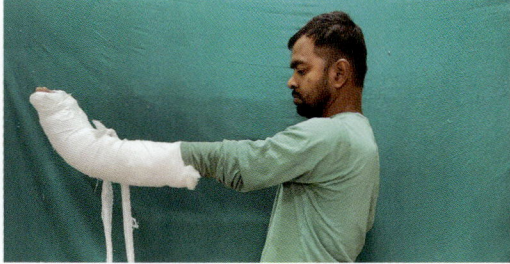

Fig. 9.17 Splintage after tendon transfer in radial nerve palsy.

Tubiana did the centralization of insertion of the ECRL.

- Apart from suturing PT to ECRB, the ECRL tendon is divided at its insertion into the base of the second metacarpal, freed up proximally up to the musculotendinous junction, rerouted beneath the dorsal retinaculum in the fourth EDC compartment, and fixed to the base of the third and fourth metacarpals with sutures and staples.

Suggested Readings

1. Davis TRC. In: Green DP, eds. Green's operative hand surgery. Vol. 1. 8th ed. Elsevier; 2022:1189–1242
2. Jones NF, Khiabini KT. In: Mathes SJ, eds. Plastic surgery: the hand and upper limb. Part 2. Vol. 8. 2nd ed. Canada: Elsevier; 2006:453–488
3. Brown AP. Tendon transfers for radial nerve palsy. In: Saunders RJ, Astifidis RP, Burke SL, Higgins JP, Mcclinton MA, eds. Hand and upper extremity rehabilitation: a practical guide. St. Louis, MO: Elsevier; 2006:189–192

10 Flexor Tendon Injury

Rimpi Jain

Learning Objectives

At the end of the chapter, the students will be able to:
1. Recall the anatomy of hand and flexor tendons.
2. Describe the clinical presentation of a patient with flexor tendon injury.
3. Demonstrate the examination of flexor tendon.
4. Understand how to decide on a particular procedure according to the timeline.
5. Perform the steps of flexor tendon repair.

Introduction

Flexor tendon injuries result not only in loss of vital functions of the hand but also impacts the patients in terms of vocational and economic disability. The repair must be targeted toward restoration of the normal gliding function and strength of the tendons as well as prevention of adhesion and loss of movement. So the hand surgeon dealing with flexor tendon injury must be well versed with the anatomy, biomechanics, nutrition, and healing process including suturing techniques and rehabilitation protocols.

History

Particulars of the patient (name, age, sex, occupation, residence, etc.); hand dominance.

Chief Complaints

- Inability to bend the fingers.
- Inability to make a fist.
- Straightening of the fingers.
- Loss of sensation in hand (in case of associated nerve injuries).
- Blackening of fingers (in case of associated vascular injury).

History of Present Illness

- Ask about the duration of injury—whether acute or chronic injury, days or months back.
- Nature of trauma—whether traumatic or iatrogenic, self-inflicted or assault.
- Ask about the position of the fingers at the time of injury.
- Type of injury (sharp, blunt, avulsion, crush).
- Place where the accident occurred (at home, work, barnyard).
- Ask about what was the condition of soft tissues at the time of accident.
- How much has his/her work been affected?
- Sometimes, the flexor tendons are only partially injured so the patient will still be able to bend his finger but will experience excessive pain or catching of the finger during any movement. So, deeply enquire into such history if you suspect a flexor tendon injury in a patient who still shows the bending of fingers.

Negative History

- Ask about history of any other injuries in the body.

- Ask about the loss of sensation in the hand/fingers.

Treatment History

- Ask about the first aid which the patient received immediately after the injury. Where and within what time frame?
- Ask whether he consulted a general practitioner or a hand surgeon.
- Enquire about whether only dressing was done or some suturing of the skin was also done.
- What were the steps taken to control the bleeding at the time of injury?

Past History

History of diabetes mellitus, hypertension, and tuberculosis, any past surgery.

Family History

The details as in other cases including the dependency of the family members on the patient if he is the only bread winner for them.

Personal History

- History of alcoholism
- History of smoking.
- Occupation (manual laborer)
- Hand dominance.
- Marital status/number of kids/appetite/diet/sleep/bladder/bowel habit.

History of Allergy

To any food or medication.

General Examination

As for other cases.

Local Examination of Hand

Exposure

Proper exposure of both the hands up to forearm should be done in adequate light and with informed consent.

Inspection

Inspection should be done of outstretched hands with palm facing upward and rested on the top of a table.

1. **Attitude**: Look for the posture of hand in resting position. Always compare with the normal:
   - In the normal resting posture of the hand, The palm forms a hollow and the fingers are in flexed position with the thumb in slight abduction and opposition (**Fig. 10.1**).
   - In flexor tendon injury, this resting posture of a normal hand is lost and the fingers will lie in a straight posture (**Fig. 10.2**).
2. **Inspect the posture or normal resting cascade of the fingers.**
   - The normal resting cascade of the fingers is described as flexion at the metacarpophalangeal (MCP) joint through 70 to 90 degrees with increasing grade of flexion from index to little finger.

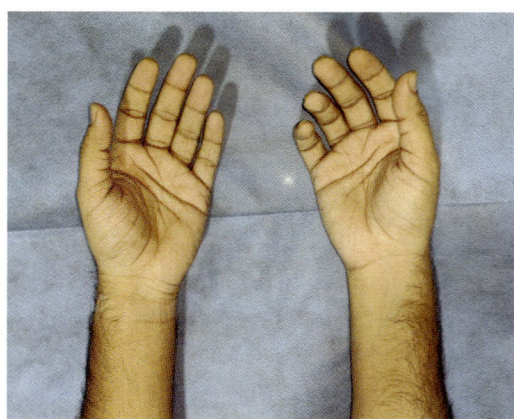

Fig. 10.1 Attitude of hands in a normal person.

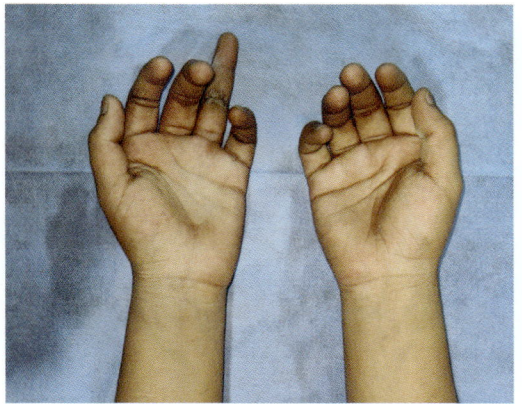

Fig. 10.2 Comparison of attitude of a normal and an injured hand (in the left hand, there is injury of both FDS and FDP of ring finger).

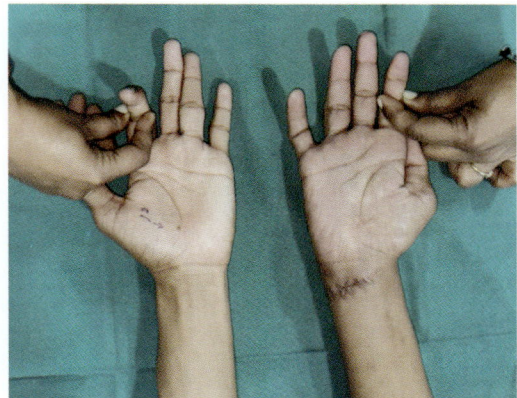

Fig. 10.3 Examination of flexor digitorum profundus (FDP) tendon (FDP in the right index finger is cut).

- This is lost in flexor tendon injury as the affected finger/s will not flex in resting position.
- When both flexor tendons of a finger are severed, the finger lies in an unnatural position of hyperextension especially compared with uninjured fingers.

3. Look for any bruising, lacerations, or scar of a sutured wound. Details of the scar in terms of location, length, width, pigmentation, hypertrophicity, etc.
4. Look for any obvious deviation of the fingers to rule out any associated fracture.
5. Examine the color of the hand/fingers to rule out any vascular injury.
6. On the skin, features of associated nerve injuries must be looked for
7.. Ask the patient to flex and extend the wrist alternatively and look at the change in affected finger movements.
   - The natural tenodesis effect on the finger movements accompanying wrist flexion and extension demonstrating the musculotendinous continuity will be lost.

Palpation

1. Temperature—any local rise due to infection.
2. Tenderness—near the scar and in the adjacent area.

3. Feel of the hand—whether dry, cool, clammy due to neurovascular injury.
4. All inspection findings must be corroborated.
5. Examine all the cut fingers for both flexor digitorum superficialis (FDS) and flexor digitorum profundus (FDP) tendon injury.
6. Test for FDP (**Fig. 10.3**):
   - The patient is asked to keep both the hands flat on the table with palm facing upward. Block the middle phalanx of the finger to be examined and ask the patient to flex the distal interphalangeal (DIP) joint of the same finger.
   - Locking the proximal interphalangeal (PIP) joint flexion is important as it is also brought by FDS and will give a false perception of intact FDP even if it is cut.
   - All the fingers are separately examined.
7. Test for FDS (**Fig. 10.4**):
   - Let the patient try to flex the PIP joint of the finger while the remaining fingers are held in extension.
   - Alternatively, the patient is asked to go pulp-to-pulp pinch between injured finger and thumb and if he can flex the PIP joint while the DIP joint extends (Boutonniere position), the superficialis tendon is at least partially intact.

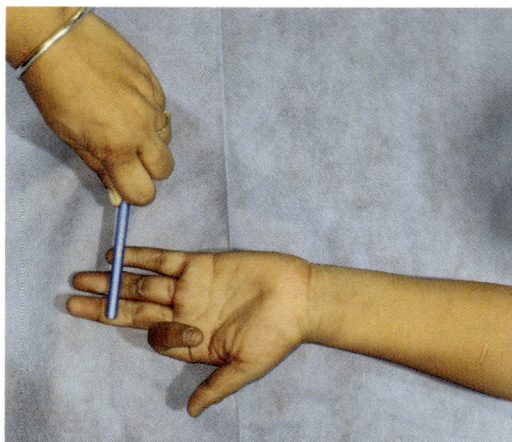

Fig. 10.4 Examination of flexor digitorum superficialis (FDS) tendon (FDS in the right ring finger is cut).

8. Flexor tendon injuries can be tentatively confirmed by several passive maneuvers:
   - Passive extension of the wrist does not produce the normal "tenodesis" flexion of the fingers.
   - On flexion of the wrist, even greater unopposed extension of the affected finger is produced.
   - On gentle compression of the forearm muscle mass, there is concomitant flexion of the joints of the uninvolved fingers.
   - Gently applying pressure on the fingertip of each digit reveals loss of normal tension.
     – Pain or weakness during resisted flexion may indicate a possible partial tendon laceration.
   - Examine the digital vessels.
   - Palpate both radial and ulnar arteries.
   - Examine for nerve injuries including digital nerves by using static two-point discrimination test separately for radial and ulnar digital nerves.

Provisional Diagnosis

A case of 7 days old zone II flexor tendon injury of right middle and ring finger.

Questions

Q1. How will you proceed? Or, what is your plan?

The plan is to do exploration and repair for which I will proceed by getting some investigations done for the patient:
- First of all, will get an X-ray of the affected hand done to rule out bony injuries.
  – Preferred X-ray views to be advised:
    ▪ Hand—anteroposterior (AP) and oblique views.
    ▪ Finger—AP and lateral views.
- Hemoglobin, complete blood count, prothrombin time/international normalized ratio (PT/INR).
- Serum electrolytes.
- Blood urea, serum creatinine.
- Viral markers (HIV1 & 2, HBsAg, HCV).

Q2. Is there any other investigation which you would like to do, if facilities are available (ultrasound sonography [USG], computed tomography [CT] scan, magnetic resonance imaging [MRI])?

In this particular case these investigations are not required as it is a clear case of sharp-cut injury and duration of injury is only 7 days. In cases which present late, a high-resolution USG/MRI would be helpful to know the gap between the tendon ends and any associated vascular injury.

Q3. What is the standard timing of tendon repair?

- If the patient is medically fit, there is no infection in the wound, and a plastic surgeon is available, it should be repaired as soon as possible.

  According to the time of presentation, tendon repair is classified into:
  – Primary repair: within 12 hours.
  – Delayed primary repair: within 10 to 14 days.
  – Secondary repair: 2 to 4 weeks.
  – Late secondary repair: after 4 weeks.

- Result of flexor tendon repair is best if it is done within hours and second best is when it is done after 10 days.
- Outcome is worst if repair is done between 4 and 7 days or after 4 weeks.

Q4. What are the principles of tendon repair?

The principles of tendon repair are:
- Atraumatic technique: The tendons and surrounding tissues should be handled as delicately as possible and kept moist in order to maximize the healing and to avoid adhesions. Only the cut ends of the tendon should be grasped by instruments and not crushed (**Fig. 10.5a, b**).
- Flexor tendon repair should be done under loupe magnification.
- Early motion after repair should be started. It increases the tendon strength, decreases adhesion, increases excursion, and improves nutrition through the pumping of synovial fluid.
- If both FDS and FDP are lacerated in zone II, both should be repaired. Repair of the superficialis tendon has following advantages:
  - Helps in protecting the vinculum longum to the profundus tendon.
  - Prevents rupture.
  - Provides a gliding interface between the profundus and underlying bone.

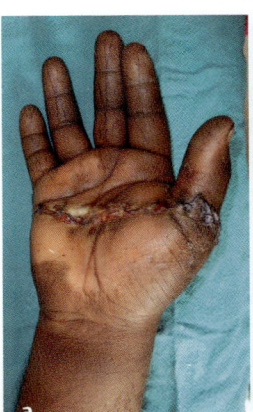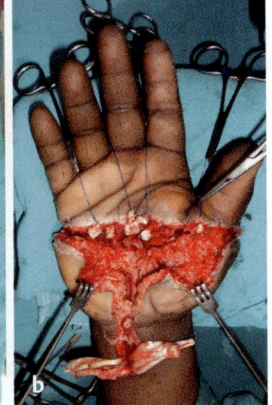

Fig. 10.5 (a, b) Atraumatic technique to hold the tendon ends in zone III.

- Improves the grip strength.
- Helps in preventing the possible secondary hyperextension of the PIP joint.
- Digital nerves and at least one artery should be repaired.
- Bony stabilization should be done before tendon repair.

Q5. Describe the anatomy of flexor tendons?

- The extrinsic flexor tendons to the hand are:
  - FDS.
  - FDP.
  - Flexor pollicis longus (FPL).
- The flexor-pronator group of muscles lies on the anterior aspect of forearm and are divided functionally and anatomically. The three functional muscle groups include the following:
  - **Pronator muscles:** Pronator teres, pronator quadratus.
  - **Wrist flexors**: Palmaris longus, flexor carpi radialis, flexor carpi ulnaris.
  - **Finger flexors:**
    - FDS.
    - FDP.
    - FPL in thumb.

According to depth, the forearm muscles are divided into three layers:
- **Superficial layer**: Pronator teres, flexor carpi radialis, palmaris longus, flexor carpi ulnaris.
- **Intermediate layer**: FDS.
- **Deep layer**: FDP, FPL, pronator quadratus.

Course of the flexor tendons:
- **Origin:** These tendons originate from muscles at about the mid forearm.
  - The tendons of the FDP originate from a common muscle belly except the index finger.
  - The tendons of the FDS originate from the separate muscle bellies, which allow more independent finger flexion.
  - The FPL tendon arises from the volar aspect of the midportion of the radial shaft and from its adjacent interosseous membrane.

- Palmaris longus is absent in about 15 to 20% of the normal population.
- **Within the carpal tunnel,** there are nine flexor tendons—four FDS, four FDP, and one FPL:
  - The FDS tendons of middle (3) and ring (4) fingers lie superficially, FDS tendons of index (2) and little (5) fingers are deep (34 over 25).
  - FDP tendons are deepest.
  - The FPL tendon is located deep and radially adjacent to the scaphoid and the trapezium.
- **Tendons enter the palm** after emerging from the carpal tunnel.
  - The digital sheath forms a closed synovial compartment and extends from the distal palm to the middle of the distal phalanx.
  - Proximally, the synovial sheath ends just proximal to the neck of the metacarpals, forming the proximal reflection of the digital flexor sheath.
  - The FDS tendons lie superficial to the FDP tendons up to the bifurcation of the FDS tendon at the midportion of the proximal phalanx.
  - Then, FDS tendon divides into two slips in the region of A2 pulley coursing laterally and then deeper to the FDP tendons.
  - Deep to the FDP tendon, the FDS slips rejoin to form Camper's chiasm (a fibrous interweaved connection between two FDS slips).
- **Insertion:**
  - FDS tendon after rejoining, distally insert on the proximal and middle parts of the middle phalanx as two separate slips.
  - The FDP tendon inserts into the volar aspect of the base of distal phalanx.
  - The FPL tendon is the only tendon inside the flexor sheath of the thumb and inserts at the distal phalanx.

Q6. What are the constituents of a tendon?
- About 70% of a tendon's dry weight is composed of type I collagen, a complex protein.
- Remaining part of the tendon is formed by ground substance, elastin, tenocytes, blood vessels, nerves, and lymphatics.

The three important structures in a tendon are:
- Primary cells responsible for collagen production are immature fibroblasts. There is cross-linkage between the tendon fibrils which forms tendon fibers. These fibers are grouped into fasciculi, which then form tendon bundles.
- The epitenon is a thin cellular layer on outer surface of the tendon that extends inward between tendon bundles and fasciculi to form the endotenon. Mature tenocytes are found within the tendon and epitenon.
- Ground substance, made up of glycosaminoglycans (hyaluronic acid, chondroitin 4-sulfate, dermatan sulfate, and heparan sulfate), glycoproteins, and noncollagenous proteins, is present in small amounts and functions to lubricate and allow tendon deformation during the application of force.

Q7. How pulleys are formed and where are they located?
- **Structure:** Pulleys are made of thickened areas of the flexor tendon sheath.
- **Components of pulley mechanism:** The transverse carpal ligament, the palmar aponeurotic pulley, and the digital pulley system make up the flexor tendon pulley mechanism that allows complete flexion of the wrist and digits without compromising extension.
  - **The transverse carpal ligament** spans the volar carpus. It maintains the transverse carpal arch and volume of the carpal canal.
  - **The palmar aponeurosis pulley** is formed by the transverse fibers of the

palmar fascia and the vertical interten-dinous septa of Legueu and Juvara that attach to the deep transverse metacar-pal ligament.

- **The digital flexor tendon sheath** has several membranous portions and a retinacular portion.
- **The fibro-osseous tunnel** and its com-plement of pulleys are integral to the function of the flexor tendons in the digits. The dorsal roof of the tunnel is formed by the:
  - MCP, PIP, and DIP volar plates.
  - The volar surface of the proximal and middle phalanges.
  - The deep transverse metacarpal ligament.
- **Function of pulleys:**
  - Pulleys play an important role in flex-ion, maintaining apposition of tendons and bones across joints, and provide fulcrum to elicit movement.
  - They prevent the bowstringing of the flexor tendons so that each joint can move independently. If bowstring-ing occurs, one joint movement will cause simultaneous movement of other joints.
  - These pulleys keep the flexor tendons closely apposed to the volar surface of the three phalanges and the three digi-tal articulations.
- **Types of pulleys (Fig. 10.6):**
  - In the fingers, there are five annular and three cruciate pulleys.
    - The annular pulleys are numbered proximally to distally: A1, A2, A3, A4, and A5.
      - The odd-numbered pulleys origi-nate from the volar plates of the MCP, PIP, and DIP joints.
      - Annular pulleys are made of thick transversely oriented fibrous bands that are relatively inflexible.
      - The A2 pulley arises from the periosteum at the proximal third of the proximal phalanx, and the

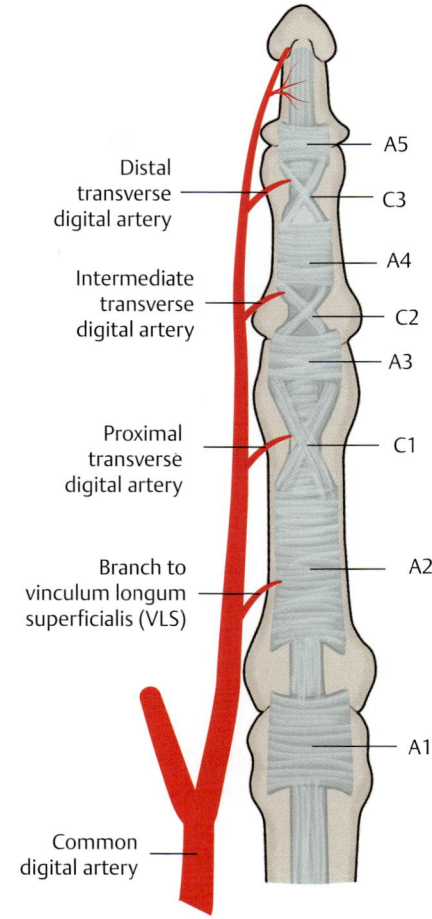

Fig. 10.6 The position of pulleys in hand.

A4 from the periosteum at the middle of the middle phalanx.
- The three cruciate pulleys are located between the annular ones, but not usually between A1 and A2.
  - The cruciate pulleys are thin and flexible, therefore allowing flex-ion-extension of the semirigid fibro-osseous canal.
- In the thumb, there are three pulleys.
  - A1 is a strong annular pulley that arises from the volar plate of the first MCP joint.
    - The FPL tendon passes through the A1 pulley and between the two sesamoid bones that are within the volar plate.

- The oblique pulley originates like an extension of the adductor pollicis from the ulnar sesamoid and the base of the proximal phalanx.
  ○ It passes from proximal ulnar to distal radial as it inserts on the radial aspect of the proximal phalanx, proximal to the condylar flare.
  ○ Its attachment proximally blends with the fibers of the A1 pulley.
- The A2 pulley in the thumb arises from the interphalangeal joint volar plate.

Q8. How does a tendon receive its vascular supply?

The nutritional supply of the flexor tendons is bimodal. It is derived from both synovial diffusion and the intrinsic tendon vascularity.

- Synovial fluid enters through small openings on the tendon surface through capillary imbibition and the pumping effect of digital motion.
  - Synovial nutrition is important in the volar 50% of the tendon.
- Intrasynovial tendon vascularity arrives through longitudinal dorsal vessels originating in the palm, the proximal synovial fold, the vincular system from the paired digital arteries, and the bone insertions at the tendon ends.

- The FDS and FDP tendons typically receive both long and short vincula within the digital sheath (**Fig. 10.7**).
- Over the proximal phalanx, both the FDS and FDP are relatively avascular; the FDP also has a relatively avascular zone over the middle phalanx.
- These areas lie deep to the major pulleys and are subjected to the greatest compressive forces during flexion.

Q9. What are the zones of flexor tendons?

There are five zones of flexor tendons (**Fig. 10.8**):

Zone I: Distal to insertion of FDS.

Zone II: Extends proximally from FDS insertion to the proximal edge of A1 pulley.

Zone III: Between the distal edge of the transverse carpal ligament and the proximal edge of the fibro-osseous canal.

Zone IV: It lies deep to the transverse carpal ligament.

Zone V: It is proximal to carpal tunnel and includes the forearm tendons and corresponding muscle bellies.

Q10. Why is zone II called "no man's land"?

The term "no man's land" for zone II flexor tendon injury was coined by Bunnell in 1918. It was so called because it was once believed that primary repair should not be done in this zone

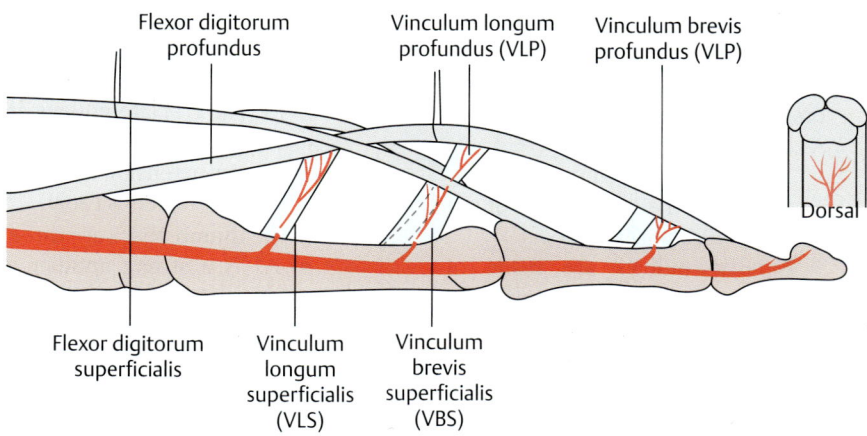

Fig. 10.7 Vincular system of flexor tendons.

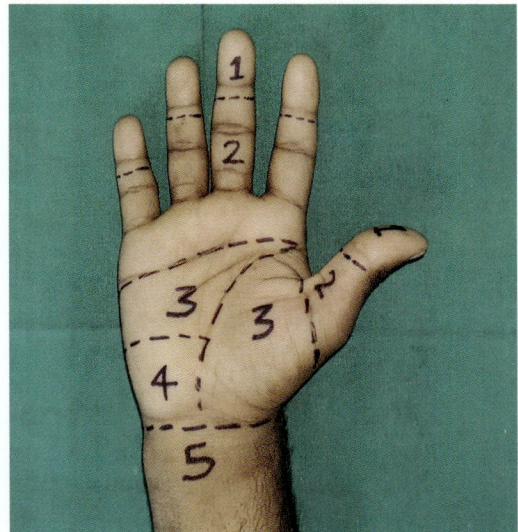

Fig. 10.8   Zones of flexor tendon.

due to constricting space of fibro-osseus tunnel which led to poor outcomes. This belief is no more there but the challenges of repair and good outcomes still exist.

Q11. What are the divisions of zone I injury and its importance?

- In zone I only FDP tendon is located.
- It is divided into:
  - Zone IA (most distal).
  - Zone IB.
  - Zone IC (most proximal).

Importance of the zones:

- When the tendon laceration is in the distal part of zone IA and IB, both the proximal and distal ends can be easily found because the vincula is connected to the proximal tendon to prevent retraction.
- When cut in zone IC, the tendon may retract more proximally.

Treatment:

- **Zone IA injuries:** The distal stump is very short.
  - The proximal tendon end can be sutured with Bunnell or modified Becker suture with 3–0 polypropylene, and an osteoperiosteal flap is raised at the base of the distal phalanx. An oblique drill-hole is made, suture is

passed through the hole and brought out through the nail, and tied over a button above the nail.

- Another method is to drill a transverse hole through the distal phalanx. After the tendon stump is sutured, the suture is led through the hole and tied to the other end, through an open approach or percutaneously.
- **Injuries in zones IB and IC:** Sufficient length of tendon stumps are present so that common end-to-end repair can be done.

Q12. What are the divisions of zone II injury and its importance?

- Zone II is divided into three parts:
  - Zone IIa—beneath A4 pulley.
  - Zone IIb—beneath C1 pulley.
  - Zone IIc—beneath A2 pulley.
- If both the FDS and the FDP are lacerated in zone II, both should be repaired.
- Tendon injuries in this area are often exposed through a Bruner skin incision and a window opening in the synovial sheath, a release, or local excision of a short part of the annular pulleys.

Q13. How will you manage zone III, IV, and V injuries?

Key aspects in zone III and V injuries:

- Zone III and V injuries are repaired by the same suture techniques as zone II.
- Both zones have a better prognosis because of the improved vascularity and lack of constricting space.
- In zone III injuries, the origin of the lumbrical should be preserved.
- Zone V injuries (spaghetti wrist) can be complicated by multiple tendon lacerations and major neurovascular injury. Myostatic contraction can occur early, and therefore zone V injuries should be repaired early within hours or days.

Key aspects in zone IV injuries:

- Zone IV injuries are often associated with median nerve and arterial injury.
- The transverse carpal ligament may need to be divided to allow tendon repair which

should be later repaired at the time of wrist closure.

Q14. How will you manage closed tendon injuries?

- Closed pulley ruptures are usually treated conservatively or may require surgical reconstruction.
- Leddy and Packer classified close tendon ruptures into following types:
  - **Type 1:**
    - Avulsion of FDP tendon from the phalanx and retraction into the palm.
    - The vincula of the FDP tendon are disrupted.
    - A tender mass is present in the palm.
    - The tendon should be reinserted within 7 to 10 days before the sheath collapses.
  - **Type 2:**
    - This is the most common type.
    - FDP tendon retracts to the level of the PIP joint.
    - The sheath is not compromised, and muscle contracture does not develop easily.
    - Repair may be attempted 1 month after injury.
  - **Type 3:**
    - A large bone fragment is attached to the FDP tendon.
    - This bone fragment frequently prevents the tendon from retraction proximal to the A4 pulley.
    - Bony fixation using a K-wire or a screw usually suffices.
  - **Type 4:**
    - The FDP tendon avulses from the bony fragment.
    - The avulsed tendon retracts beyond the middle phalanx and even into the palm.
    - In treating such injuries, the bony fragment is attached into the distal phalanx first, then the avulsed tendon is advanced.

Q15. What will you do in case of partial tendon laceration?

- **Laceration <60% of the diameter of the tendon:**
  - It does not require repair by core sutures.
  - The cut portion of the tendon can be repaired with epitendinous stitches to smoothen the tendon surface and to strengthen the tendon.
- **Laceration of 60 to 80%:** It requires at least an epitendinous repair and is better repaired using a two-strand core suture through the cut portion.
- **Laceration of 80 to 90%:** It is treated as a complete laceration.

Q16. What are the contraindications of primary repair of tendons?

Following are the contraindications:
- Severe contamination of the wound.
- Loss of soft tissue coverage.

Q17. What are the various incisions for flexor tendon surgery?

- The finger's position when the tendon was lacerated will determine the position of the cut ends.
  - If the finger is injured in flexion, the tendon ends will retract distally when the finger is extended in the operating room. Thus, more distal exposure will be required.
  - If the finger is injured in extension, the distal tendon ends will not retract distally and the level of injury will correspond to the skin laceration.
- Incisions should be planned to retrieve the cut ends, to maintain vascularity to the skin flaps, to address other injuries and to avoid crossing flexion creases at angles greater than 45 degrees to prevent unsightly and contracted scars. The commonly used are: zigzag (Brunner) or midaxial incisions and midlateral incisions (**Fig. 10.9**).

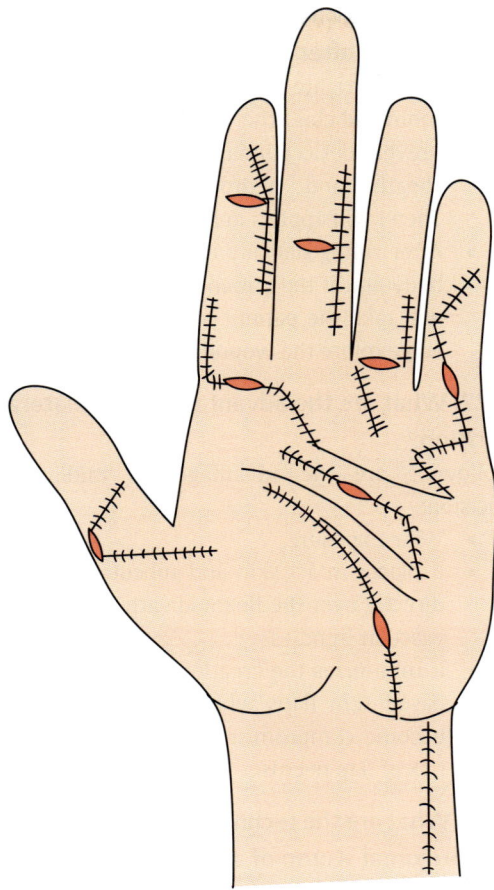

Fig. 10.9 Incisions for flexor tendon surgery.

Q18. What are the suture techniques used for flexor tendon repair?

- The most common technique used is modified Kessler technique for core suture (**Fig. 10.10**).
- The core suture is usually a 3–0 or 4–0 nonabsorbable monofilament or braided polyester used in conjunction with an epitendinous 5–0 or 6–0 nonabsorbable monofilament.

Q19. What suture material should be used for tendon repair?

- Core suture is usually a 3–0 or 4–0 nonabsorbable monofilament.
- Prolene is most commonly used.
- If we consider suture strength, knot holding ability, stretch, and tissue reactivity then stainless-steel sutures are ideal, but stainless steel is difficult to work with and can disturb the flexor tendon.

Q20. What are the advantages and disadvantages of Prolene suture?

Advantages:
- High tensile strength.
- Low tissue reactivity.
- High infection resistance.

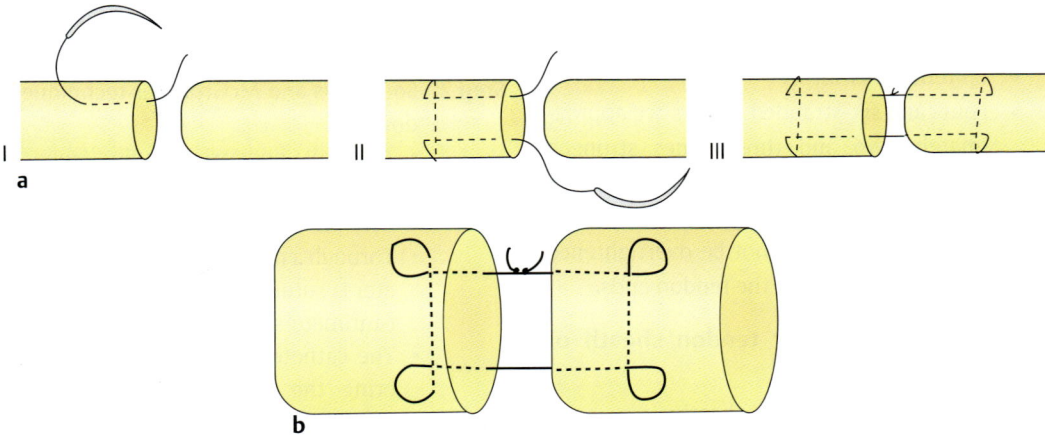

Fig. 10.10 (**a, b**) Modified Kessler technique.

- Low coefficient of friction.
- High plasticity.

Disadvantages:
- Poor knot security.
- Low elasticity.
- Expensive.

Q21. Where should the core sutures be placed?

Core sutures should be placed volarly to protect the dorsal intrinsic tendon vascularity.

Q22. What is the purpose of epitendinous suture?

- Epitendinous sutures smoothen out the final repair.
- Increase the repair strength by 10 to 50%.
- Prevent gapping.

Q23. When does the strength of tendons return?

The weakest point occurs 4 to 5 days after the repair. After 19 days, the strength of the repair increases directly proportional to the stress applied.

Q24. How are tendon repair techniques classified?

- Core suture
  - Two strand
  - Four strand
  - Six strand
- Epitendinous suture
- Four- and six-stranded repairs are approximately two and three times stronger, respectively, than two-stranded flexor tendon repairs.
- Core sutures should not be overtightened to avoid bunching of the tendon ends.

Q25. Should we repair tendon sheath or not?

Yes, we should repair tendon sheath:
- To limit adhesion formation.
- To facilitate synovial nutrition.
- To help remodel the tendon repair site.
- To improve tendon sheath biomechanics.

Q26. How will you manage the case immediately after the injury?

- I will irrigate the wound in emergency room and close the wound loosely so as to prevent desiccation of underlying tendons, sheath, and neurovascular structures. Then I will apply a dorsal splint.
- After ruling out any other injuries to the body and if the patient is fit for surgery, I will take the patient to operation theater and explore the wound.

Q27. What are the advantages of midlateral incision?

Following are the advantages of midlateral incision:
- Wide exposure.
- It places intact skin and subcutaneous fat directly over the flexor sheath and neurovascular bundles.
- It minimizes the creation of small distally based skin flaps whose perfusion might become compromised and be at a higher risk of flap necrosis.

Q28. What are the techniques for identifying the proximal stump of a tendon?

Step 1: Flex the wrist and fingers: Distal milking of the tendon stump is done along its course.

If not

Step 2: Sourmelis and McGrouther technique is done:
- A small pediatric feeding tube is passed from the wound into the palm beneath the annular pulley system.
- Through a mid-palm incision, the catheter is sutured to both tendons several centimeters proximal to A1 pulley.
- The catheter is pulled distally, delivering the tendon stumps into the distal repair site.

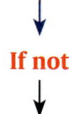

If not

Step 3: Extend the incision: An incision is made just distal to the transverse carpal ligament to isolate the tendon stump.

Q29. Which tendon is repaired first: FDS or FDP?

FDS tendon is repaired first because of the following benefits:

- It will protect the vinculum longum to FDP.
- It will provide a gliding interface between the FDP and underlying bone.
- It will improve grip strength.

Q30. What are the mechanisms of healing after tendon repair?

Tendon healing repair:

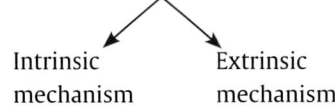

Intrinsic   Extrinsic
mechanism   mechanism

- **Intrinsic healing:** Occurs through tenocytes of the epitenon and endotenon, nourished by the intratendinous blood supply and by synovial diffusion.
- **Extrinsic healing:** Divided into three phases:
  - Inflammation: 48 to 72 hours.
  - Proliferation: 5 days to 4 weeks.
  - Remodeling.

Q31. What are the factors influencing the strength of tendon repair surgery?

Following are the factors which affect the strength of a surgical repair.

- **Number of suture strands across the repair sites:** Strength is roughly proportional to the number of core sutures.
- **Tension of repairs:** Slight tension in the core sutures is necessary to resist gapping at the repair site.
- **Types of tendon suture junction:** A locking tendon suture junction is generally better than a grasping junction in terms of holding power.
- **Diameter of suture locks in the tendons:** Diameter of the suture locks must reach or exceed 2 mm.

- **Suture caliber (diameter):** Improved repair strength by increasing suture calibers. Clinically, the caliber of suture used in adults is either 3–0 or 4–0.
- The material properties of suture materials.
- **Peripheral sutures:** Peripheral sutures serve to "tidy up" the approximated tendon stumps.
- **Curvature of tendon gliding paths:** The repair strength decreases as tendon curvature increases. Surgical repair in a tendon under a curvilinear load is weaker than that under a linear load; the repair strength decreases as the curvature increases.
- Holding capacity of a tendon, affected by varying degrees of trauma and posttraumatic tissue softening, plays a vital role in repair strength.

Q32. Which zone has most favorable results?

Zone III has most favorable results as it is least rigid zone; therefore, repair is easy.

Q33. How do you check whether tendon repair is gliding under the pulley?

After tendon repair, it is checked by passive digital flexion and extension. Failure to evaluate tendon glide after repair may lead to substantially decreased digital range of motion.

Q34. What is the postoperative position of the hand?

A protective splint is applied to immobilize fingers with wrist in 20 degrees of flexion, MCP joints flexed to 70 degrees, and the interphalangeal joints in relative extension.

Q35. Why the FDP tendon wound not retract proximally?

Because it is attached to lumbricals.

Q36. What is the role of MRI in tendon injury?

MRI can distinguish postoperative adhesions from ruptures with 100% accuracy, whereas clinical examination is only 60% accurate. MRI will localize retracted tendon ends. It may also be useful for the diagnosis of partial tendon lacerations and the differentiation of isolated adhesion from elongated callus.

Q37. What is the postoperative rehabilitation after flexor tendon injury?

There are several protocols but the commonly followed is:

Kleinert (**Fig. 10.11**): Wrist is placed in palmar flexion of 30 to 40 degrees and MCP joint in 60 to 70 degrees of flexion with a dorsal protective splint. It uses active extension with passive flexion by a dorsal extension blocking splint with rubber bands running from the fingernails to the volar wrist or forearm. The rubber bands keep the patient from flexing the digits against resistance.

- After 3 to 4 weeks dorsal splint is removed, but rubber bands are maintained and attached to a volar wrist cuff.
- Wrist range of motion exercises are started and finger exercise continued.
- Gentle active flexion started around 4 weeks.
- At 6 weeks place and hold exercises as well as blocking exercises are commenced.
- Passive extension initiated at 8 weeks.

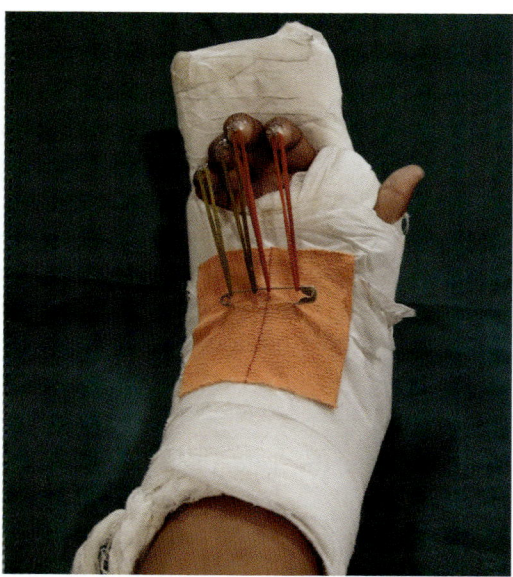

Fig. 10.11 Application of Kleinert.

Disadvantage: It causes flexion contracture of the fingers.

Q38. Why all fingers are kept in rubber band traction?

All fingers should be placed in rubber band traction.

- To ensure added FDP protection.
- To promote better tendon excursion.
- To decrease the risk of PIP contracture.

Q39. How to assess the outcomes after surgery?

There are several criteria:

- Strickland and Glogovac criteria are the most commonly used methods.
- The Moiemen and Elliot criteria are specifically used in cases of zone I repair to evaluate the active range of flexion of the DIP joint.
- The total active range of motion (TAM).
- Buck-Gramcko method.

Q40. What are the complications of tendon repair?

Early complications:

- Infections.
- Wound healing problems.
- Tendon rupture or pulley rupture.
- Poor tendon glide in the sheath.

Late complications:

- Tendon rupture.
- Tendon adhesions.
- Joint contracture.
- Pulley dysfunction with resultant bowstringing.

Q41. What is Quadriga phenomenon?

Quadriga phenomenon manifests as a decrease in flexion of an adjacent normal finger due to shortened FDP in the affected finger because of the common muscle belly of small, ring, and middle finger slips of FDP. "**Quadriga**" refers to a Roman chariot with four horses driven through a common rein by the driver. If the rein to one horse is shortened, then the others horses will also have a shortened rein experience.

Causes:
- Too distal advancement of one FDP during repair in zone I.
- Too short tendon graft.
- FDP sutured to the extensor tendon in a distal finger amputation.
- FDP adheres to the proximal phalanx in an amputation.

Treatment:
- Release of adhered FDP in injured digit.
- Lengthening of the tendon.
- Tenolysis.

Q42. What is lumbrical plus finger?
- If the tendon graft is too long then a lumbrical plus finger may occur.
- If the graft is too long, excessive traction is exerted on the lumbricals muscle which is pulled proximally.
- This will paradoxically lead to extension at the interphalangeal joints and finger will stick out while attempting to hold an object.
- This problem can be avoided by ensuring proper length at the time of placement of the graft.

Q43. What are the indications of secondary tendon reconstruction?
Following are the indications:
- Tendon injuries not treated within 1 month after injury.
- Rupture of the tendon repairs at primary or delayed primary stages.
- Tendon injuries not indicated for primary repair.
- Badly scarred digits.

Q44. What should be the criteria for secondary tendon reconstruction?
- Supple passive motion of the hand.
- Good soft tissue condition.
- Sufficient time after initial tendon injury: at least 3 months.

Q45. What are the contraindications for secondary tendon reconstruction?
- Limited joint motion.
- Presence of soft tissue wounds or defects and fractures which are not well-healed.

Q46. What are the indications of free tendon grafting?
Tendon grafting is indicated in following cases:
- When the lacerated tendons are not treated during primary or delayed primary stage.
- When the primary repairs have ruptured and cannot be re-repaired directly.
- In cases with severe contamination, infection, lengthy loss of tendon substance, extensive destruction of the pulleys, or accompanying injuries.

Q47. What is the indication of staged tendon reconstruction?
- Patients who have serious scarring in the tendon bed.
- Failed previous efforts at secondary flexor tendon procedures.

Q48. What is the ideal timing of tendon grafting?
Three months after injury.

Q49. What are the donor sites for tendon graft?
The donor sites are:
- Palmaris longus tendon (15 cm).
- Plantaris tendon (25 cm).
- Long-toe extensor.
- Toe flexor.

Q50. What incision is used for tendon grafting?
Volar Bruner's incision or the midaxial approach.

Q51. What are the stages of tendon reconstruction?
Stage 1 (Fig. 10.12a–c):
- All scar from the tendon bed is excised through a volar zigzag incision which is continued to the lumbrical origin in palm.
- The scarred tendon is excised with a 1-cm stump of the profundus tendon retained at its distal insertion.

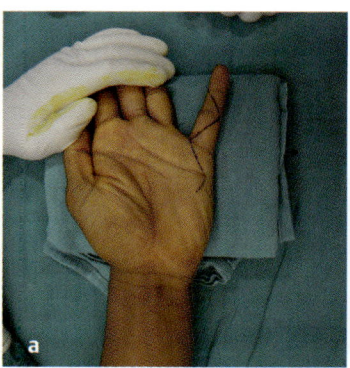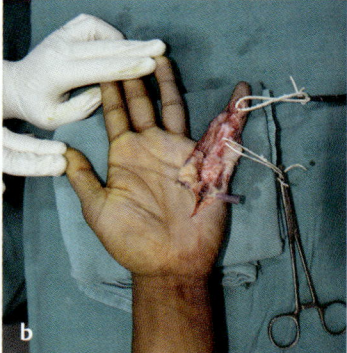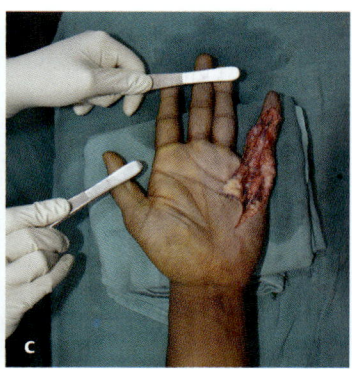

Fig. 10.12 (a–c) Steps in Stage 1 of tendon reconstruction—volar zigzag incision, reconstruction of pulleys, and placement of silicon tendon implant.

- A2 and A4 pulleys should be reconstructed.
- A tunnel is maintained by inserting a Dacron-reinforced silicone tendon implant which helps to stimulate the formation of a mesothelium-lined pseudosheath.

Stage 2:
- It is done after 3 months through small incision adjacent to the distal implant–tendon junction.
- The implant is disconnected from the tendon and a free tendon graft is harvested and inserted into the pseudosheath tunnel.
- Care is taken not to open the pseudosheath proximal to the DIP joint and to avoid injury to any pulleys.

Q52. What are the indications of tenolysis?

Indications of tenolysis are:
- It is indicated when the passive range of digital motion greatly exceeds the range of active flexion several months after direct end-to-end tendon repair or tendon grafting.
  - This can be expected when there has been severe damage to the peritendinous tissues or compound injuries (such as digital or palm replantation). Adhesion formation is more common in these cases.

Q53. What are the prerequisites of tenolysis?

The prerequisites are:
- All fractures should be healed.
- Skin and subcutaneous tissues should be soft and pliable and there should be minimal reactions around the incision scars.
- There should be no joint contractures and a near-normal passive range of digital motion has been achieved.

Q54. What is the optimal time of tenolysis?

A waiting period of minimum 3 months must be there to allow necessary healing and revascularization of tendons, so as to avoid endangering tendon strength. At 4 to 6 months, patient's final function can be assessed reliably.

Suggested Readings

1. Tang JB. Flexor tendon injuries and reconstruction. In: Chang J, Neligan PC, eds. Plastic surgery: hand and upper extremity. Vol. 6. 4th ed. Canada: Elsevier; 2018:188–226
2. Williamson DG. Flexor tendon injuries and reconstruction. In: Mathes SJ, Hentz VR, eds. Plastic surgery: the hand and upper limb. Part 1. Vol. 7. 2nd ed. Saunders Elsevier; 2006:358–416

11 Extensor Tendon Injuries
Veena K. Singh

Learning Objectives

At the end of this chapter, the students will be able to:
1. Recall the anatomy of extensor mechanism of the hand and fingers.
2. Describe the clinical presentation of a patient with extensor tendon injury.
3. Demonstrate the examination of extensor tendon injury.
4. Understand how to decide on a particular procedure according to the timeline.
5. Perform the steps of extensor tendon repair.

Introduction

Extensor tendon injury is commonly associated with fracture, skin avulsion, joint or nerve injury, which easily disrupts the delicate balance between the static and dynamic forces acting on extensor mechanism. The superficial location of the tendons and easy access deceives into difficult surgical management and poor outcomes. There should be clear understanding of the anatomy, dynamic functionality, repair techniques, and appropriate rehabilitation protocol.

History

Particulars of the patient (name, age, sex, occupation, residence, etc.) and hand dominance.

Chief Complaints

- Inability to straighten the fingers (one or more fingers).
- Weakness in straightening the fingers.
- Presence of a scar or deformity of the fingers.

History of Present Illness

- Ask about the duration of injury—whether acute or chronic injury, days or months back.
- Exact details of the trauma—whether traumatic or iatrogenic, self-inflicted or assault.
- Type of injury (sharp, blunt, avulsion, crush).
- Any associated fracture or injuries anywhere else in the body.
- Details of any associated bleeding.
- First aid received and any surgical intervention for fractures, bleeding, or any attempt at tendon repair.
- Details of splintage, if any.
- Details of physiotherapy.
- Any history suggestive of loss or decreased sensation.
- Pain, if any, and its details.
- What day-to-day functionality of the hand is lost due to the injury and what are the daily works which the patient is unable to do at present but could perform earlier.

Past History

History of diabetes mellitus, hypertension, and tuberculosis, and any past surgical intervention.

Personal History

History of smoking and alcohol or any other addiction.

Family History

The details as in other cases including the dependency of the family members on the patient if he is the only breadwinner for them.

History of Allergy

Allergy to any food or medication.

Examination

General Examination

Same as for other cases.

Local Examination of Hand

Exposure

Proper exposure of both the hands and forearm up to the elbow should be done in adequate light and with proper explained informed consent.

Inspection

- Inspection should be done of outstretched hands with palm facing upward and rested on the top of a table.
  - Attitude: Look for the posture of hand in a resting position. Always compare with the normal.
    - The normal resting posture of the hand is that the palm forms a hollow and the fingers are in flexed position with the thumb in slight abduction and opposition.
    - In extensor tendon injury, this resting posture of a normal hand is lost and the injured fingers will lie in more flexed posture.
    - Ask the patient to turn round his hand with palm facing downward and ask him to stretch the fingers. The affected finger/s will not be able to straighten as the other fingers (**Fig. 11.1**).
  - Site of injury: Look carefully to locate the site of injury and the presence of scar.
  - Details of the scar in terms of site, size, color, thickness.
  - Look for any obvious deviation of the fingers to rule out any associated fracture.
  - Atrophy: Look carefully at the forearm and identify any wasting if present. Always compare with the normal limb.

Palpation

- Temperature: Any local rise due to infection.
- Tenderness: Near the scar and in the adjacent area.
- All inspection findings must be corroborated.

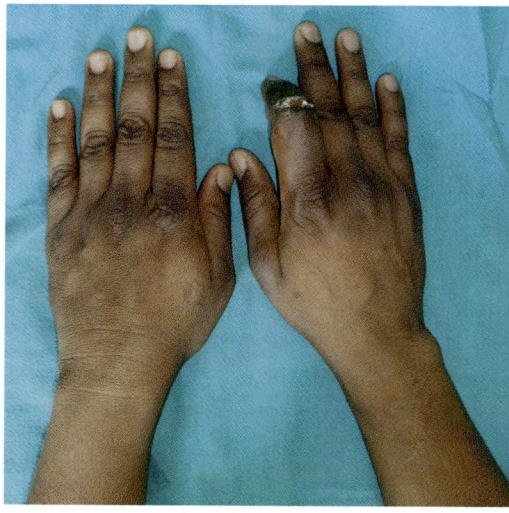

Fig. 11.1 Attitude of fingers.

- Examine using static two-point discrimination test separately for radial and ulnar digital nerves.

Movements

- Extension:
  - Wrist joint
  - Metacarpophalangeal (MCP) joint
  - Proximal interphalangeal (PIP) joint
  - Distal interphalangeal (DIP) joint

  Active and passive range of movement (and against resistance also) in terms of present or restricted

- Range of movement (ROM) at each joint in terms of degrees.

X-ray hand—anteroposterior (AP) and oblique views—if available, must be seen to rule out any associated fracture.

Provisional Diagnosis

A case of 4 weeks old Zone VI extensor tendon injury of the left hand without any associated fracture or neurovascular injury.

Questions

Q1. How will you proceed?
The plan is to explore and repair for which we will have to get some investigations done:

- First of all, an X-ray of the affected hand will be done to rule out bony injuries.

- Preferred X-ray views to be advised:
  - Hand: Anteroposterior (AP) and oblique views.
  - Finger: AP and lateral views.
- Hemoglobin, complete blood count, prothrombin time/international normalized ratio (PT/INR).
- Serum electrolytes.
- Blood urea, serum creatinine.
- Viral markers (human immunodeficiency virus [HIV] 1 & 2, hepatitis B virus surface antigen [HBsAg], hepatitis C virus [HCV]).

Q2. How will you demonstrate the extension of fingers at MCP joints?
- Ask the patient to flex the MCP joints of all fingers with wrist in neutral position.
- Observe from the sides of the fingers and ask the patient to extend the MCP joints (**Fig. 11.2**).
- Ask him to hyperextend (straighten) the fingers.

To test the extension at an individual finger:
- Ask the patient to keep their hand on a table top with palm facing downward.
- Extensor tendon of each finger must be checked individually by asking the patient to hyperextend the fingers against resistance (**Fig. 11.3a, b**).
- Extension of index finger and little finger must be tested separately by asking to hyperextend the index/little finger while blocking the other fingers. This checks

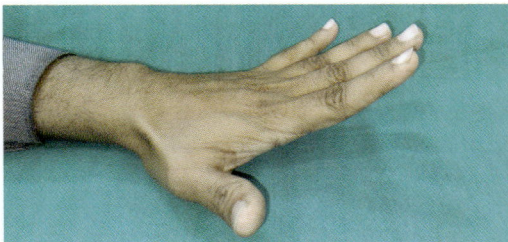

Fig. 11.2 Examination of extension at metacarpophalangeal (MCP) joint.

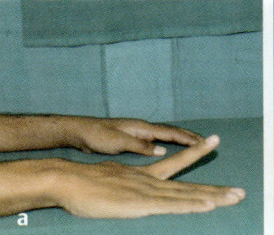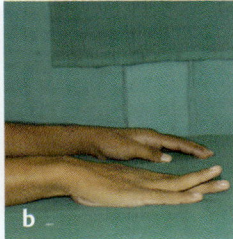

Fig. 11.3 **(a, b)** Examination of extension at metacarpophalangeal (MCP) joint of individual finger.

the action of extensor indicis proprius (EIP) and extensor digiti minimi (EDM) by blocking the action of extensor digitorum communis (EDC) (**Fig. 11.4a, b**).

- Extensor pollicis longus (EPL): Place the hand on the table and hold the distal phalanx of the thumb to keep the IP joint in flexed position. Ask the patient to extend his thumb while continuing force application to maintain the flexion at IP joint. (Refer to the Chapter 9 on "Radial nerve palsy.")

Q3. How will you classify the extensor tendon injuries?

The extensor tendon injuries are classified into nine zones based on the unique anatomic features and mechanical properties of each zone (**Fig. 11.5**):

- The rationale for such classification is based on its clinical importance and the surgical outcomes.
- Kleinert and Verdan proposed eight zones and ninth was added by Doyle (**Table 11.1**).

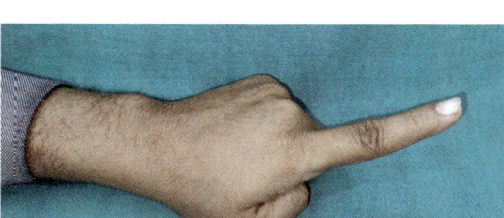
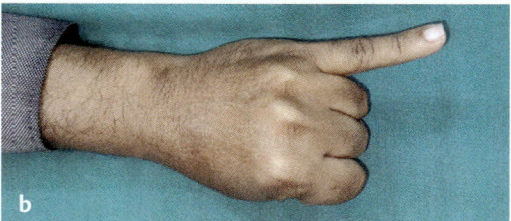

Fig. 11.4 (a, b) Examination of extensor indicis proprius (EIP) and extensor digiti minimi (EDM).

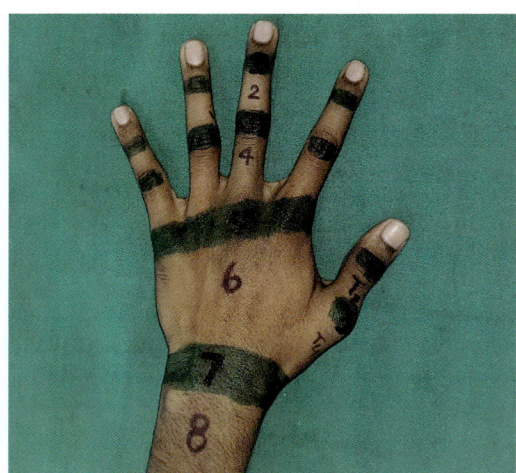

Fig. 11.5 Markings of zones of extensor tendon injury.

Table 11.1   Proposed nine zones

Zone	Areas (in fingers)	Thumb
I	DIP joint	IP joint
II	Middle phalanx	Proximal phalanx
III	PIP joint	MCP joint
IV	Proximal phalanx	Metacarpal
V	MCP joint	CMC joint
VI	Metacarpal	———
VII	Dorsal retinaculum	Dorsal retinaculum
VIII	Distal forearm	Distal forearm
IX	Proximal forearm	Proximal forearm

Abbreviations: CMC, carpometacarpal; DIP, distal interphalangeal; IP, interphalangeal; MCP, metacarpophalangeal; PIP, proximal interphalangeal.

Q4. What incisions will you place to expose the injured tendon?

- Longitudinal incisions are given over the dorsum of fingers as the skin is loose and less glabrous (**Fig. 11.6**).
- Advantages of a longitudinal incision is that it protects the venous and the lymphatic drainage and gives a wide exposure to the whole extensor mechanism.
- Lazy **"S"-** or **"C"**-shaped incisions avoiding the crossing of extension creases are also used.

Q5. How will you identify the tendons and what is their arrangement?

- At the wrist, muscle fascia of extensor tendons fuses together to form extensor retinaculum.
- Vertical septa divide the space under the extensor retinaculum into six compartments (**Fig. 11.7**):
  - First compartment contains:
    - Abductor pollicis longus (APL)—Inserts into thenar muscles fascia and base of thumb.

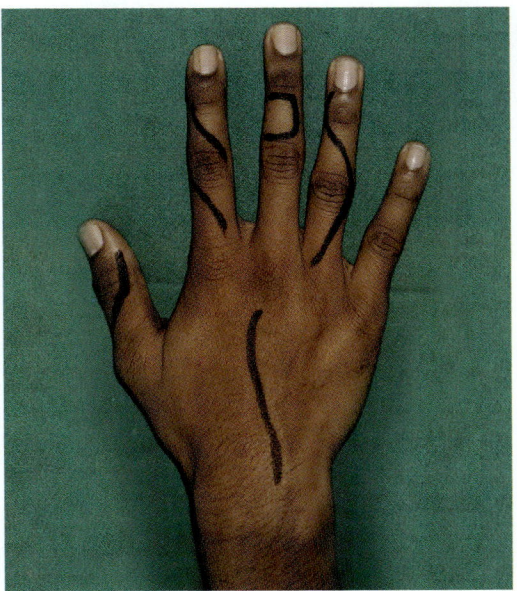

Fig. 11.6 Incision marking for exposing the extensor tendons.

- Extensor pollicis brevis (EPB): Fuses with extensor hood over MCP joint and inserts at base of proximal phalanx of thumb.
  - **Second** compartment contains:
    - Extensor carpi radialis longus (ECRL): Inserts on the radial aspect of metacarpal of index finger. It is a radial deviator of wrist in extension.
    - Extensor carpi radialis brevis (ECRB): Inserts on the base of metacarpal of middle finger. It brings extension of wrist in central axis.
  - **Third** compartment contains:
    - EPL: Passes over the Lister's tubercle, ulnar to EPB at MCP joint and becomes a flat tendon to continue toward its insertion at the base of thumb distal phalanx.
  - **Fourth** compartment contains:
    - EIP: Fuses with extensor hood over MCP joint and passes ulnar to the EDC tendon of index finger.
    - EDC
  - **Fifth** compartment contains:
    - EDM: Tendon with independent extensor action.

Note: Both EIP and EDM lie ulnar to EDC slip.
  - **Sixth** compartment contains:
    - ECU: Inserts on the ulnar aspect of the metacarpal of little finger.
      - Brings ulnar deviation of the wrist in extension.
      - Gets paralyzed in posterior interosseous nerve (PIN) palsy.
- Importance of the extensor retinaculum: It prevents the:
  - Dorsal bowstringing of extensor tendons when wrist is extended.
  - Volar bowstringing of tendons in the first compartment when wrist is flexed.
  - Volar forearm in pronation.

Note: Bowstringing shortens the tendon path which relatively lengthens the muscle tendon unit which then becomes less efficient in applying power to a joint distal to it.

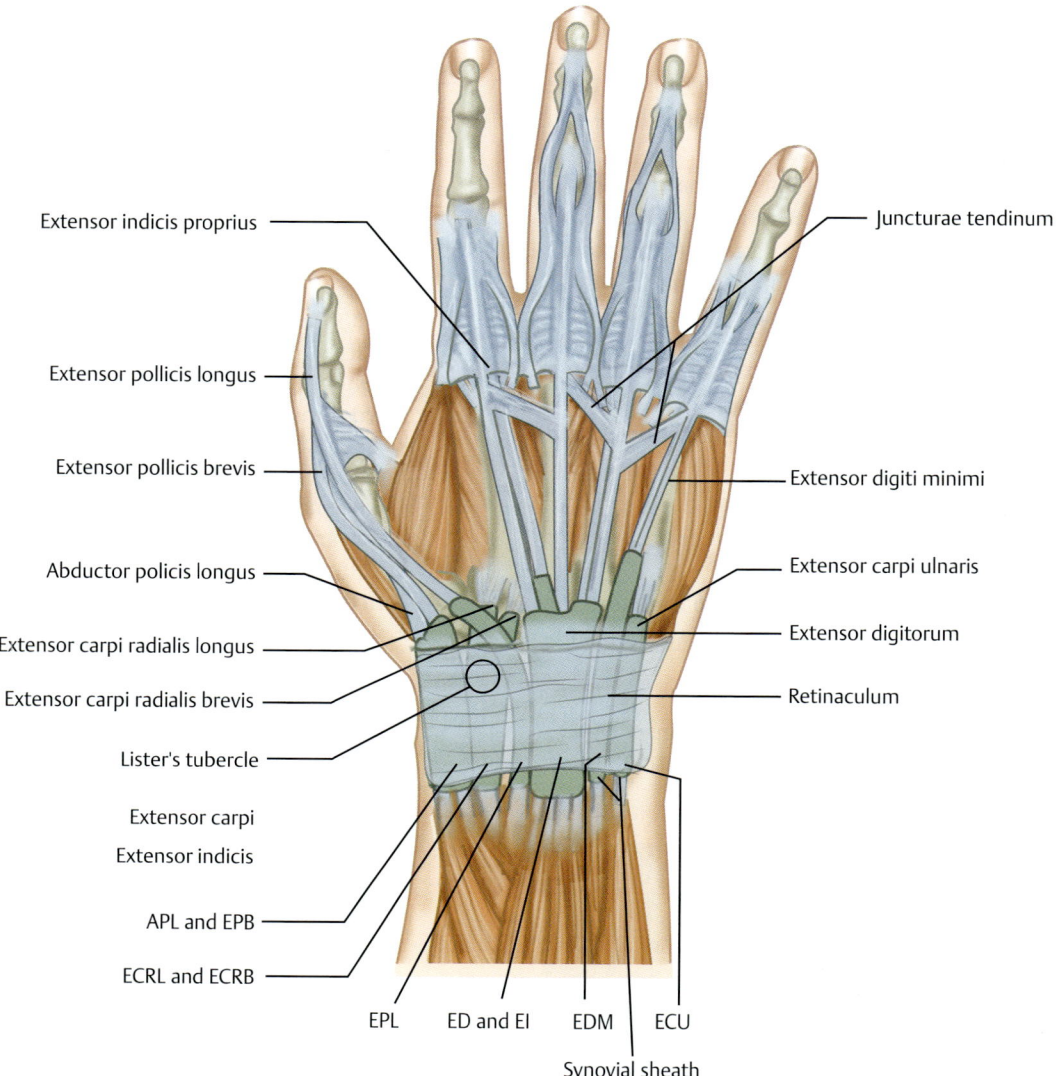

Fig. 11.7 Extensor compartments.

Q6. What is Landsmeer ligament?

Landsmeer ligament is the other name of oblique retinacular ligament (ORL).

- It connects the proximal phalanx to the distal phalanx.
  - It passes volar to the proximal phalanx and dorsal to the distal phalanx.
  - It originates from proximal phalanx and inserts on to the base of the distal phalanx (**Fig. 11.8**).
- It is a ligament, and hence, no contractile property is there.

- Its function is related to the PIP joint extension and its tenodesis effect.
  - When PIP is in flexion, ORL is relaxed.
  - When PIP is in extension, it tightens and extends the DIP joint.
  - Test to check the effect of tenodesis effect of PIP joint extension on ORL— **by doing passive flexion of DIP joint when:**
    - PIP joint is in flexion (DIP joint can be flexed easily).
    - PIP joint is in extension (DIP joint can't be flexed).

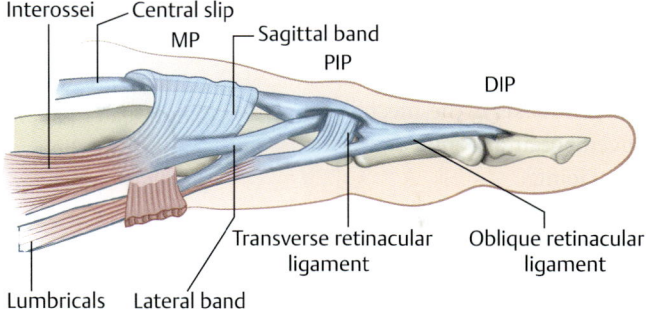

Fig. 11.8 Anatomy of Landsmeer ligament.

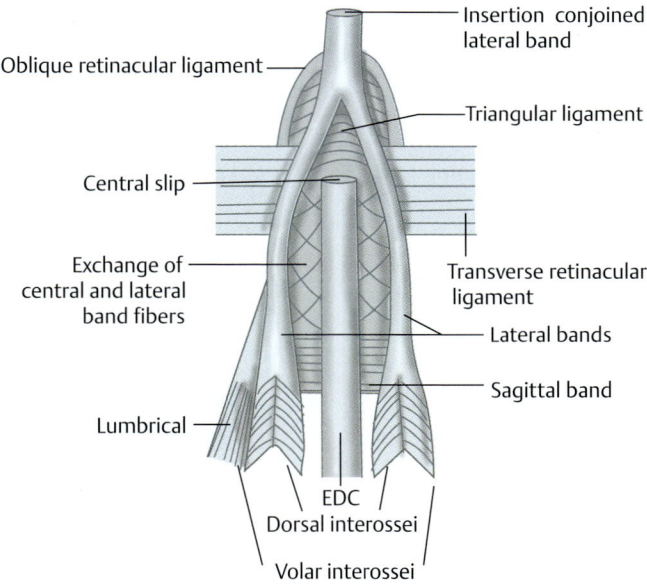

Fig. 11.9 Anatomy of extensor expansion.

Q7. How does the extensor mechanism work?

Anatomy of extensor mechanism:

- When all the long extensors reach the MCP joint they flatten to form the dorsal hood and envelop the dorsum of proximal and middle phalanges (**Fig. 11.9**).

  ↓

- The central slip of extensor tendon is stabilized over the head of metacarpals by **sagittal bands**. The central slip inserts into the base of the middle phalanx and brings PIP joint extension.

  ↓

- The two lateral bands are the tendinous continuity of interossei and lumbrical which inserts into the base of distal phalanx as **conjoined lateral bands**.

  ↓

- The lateral bands are connected to the central slip by **triangular ligaments** which prevent the volar displacement of the lateral bands.

Functionality of extensor mechanism: The dynamic tenodesis effect along with the muscle power is responsible for the extension at fingers. **Dynamic tenodesis** is the mechanism by which movement at one joint transmits power to a distal joint.

- Sequential events in extension of fingers:

Flexion at wrist leads to relaxation of flexor tendons and tightening of extensor tendons

↓

Both lead to extension of the MCP joints

↓

This tightens the intrinsic tendons

↓

Leading to extension of PIP joint

↓

This tightens the lateral bands and oblique retinacular ligament (ORL)

↓

Leading to extension of DIP joint

- The long extrinsic are the prime extensor at MCP joint. They also extend the IP joint when hyperextension at MCP joint is prevented which is brought by intrinsic.
- The intrinsic muscles contribute to IP joint extension by following mechanisms:
  - The intrinsic muscles of the hand bring flexion at MCP joint and prevent hyperextension. This allows the extrinsic to exert extension force at IP joints.
  - The intrinsic muscles also exert active extension at IP joints through the lateral bands. The intrinsic muscles playing a role in IP joint extension are interossei, lumbricals, thenar, and hypothenar muscles. The interossei, abductor pollicis brevis (APB), and adductor pollicis have two insertions: first, at the base of proximal phalanx which leads to

flexion at MCP joints and also abduction and adduction movement of the fingers. A second insertion in the lateral bands lead to IP joint extension.

- Lumbricals help in IP extension by a third mechanism—because of its origin from the radial side of the flexor digitorum profundus (FDP) tendon, its contraction will pull the FDP tendon distally which relaxes the antagonist to extension.

Q8. What are the suturing techniques for injured extensors tendons?

Suturing techniques of injured tendons depend on the zone of injury:

- In Zone I to V, distal to the MCP joints, the extensor tendon is wide and flat whereas it is narrow and thick in Zone VI to VIII.
- There are two main suturing techniques:
  - Core-grasping suture (**Fig. 11.10**).
  - Cross-stitch suture (**Fig. 11.11**).
- Suturing options by zone:

Zone	Suture technique	Suture material
I and II	Splint only	None
	Skin with tendon	5–0 monofilament
	Tendon suture	6–0 monofilament
	Pull-out tendon	4–0 monofilament
III–IV and V	Grasping tendon suture	4–0 braided
	± Simple or cross stitch	6–0 monofilament
VI, VII, VIII	Grasping core tendon with epitenon	4–0 braided
	Multiple slips to same digit sutured together	4–0 braided

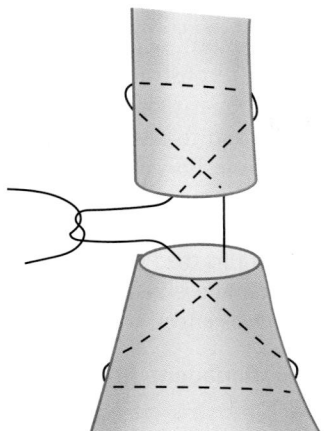

Fig. 11.10 Techniques of extensor tendon repair: core-grasping suture.

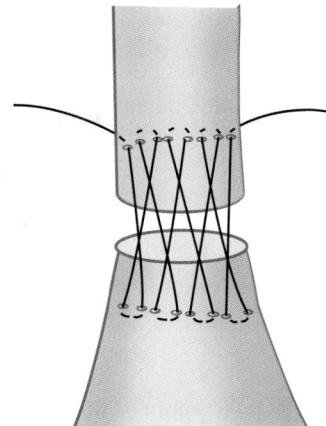

Fig. 11.11 Techniques of extensor tendon repair: cross-stitch suture.

Q9. What is the management of injury in Zone I?

Features of Zone I injuries (DIP level):

- Injury in Zone I results in loss of extension at DIP joint.
- Also known as mallet finger, baseball finger, dropped finger, or extension lag.
- The mechanism of injury usually involves a sudden flexion force on the straight/extended DIP joint.
- Always get an X-ray done to rule out the avulsion fracture at dorsal base of distal phalanx.

Treatment:

- Acute mallet injury: Closed injuries:
  - Conservative management with immobilization of DIP joint using a splint for 6 weeks.
  - Static splintage may be extended to 8 weeks treatment.
  - Indications for surgery:
    - Open injuries.
    - Closed injuries in a person unable to work with a splint.
    - A large dorsal fracture fragment with palmar subluxation of distal phalanx.
  - Surgical options may be:
    - Suturing the skin alone and providing an extension splint.
    - Pull-out suture with K-wire inserted through DIP joint to keep it in extension. Sutures and K-wire can be removed after 3 weeks followed by splintage for 6 to 8 weeks.
- Chronic mallet injury:
  - Requires no treatment: Up to 30 degrees of extension lag at DIP joint is acceptable as far as functional disability is concerned.
  - If severe functional disability, then it requires surgical intervention.
    - The injured part of tendon is explored and sutured after advancement of 2 to 3 mm.
    - A K-wire is inserted for DIP joint immobilization which is removed after 3 weeks followed by a static splint application.
  - Joint fusion: It is done when DIP joint is painful and arthritic with fixed deformity.
- Swan-neck deformity (**Fig. 11.12**):
  - Can be a result of mallet injury. It is the characteristic appearance of the finger with hyperextension at PIP joint and flexion at DIP joint.

– Pathophysiology of swan-neck deformity:

Injury to extensor tendon insertion on distal phalanx

↓

Disruption in extension of DIP joint

↓

Concentration of extensor forces at PIP joint causing persistent PIP extension

↓

Volar plate at PIP joint becomes lax

↓

Swan-neck deformity occurs as PIP joint goes into hyperextension

↓

At a critical point of hyperextension at PIP joint, it does not flex anymore

↓

Dorsal displacement of lateral bands occur

↓

When patient tries to flex the PIP joint, the DIP joint flexes initially, tightening the lateral bands which further hyperextend the PIP joint

↓

Gradually, the flexors exceed the extension pull which snaps the PIP joint into flexion causing a "snapping PIP joint"

– Treatment of swan-neck deformity:
  - Reconstruction of ORL: Littler's spiral ORL reconstruction:
    ○ Uses palmaris longus (PL) graft.
    ○ PL is fixed to distal phalanx and goes from dorsal to volar aspect spiraling around proximal phalanx where it is fixed.
    ○ It restrains the PIP joint hyperextension and extends DIP joint by tenodesis effect.

Q10. What is the management of injury in Zone II?

- In this zone, there are lateral bands and each one of them can extend the DIP joint.
  – Lacerations <50% of tendon: Skin closure only.
  – Lacerations >50% of tendon: Repair to be done.
    - In case of tendon gap, a graft might be required.
    - Only 2 to 3 mm of tendon excursion required for DIP joint flexion at middle phalanx level.

Q11. What is the management of injury in Zone III?

Features of Zone III injuries:

- In this zone, central tendon inserts on the base of middle phalanx.
- This zone is unique as it is the zone of central tendon and lateral bands.
- Boutonniere deformity (flexion at PIP joint and hyperextension at DIP joint) is encountered in zone III injuries (**Fig. 11.13**).

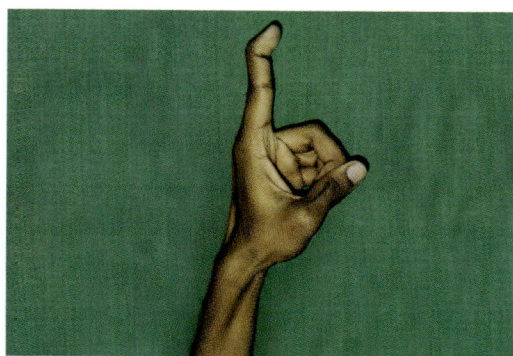

Fig. 11.12 Swan-neck deformity.

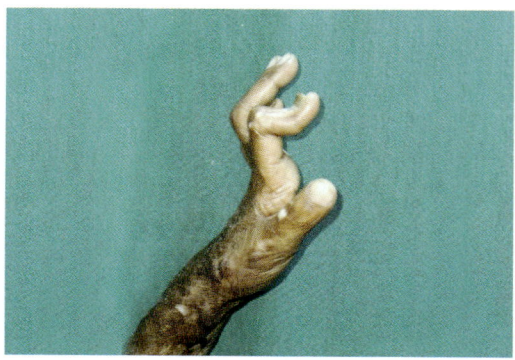

Fig. 11.13 Boutonniere deformity.

Pathophysiology of boutonniere deformity:

Disruption of central tendon

↓

Initially injured lateral bands are dorsal only and keep extending the PIP joint

↓

Triangular ligament stretch and lateral bands displace in volar direction

↓

With time, head of proximal phalanx "button holes" through the extensor mechanism leading to boutonniere deformity

- Treatment:
  - Acute closed boutonniere injury:
    - Extension splint for 6 weeks.
  - Open boutonniere injury:
    - Repair of central tendon with a grasping suture with PIP joint in extension for 6 weeks.
    - If a portion of central tendon is absent, a tendon graft may be used.
    - Both lateral bands are split longitudinally and central portions are sutured.
  - Chronic fixed boutonniere:
    - In a long-standing deformity, the oblique retinacular ligament (ORL), the transverse retinacular fibers, collateral ligaments, and the volar plate become tight.
    - Aggressive physiotherapy to achieve full passive ROM is required.

↓

If fails

↓

First stage: Release of collateral ligaments and volar plate

Second stage: Surgical reconstruction of the tendon

The reconstruction of tendon is done in sequence:

Most lateral part of lateral bands (ORL) is dissected from the lateral bands

↓

Ask the patient to extend the PIP joint as the freed ORL can bring PIP joint extension by tenodesis

↓

If patient cannot actively extend PIP joint

↓

Divide the lateral bands distal to the insert or of central slip

↓

It improves active DIP flexion

↓

If still does not allow active PIP joint extension

↓

Lateral bands are sutured to the central slip in a dorsal position

↓

It leads to improvement of PIP joint extension

↓

PIP joint is immobilized with a K-wire for 2 weeks followed by static dorsal PIP joint splint

Q12. What is the management of injury in Zone IV?

- Partial lacerations <50% of the tendon: Does not require repair with sutures.
- >50% of tendon width injuries:
  - Repaired with a grasping suture and a simple running or cross-stitch suture.
  - Hand is immobilized for 4 weeks with wrist extended, MCP joints flexed, and IP joints extended.
- In thumb, Zone IV involves tendons of EPL and EPB and should be carefully examined so as not to miss the diagnosis and are repaired using core sutures (**Fig. 11.14 a, b**).

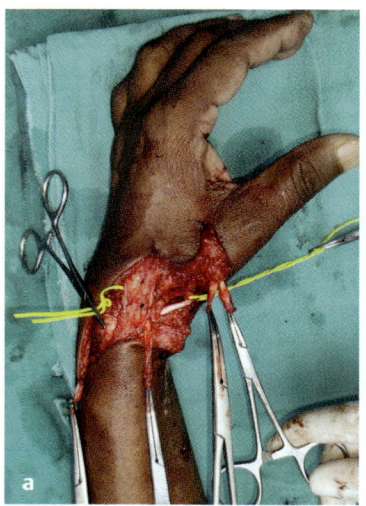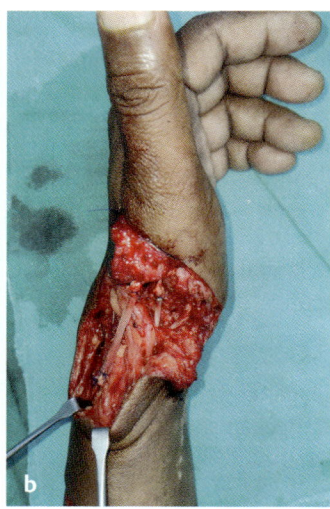

Fig. 11.14 (a, b) Extensor tendon injury in Zone IV of thumb.

Q13. What is the management of injury in Zone V?

- Zone in which lies the central tendon and sagittal bands.
- The central tendon is like a broad hood over the MCP joint and stabilized by the sagittal bands which prevent the radial/ulnar subluxation.
- Features of injury in Zone V:
  - Partial injuries are common owing to the expanded configuration of the central tendon in this zone.
  - These injuries have a tendency to get missed when finger is examined in extended position.
  - So, to reveal the partial injuries, tendon must be examined with digit in flexion and asking the patient to extend the MCP joint against resistance.
- Treatment:
  - The extensor tendons do not retract at much due to juncture tendinous and sagittal bands.
  - Repair is done with a grasping suture, and hand is splinted in wrist extension with 30 degrees of MCP joint flexion.
  - If there is associated sagittal band lacerations, it must be repaired simultaneously with immobilization of MCP joint in extension for 3 weeks.

- Human bites over the MCP joints (knuckles) must be left open after debridement as treated with systemic antibiotics.

Q14. What is the management of injury in Zone VI?

- As in Zone V, tendon injuries in Zone VI can be missed as the juncture distal to the site of laceration can provide some MCP joint extension and intrinsic continues to extend the IP joints.
- Grasping suture is used to repair the tendon but if multiple small tendon slips are cut, then slips to a single finger can be sutured together.

Q15. What is the management of injury in Zone VII?

- Features of injuries in Zone VII:
  - This is the area of dorsal retinaculum and repair of tendon injuries in this zone requires opening up of extensor tendon (**Fig. 11.15a, b**).
  - Sensory examination of dorsal nerves must be done and repair should be done in case of injury to avoid neuroma formation.
- Treatment:
  - Attrition ruptures of EPL tendon at Lister's tubercle are seen in rheumatoid

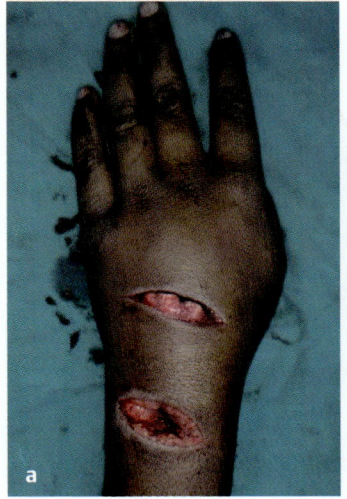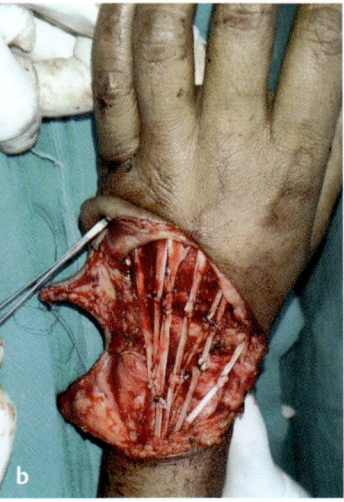

Fig. 11.15 **(a, b)** Extensor tendon injury in Zone VII.

arthritis and distal radials fracture. Since the ends are frayed, a tendon graft is required.

- For EPL injuries, EIP to EPL transfer is a viable option. EIP is divided at the MCP joint where it lies on the ulnar side of EDC and passed subcutaneously and sutured to EPL at the MCP joint of thumb in full extension of thumb and wrist in flexion.
- In case of EDC rupture, the distal end of ruptured tendon is sutured to the intact adjacent extensor.
- In case of multiple EDC ruptures, EIP can be used for transfer.

Q16. What is the management of injury in Zone VIII and IX?

- Features of injuries in Zone VIII and IX:
  - May have a combination of injured tendon, muscle, or nerves, especially motor branches.
  - Motor branches to hand extensors are present in the forearm in two groups:
    - Proximal–superficial group: ECRB, ECRL, EDC, EDM, ECU.
      - ○ Originate and receive motor branch near the lateral epicondyle.

- Distal-deep group: EIP, ABPL, EPB, and EPL.
  - ○ Originate in distal half of forearm.
  - ○ So, a proximal forearm injury with loss of distal group function is more likely to be a motor nerve injury rather than a tendon injury.
- Treatment:
  - While exploring the PIN, the safer plane of dissection is between ECRB and EDC to avoid injury to intact motor branch. Since the supply of distal-deep muscle is deeper to ECRB-EDC plane, it is preserved during surgical exposure of PIN.
  - Musculotendinous lacerations are sutured with a grasping tendon and immobilized in a POP cast for 4 weeks.

Suggested Readings

1. Tang JB. Flexor tendon injuries and reconstruction. In: Chang J, Neligan PC, eds. Plastic surgery: hand and upper extremity. Vol. 6. 4th ed. Canada: Elsevier; 2018:188–226
2. Williamson DG. Flexor tendon injuries and reconstruction. In: Mathes SJ, Hentz VR, eds. Plastic surgery: the hand and upper limb. Part 1. Vol. 7. 2nd ed. Saunders Elsevier; 2006:358–416

12 Dupuytren's Disease (DD)
Veena K. Singh

Learning Objectives

At the end of this chapter, the students will be able to:
1. Describe the clinical presentation of Dupuytren's disease of hand.
2. Understand the pathophysiology of Dupuytren's disease.
3. Understand the planning and management of deformity in Dupuytren's disease.
4. Demonstrate the markings for surgery.

Introduction

Dupuytren's disease (DD) involves the fascial structures of the palm and digits. It is insidious in onset, progressive in nature, and characterized by the formation of nodules and cords leading to contracture. It mainly involves the metacarpophalangeal (MCP) and interphalangeal (IP) joints of one or both hands. Due to its occurrence in older patients and progressive nature, it is very important for the plastic surgery trainees to understand its pathophysiology, prognosis, and management plan.

Chief Complaint

- Inability to straighten the finger/s of one or both hands.
- Swelling over the middle or distal region of the palm.
- Presence of cord-like structure or thickening of the palmar skin.
- Presence/Absence of skin pits or distortion of creases over palm.

History of Present Illness

1. Onset: What started first—swelling (nodules) or skin pits or distortion of the palmar crease.
   - These are the early signs of DD and usually involves the ulnar part of the palm.
- **Nodules** may be felt as painless, firm to hard swelling under the palmar skin along the axis of the fingers (might be mistaken for a skin callus in laborer's hand).
- **Skin pits** are also the early signs of the disease and usually present just proximal to a nodule. These are caused due to adhesions between the longitudinal and vertical fibers of the palmar fascia. These may later disappear.
- **Distortion of palmar creases** may be seen as deepened or broadened skin creases on the palm (Hugh Johnson sign).
- These lesions are manifestations of early stage of disease and do not cause any functional impairment except feeling of tightness or mild pain on stretching the fingers.
2. **Progression:**
   - Over how many months/years.
   - Slowly/rapidly progressive.
   - Appearance of longitudinal cords starting from palm up to the fingers leading to pulling up the fingers in gradual flexion.
   - At this stage, patient usually complaints of inability to straighten the fingers.
3. Any history of trauma to the hand/fingers.
4. History of any such lesions on the dorsum of the hand or on the sole or in the skin over penis.
5. History regarding the severity of functional impairment of day-to-day activities.

Past History

- Medical history of type II diabetes mellitus, hypertension, epilepsy, Koch's must be taken.
- Surgical history is important in cases of recurrence of disease in the same or other hand.

Personal History

- History of alcoholism
- History of smoking.
- Occupation (manual laborer)
- Hand dominance.
- Marital status/number of kids/appetite/diet/sleep/bladder/bowel habit.

Family History

- Similar cases in the family including parents/siblings.
- Reported positive family history in 10 to 30% of the cases.
- It is important in cases of Dupuytren's diathesis characterized by:
  - Positive family history.
  - Bilateral hands involvement.
  - Presence of ectopic lesions like knuckle and plantar lesions.
  - Early age at onset.
  - Presence of associated diseases like diabetes.
  - May/may not be associated with isolated involvement of little fingers and proximal IP (PIP) joint.
  - Recurrence is more common.

Treatment History

- Any nonsurgical intervention for the same.
- History of physiotherapy of smaller joints of the hand.

History of Allergy

To any drug/food.

General Physical Examination

- Remains same as in other cases.
- In addition to routine general physical examination, look for ectopic lesions.

Knuckle Pads (Garrod's Nodules)

- Fibrous process over the dorsal aspect of PIP joints.
- They are firm and painless and do not cause limitation of finger flexion.
- Usually adhered to the overlying skin and underlying extensors.

Plantar Lesions (Ledderhose's Disease)

- They manifest as nodules/swellings over the sole in the instep area.
- Usually adhered to plantar fascia but free from skin.
- Their presence is referred to as Ledderhose's disease.
- Usually do not cause any discomfort except for mild pain during walking.

Peyronei's Disease

- It manifests as plaque on the dorsum of penis.
- May range from small lesion to a broad sheet.
- Involvement of tunica albuginea of the corpora cavernosa of the penis.
- The chief complaint of the patient is painful erection with bending of the penis otherwise it is painless.
- Less common than knuckle pads or plantar lesions.

Rare incidences of tensor fascia lata involvement, gum involvement, or Achilles tendon involvement.

Local Examination

- Proper consent.
- Adequate light.

- Exposure of both hands rested on a table top from elbow to finger tips with palm facing upward.

Inspection

1. **Attitude of the hand.**
2. **Deformity description** (**Fig. 12.1**): Like flexion deformity at which joints and in how many fingers:
   - U/L or B/L.
3. **Presence of:**
   - Pits ⎤
   - Nodules ⎬ Location, extent, and detailed description.
   - Distortion of palmar crease ⎦
   - Cords (**Fig. 12. 2**):
     - Usually lie along the long axis of the digits.
     - It is not adherent to the palmar skin.
     - It arises from proximal palm and extends up to the distal palmar crease or laterally on each side of the MCP joint. At the distal end, it merges with the dermis of the skin.
     - At a later stage, it usually runs longitudinally along the central axis of a digit and in most cases, it ends distal to the PIP joint either centrally or laterally on each side of the joint.

- Any other swelling around the cords (apart from nodule)-may be the displaced neurovascular bundles.

4. **Position of MCP, PIP, and distal IP (DIP) joints:**
   - Whether in flexion contracture since the palmar and digital cords lead to progressive joint contractures.
   - **MCP joint** is the first one to get affected. Due to progressive contracture, hyperextension at MCP joint may be restricted.
     - Flexion contracture occurs up to 60 degrees and usually leads to minimal functional impairment.
   - **PIP joint:**
     - As the disease progresses, PIP joint flexion contracture may occur and in severe cases, there is complete loss of extension.
     - This leads to a functional disability of the hand and patient is unable to perform his day-to-day activities and might hurt the fingers also.
     - Since there is no fixed contracture, the full active flexion is preserved.
   - **DIP joint:**
     - Not affected by the disease.
     - May go into hypertension as a result of long-standing flexion contracture of PIP joint.

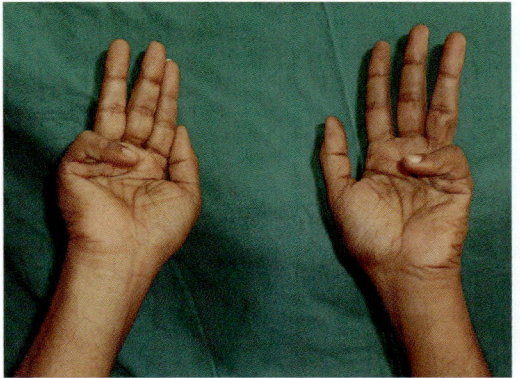

Fig. 12.1 Dupuytren's disease of little finger in both hands.

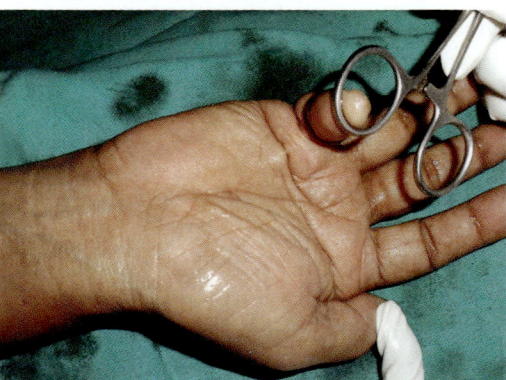

Fig. 12.2 Clinical appearance of a longitudinal cord.

5. **Abnormalities in the nail or skin:** Skin maceration or nail incrustation might be present.

Palpation

1. Feel of the palmar skin.
2. Palpation of pits, nodules, palmar creases, cords, any other swellings.
   - All inspectory findings are corroborated.
   - In case any soft, pulpy swelling is present on either side of the cord at the level of MCP joint, it may indicate the distortion of neurovascular bundle location (Short-Watson sign). It might dislocate to a more superficial and medial position by the longitudinal cord. In case it is present, one needs to be careful during surgery (Short-Watson sign).

Movements and Measurements

- At MCP, PIP, and DIP joint.
- Active and passive range of movement (ROM).
- Using a goniometer, the angles at each joint must be measured.

Provisional Diagnosis

A case of DD involving the MCP and PIP joint of ring finger of right hand in a patient of 60 years with associated history of diabetes mellitus for a duration of 6 months.

Questions

Q1. What is the differential diagnosis?
- In presentation with isolated nodule, other diagnosis like epidermoid cyst, callosities, or fibrous conditions, e.g., nodular fasciitis, desmoid fibroma may be kept in mind.
- In presentation with contracture, differential diagnosis may include:
  - Congenital flexion contracture (camptodactyly).
  - Posttraumatic contracture.

Q2. What are the risk factors for DD?
Risk factors for DD are:
- Diabetes mellitus: DD patients having diabetes mellitus usually present with mild, nonprogressive disease limited to palmar nodules.
- Epilepsy.
- Alcoholism.
- Associated trauma: Several studies have shown that in manual laborers, microruptures of the palmar fascia stimulate hypertrophic healing, leading to contracture.
- Male gender.
- Middle aged to elderly patients.
- Ring and little fingers are more commonly affected.

Q3. How will you assess the severity of the disease?
Tubiana scoring system is used to assess the lesions in DD:
- The hand is divided into five rays.
- For each digit, total flexion deformity/contracture over MCP, PIP, and DIP joint is measured.
- A number is allocated, which changes when there is increment of 45 degrees in the deformity.
  - "N" is the notation for nodule in cases where there is no deformity.
  - Letter "P" stands for palmar lesions.
  - Letter "D" stands for digital lesions.
  - Letter "H" stands for fixed hyperextension of DIP joint.
  - Letter "R" stands for recurrence in a previously operated ray.
  - Letter "E" stands for extension of disease in an unoperated ray.
  - Letter "A" stands for amputation.

Score:
0—no lesion.
"N" (score=0.5)—Palmar/digital nodule without flexion deformity.
1—Total flexion deformity 0–45 degrees.
2—Total flexion deformity 45–90 degrees.
3—Total flexion deformity 90–135 degrees.
4—Total flexion deformity >135 degrees.

- The total score of the hand is the sum of scores at individual digit and gives the status of hand.
- It allows an objective assessment of the disease progression over time and in the postoperative period.

Q4. What is the normal anatomy of palmar and digital fasciae?

Palmar fascia consists of two layers (**Fig. 12.3a, b**):

- Deep anterior fascia (the deeper layer) which covers the interosseous muscles (not affected in Dupuytren's).
- Superficial fascia (or midpalmar superficial aponeurosis) forms a triangular layer with its apex in continuation with palmaris longus: This is the layer which gets involved in Dupuytren's.

The **superficial fascia** has three types of fibers:

- **Longitudinal fibers:** These fibers run superficial to the flexor retinaculum and flexor tendons and form the pretentious bands. Distally, the longitudinal fibers have three types of insertion:
  - The superficial fibers terminate into the deep surface of dermis around the distal palmar crease. Involvement

of these fibers in the initial stage of Dupuytren's form palmar skin pits.
  - The intermediate fibers pass on to the fingers and form retrovascular fascial structures.
  - The deepest fibers divide around the flexor tendon sheath and insert at MCP joint on each side.
- **Transverse fibers:** These fibers have two different sets in the superficial fascia: proximal and distal.
  - Proximal fibers (also known as proximal transverse ligament):
    - These fibers form a 1.5-cm-wide fibrous band and end distally at distal palmar crease.
    - They lie deep to pretentious bands but superficial to the neurovascular bundles and are not involved in disease process. This is the reason why dissection of longitudinal bands up to the distal palmar crease is safer.
  - Distal transverse fibers (also known as natatory ligament).
    - Its proximal edge runs over the base of proximal phalanges, extending from radial border of the index finger to the ulnar border of the little finger.

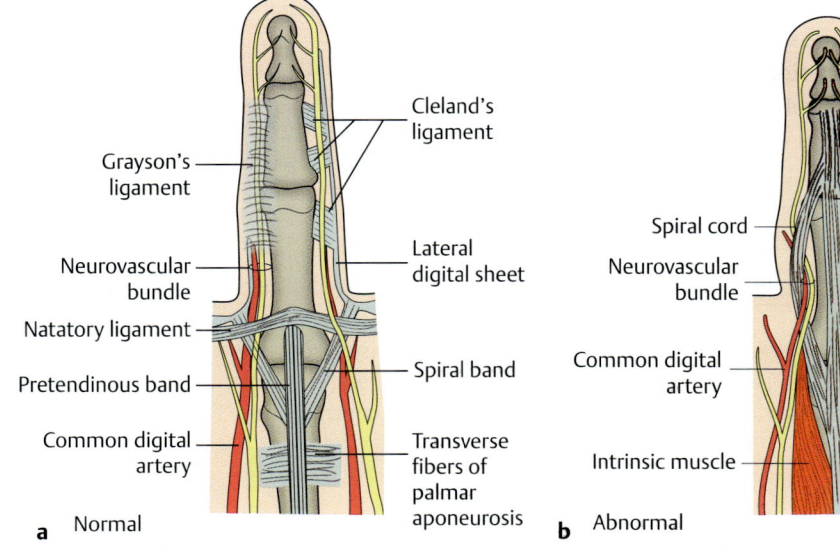

Fig. 12.3 (a, b) Anatomy of normal and pathologic palmar and digital fascial structures.

- Its distal edge extends into the digital fascia and the interdigital skin folds.
- **Vertical fibers:**
  - These fibers run between the superficial and deep fascia.
  - They form eight vertical septa on either side of longitudinal compartments containing either flexor tendons or lumbricals along with the neurovascular bundles.

Digital fascia:
- A circular fascial covering is present which consists of:
  - Volar part which is superficial to the flexor tendon sheath.
  - Dorsal part which lies superficial to the extensor tendons.
- Both volar and dorsal parts unite along the medial and lateral aspects of the finger to form a sheath around the neurovascular (N-V) bundle.
- These lateral structures are:
  - **Cleland ligament:** Lies dorsal to N-V bundles and arises from IP joints on each side and spreads out toward the lateral skin.
  - **Grayson Ligament:** Lies volar to N-V bundles and arises from flexor tendon sheath on volar aspect and spreads out laterally into the skin.
  - **Transverse retinacular ligaments:** Arise from the volar aspect of PIP joint capsule and pass dorsal to the Cleland ligament to get attached to the lateral margin of the extensor apparatus.

Thumb and first web space:
- Two transverse structures cross the first web space:
  - Distal commissural ligament of Grapow.
  - Proximal commissural ligament.

Q5. What is the pathologic anatomy of the fasciae in Dupuytren's?

The pathologic anatomy of palmar and digital fasciae in DD consists of two types of pathologic fibrous tissue:
- Nodules.
- Cords.

Palm of the hand:
- The palmar cords develop along the course of pretendinous bands.
  - They extend up to either the proximal or middle phalanx to form "Central cord."
  - Sometimes they combine with lateral digital cord (spiral cord) and displace the N-V bundles to a more superficial and medial position leading to risk of damage during surgery.

Fingers:
- Four types of cords contract at the PIP joint as described by McFarlane et al.
  - Central cord: It is the continuation of palmar longitudinal cord and extends up to PIP joint on either side.
  - Lateral cord: Arises from natatory ligament to the lateral skin of DIP joint. It lies between the skin and N-V bundle.
  - Spiral cord: It may be an elongation of palmar central cord or originate from the terminal part of an intrinsic tendon (**Fig. 12.4**).
    - Proximally, it lies posterior to N-V bundle then lies lateral and superficial and then volar to N-V bundle in the distal part.
    - It inserts into flexor sheath or phalanx.
    - These spiral cords are usually involved in severe PIP contractures.
  - Retrovascular cord:
    - Arises from the retrovascular structures, (e.g., Cleland ligament).
    - It contracts both PIP and DIP joint.

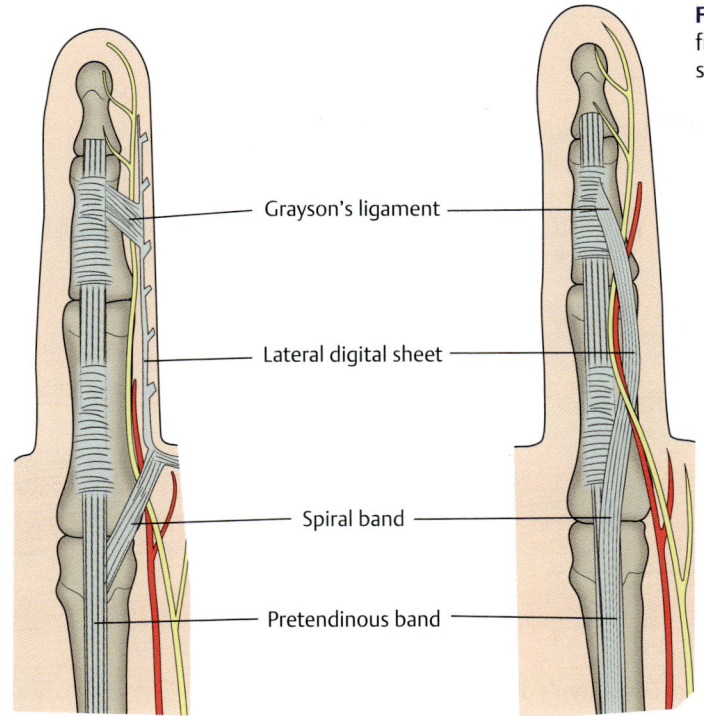

Fig. 12.4 Formation of spiral cord from normal fascial palmodigital structures.

Grayson's ligament

Lateral digital sheet

Spiral band

Pretendinous band

Q6. What are the nonsurgical options and when you will go for it?

The nonsurgical management may include:

- Physiotherapy:
  - Splints.
  - Ultrasonic therapy.
- Radiotherapy.
- Steroid infections.
- Vitamin E.
- Enzymatic fasciotomy—a combination of trypsin and hyaluronidase.

Q7. What are the options for surgical management and when will you go for it?

Indications for surgical treatment are:

- Do not operate in absence of contracture.
  - In cases of nodules, local steroids injections may be given.
  - A **"table top" test** is performed to confirm the presence of contracture in early stage. The patient is asked to put his palm of the hand and fingers flat on a table. If a contracture is there, the palm and fingers will not be in complete contact with the table.
- Early surgery is indicated if PIP joint contracture is present.
  - Long-standing PIP joint contracture may lead to stiffness of the joint to contracture of collateral ligaments.

Selection of surgical procedures:

- The aim of the surgery is not only to correct the deformity but also to prevent the recurrences.

For patients with risk factors for early recurrence (**Fig.12.5**):

- <45 years
- Rapidly progressive disease
- Strong risk for diathesis

⎱ Dermofasciectomy in the first stage.

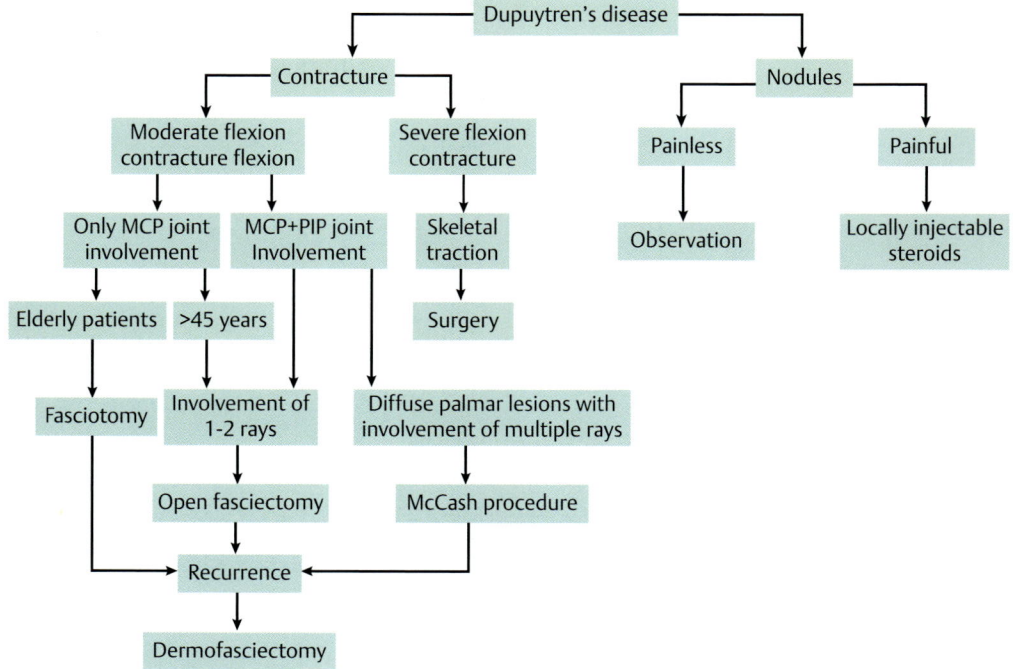

Fig. 12.5 Algorithm for management of Dupuytren's disease.

The surgical options are:
- Fasciotomy (also known as aponeurotomy):
  - Subcutaneous Fasciotomy.
  - Open Fasciotomy.
  - Needle Fasciotomy.
- Fasciectomy.

Q8. What is the difference between Fasciotomy and Fasciectomy?
- Fasciotomy: Severing of the contracture bands or cords without excision.
- Fasciectomy: Excision of the Dupuytren's cord tissue in one or more rays.

Q9. What are the types of fasciotomy?
- Needle fasciotomy:
  - Local anesthetic agent, lidocaine, is injected into the skin overlying the diseased cord.

A 25-gauge needle is used to divide the cord by pricking in multiple areas of the cord. Needle should be inserted up to bevel deep only to avoid injury to the neurovascular bundle.

The MCP joint is stabilized and the finger is brought forcefully but smoothly into extension.

↓

A crack sound is made when cord ruptures.

↓

Several sittings may be required in combination with physiotherapy to achieve full extension of the involved finger.

Injections containing collagenase from *Clostridium histolyticum* is also used to soften the cord and then manipulate the finger for breaking the cords.
- With this method, complications like skin breakage, transient dysthesias, and local infections can occur.

- Only indicated in the early stages of disease in elderly or unhealthy patients.
- Subcutaneous fasciotomy:
  - It is done through a skin stab incision using a number 11 scalpel blade.
  - Blade is stabbed in line with the cord and then turned perpendicular to severe the diseased cord.
  - Finger is then forcefully extended with continuous gentle manipulation.
- Open fasciotomy:
  - The diseased cords are divided under direct vision through a skin incision placed longitudinally along the side of the cord.

Q10. What are the steps in fasciectomy?

Fasciectomy can be:
- Limited (partial or regional fasciectomy):
  - Surgical excision of all diseased abnormal fibrous tissue.
  - It is the standard and most popular method of treatment for DD.
  - There are various methods of skin closure after limited fasciectomy.
    - By direct closure of skin or with Z-plasty flaps.
    - By open technique (McCash) and secondary healing of the wound.
    - By placing a skin graft over the residual skin defect after straightening of the finger.
- Radical (extensive fasciectomy):
  - Surgical excision of all the palmar fascia including the normal and diseased tissues both.
  - **Steps:**
- Skin incisions are carefully planned as there are various options (**Fig. 12.6**):
  - Bruner's incisions are commonly followed.
  - Skin incisions should be such that if possible, lengthening of the skin can be planned whenever required (**Fig. 12.7a, b**).

- Well-vascularized skin flaps are raised along with the subcutaneous fat and elevated away from the diseased cord.
- Fasciectomy is done from proximal to distal by freeing the diseased fascia on its both sides and from under surface and divided under direct vision.
- At the finger level, the N-V bundles become superficial and so protected carefully before excision of the diseased tissue.
- All macroscopically involved fibrous tissue are excised as far as the distal phalanx.
- In long-standing deformities of PIP joint, there might be:
  - Shortening of flexor tendon sheath which can be lengthened by one or two transverse incisions at proximal phalanx and PIP joint level.

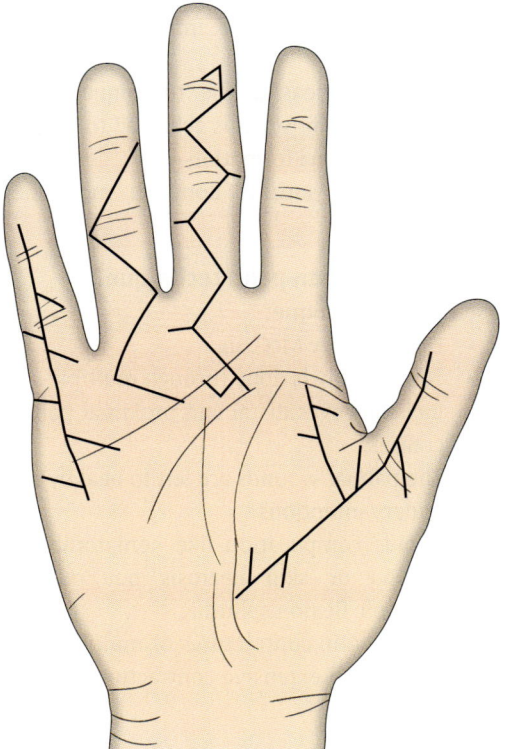

Fig. 12.6 Incisions for fasciectomy in Dupuytren's disease.

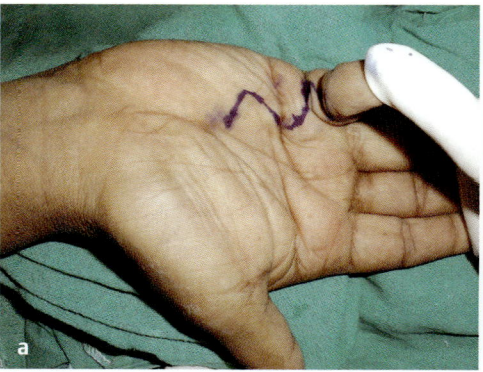 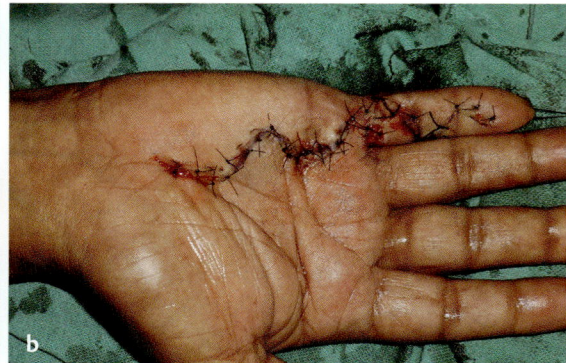

Fig. 12.7 (a, b) Lengthening of skin after release.

- PIP joint contracture, which can be corrected by division of volar plate check in ligaments.
  - Once the finger extension is achieved, do "central slip tenodesis" test to check if there is attenuation of the central slip of the extensor mechanism which will require PIP joint immobilization for 3 weeks.
  - After releasing the tourniquet, complete hemostasis is achieved to prevent hematoma formation.
  - Skin closure is done as mentioned above.

Q11. What is open palm technique?
Open palm technique:
- Described by McCash.
- Fasciectomy is done through multiple skin incisions over distal and proximal palmar creases.
- The palmar wounds are left to heal by secondary intentions.
- Avoids complication like hematoma formation or skin necrosis but requires dynamic flexion splinting.
- Indicated in contractures of multiple MCP joints with extensive contracture of distal palmar skin.

Q12. What is dermofasciectomy?
Dermofasciectomy is the excision of skin with the underlying diseased cord and covering the created open wound with skin grafting.
- Indication:
  - Young patients.
  - Rapidly progressive disease.
  - Strong diathesis.

Q13. What are the postoperative complications?

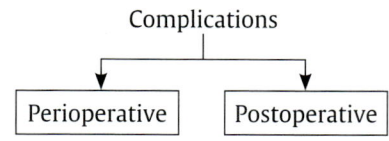

Complications

Perioperative	Postoperative

- Injury to N-V bundles

- Hematoma
- Skin necrosis and wound dehiscence
- Injection
- Joint stiffness
- Reflex sympathetic dystrophy (or, sympathetic mediated pain)
  - More frequent in women
  - Increased sympathetic flare reactions

Q14. What is the postoperative protocol and physiotherapy?

Postoperative care will include the following:

- Compressive bulky dressing.
- Limb is elevated.
- First dressing on the seventh to eighth postoperative day followed by a lighter dressing and physiotherapy.
- Physiotherapy:
  - Necessary in cases of PIP joint contractures.
  - Active and passive flexion of involved fingers.
  - Gradual finger extension is allowed after 3 weeks.
  - Early dynamic splinting is given if joint procedures have been performed.

Q15. What are the salvage procedures?

There are few salvage procedures in a severely contracted finger.

- **Skeletal traction**: By applying an external fixator to the involved finger with progressive continuous extension which is usually achieved after 2 to 3 weeks of traction.
- **Wedge osteotomy:** A dorsal wedge from the proximal phalanx is removed so that a more functional range of motion is achieved at PIP joint.
- **Total anterior (volar) tenoarthrolysis:** The flexor apparatus and the volar plate of PIP and DIP joint are detached from the underlying bone through a lateral incision in the affected digit.
- **PIP joint arthrodesis:** PIP joint is arthrodesed in a more functional position in case of a severely contracted PIP joint.

- **Amputation:**
  - In severely contracted fingers with recurrence and neurovascular deficits.
  - Most commonly done in little finger.

Q16. Why is counseling of the patient required before taking up for surgery?

Preoperative patient counseling is of utmost importance:

- Need of aggressive postoperative physiotherapy to achieve the normal range of motion of joints.
- Recurrence of the disease in the operated part or elsewhere in the same or contractual hand.

Q17. How will you manage recurrences?

Recurrence is defined as the reappearance of the diseased tissue in the same area where previous fasciectomy was done.

- Management of all recurrences do not require re-surgery which is done only in young patients with a recurring contracture of PIP joint.
- Recurrence of DD can be possibly managed by dermofasciectomy with skin grafting which is the surgical technique of choice in Dupuytren's diathesis and patients with several risk factors.

Suggested Readings

1. Watt AJ, Huang JI. Management of Dupuytren's disease. In: Neligan PC, ed. Plastic surgery: hand and upper extremity. Vol. 6. 4th ed. Canada: Elsevier; 2018:372–388
2. Leclercq C. In: Mathes SJ, Hentz VR, eds. Plastic surgery: the hand and upper limb. Part 1. Vol. 7. 2nd ed. Saunders Elsevier; 2006:729-758

13 Post-Burn Contracture (PBC) Hand

Rimpi Jain and Veena K. Singh

Learning Objectives

At the end of this chapter, the students will be able to:
1. Describe the clinical presentation of post-burn contracture of hand.
2. Understand the underlying pathophysiology of the deformity.
3. Demonstrate the clinical examination of a burned hand.
4. Demonstrate the markings for release of contracture.
5. Perform the various surgical procedures for correction of the deformity.

Introduction

Hands make up generally 1% of our body surface zone, both in the grown-ups and youngsters. Burns involve hand in around 80% of cases and deformities of hand is a common problem foreseen while managing late burn patients. Detailed preoperative assessment and planning is crucial to look for the cause of contracture, which may include post-burn scar, tight musculotendinous units or joint damage. Meticulous examination of the hand, understanding patient's expectations and counseling about realistic ones, motivating for postoperative care—all are equally crucial in the preoperative work-up of chronic burn deformities of hand.

History

Particulars of the patient (name, age, sex, occupation, residence, etc.); hand dominance.

Chief Complaints

- Deformity of the hand due to burn injury.
- Inability to straighten the fingers/thumb.
- Wound over the hand or fingers.

History of Present Illness

- Ask about the mode of injury—accidental or rescuer burns.
- Cause of injury—whether it was due to flame burn, scald burn, or electric burn.
- Ask about the duration of burn.
- Duration of contact with the source.
- Whether hands were immersed in water or not immediately after the burns.
- Condition of wound after burn—color of the wound and blisters were there or not.
- Whether swelling was present in the hand, after how much duration, and for how long.
- Whether daily activities have been affected and to what extent.
- Detailed history of the wound should be taken, for example, wound developed after how many days of burn injury, dressing done by the patient or doctor, dressing continued or not, how frequently the dressings were changed, material used for dressings, if there is any recurrent breakdown of the wound once healed.

Negative History

- Ask about loss of sensation in the hand.
- History of burn in any other part of the body.

Treatment History

- Ask about the treatment that the patient has received after the injury.
- Whether debridement was done or not.
- Fasciotomy done or not.
- Whether infection was there. If yes what was done for it?
- Ask about the duration of healing of wound.
- Whether physiotherapy was done or not.
- Any use of splintage.

Past History

History of diabetes mellitus, hypertension, tuberculosis, or any other medical illness.

Any surgery done in the past for the current problems.

Personal History

History of addiction including alcoholism, smoking, marital status, number of kids, employment status; in case of females ask for last date of menstrual period (LMP).

Family History

Number of family members dependent on the patient.

History of Allergy

Allery to food or medications.

General Examination

- General physical examination as for other cases.

- Always check the availability of donor sites (thigh, legs, back) for graft.
- Look for healed scars or wound over other areas in the body.

Local Examination of Hand

After proper consent, with adequate exposure and light.

Adequate exposure - exposure of affected limb from shoulder level upto the finger tips. The affected limb has to be rested on a table with forearm slightly raised and rested on elbow.

Inspection

- Attitude of the hand.
- Describe in detail the deformity at the wrist joint, metacarpophalangeal (MCP) joint, proximal interphalangeal (PIP) joint, and distal interphalangeal (DIP) joint (**Fig. 13.1a–c**). Usually there is flexion deformity at the wrist and fingers and extension deformity at MCP joint.
- Extent of the contracture band—proximal, distal, and lateral extents.
- Extent of scar and its characteristics (Vancouver burn scar scale).
- Condition of the skin adjacent to the contracture/scar, whether hypopigmented or hyperpigmented.
- Examine the remaining normal skin of palm and dorsum.
- Examine the condition of nails.
- Look if any finger is amputated and at what level.
- Examine web space and look for any syndactyly.

Classification of Burn Scar Contractures (McCauley)

- **Grade I**: Symptomatic tightness but no limitation in range of motion.
- **Grade II**: Mild decrease in range of motion without significant impact on activities of daily living; no distortion of normal architecture.

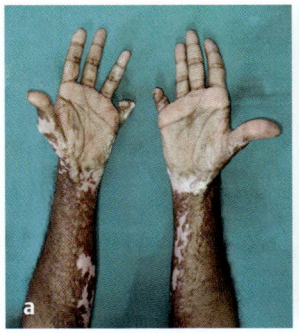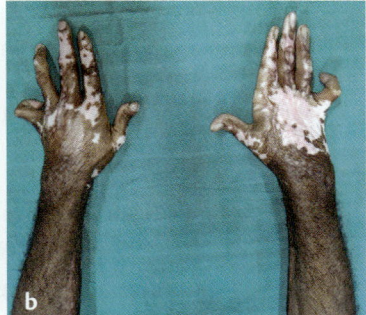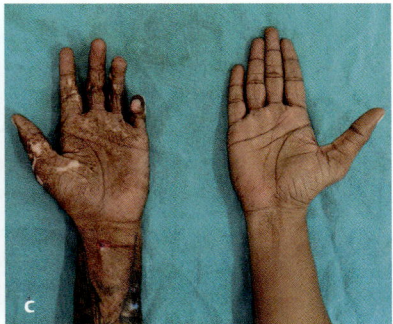

Fig. 13.1 **(a–c)** Post-burn contracture of wrist, thumb, and fingers.

- **Grade III**: Functional deficit noted, with early changes in normal architecture of hand.
- **Grade IV**: Loss of hand function with significant distortion of normal architecture of the hand.

Subset classification of Grade III and Grade IV contractures:

- A: Flexion contractures.
- B: Extension contractures.
- C: Combination of flexion and extension contractures.

Palpation

- Temperature: Check whether locally raised (indicates ongoing infection).
- Tenderness: Check over the scar. Also, over the wound and surrounding skin.
- All findings on inspection need to be corroborated.
- Consistency of the scar—whether firm or hard.
- Presence of blanching: Apply digital pressure over the scar for 2 to 3 seconds and see whether the scar blanches (becomes pale or white). Look for the return of color once pressure is released. If it takes longer time for the scar to return to its original color, it indicates an immature scar. The blanching is due to the temporary

obstruction of blood flow to that area. This causes that area to become slightly pale as compared to normal skin.

- Measure the scar in both dimensions: longitudinal and transverse.
- In case of hypertrophic scar, measure the thickness also.
- Examine sensations of the hand and fingers.
- Look for capillary refill time at the nailbed or pulp of the fingers.
- Palpate both the radial and ulnar arteries.

Movements

Document ROM at each joint in a tabular fashion.

Movement (Range of Motion)		
Elbow	Flexion	Active
		Passive
	Extension	Active
		Passive
Wrist	Flexion	Active
		Passive
	Extension	Active
		Passive
	Ulnar deviation	Active
		Passive
	Radial deviation	Active
		Passive

			MCP joint	PIP joint	DIP joint
1	Thumb	Flexion	Active Passive	Active Passive	
		Extension	Active Passive	Active Passive	
2	Index finger	Flexion	Active Passive	Active Passive	Active Passive
		Extension	Active Passive	Active Passive	Active Passive
3	Middle finger	Flexion	Active Passive	Active Passive	Active Passive
		Extension	Active Passive	Active Passive	Active Passive
4	Ring finger	Flexion	Active Passive	Active Passive	Active Passive
		Extension	Active Passive	Active Passive	Active Passive
5	Little finger	Flexion	Active Passive	Active Passive	Active Passive
		Extension	Active Passive	Active Passive	Active Passive

Measurements

With the help of a goniometer, measure the degree of contracture at each joint (**Fig. 13.2**).

Provisional Diagnosis

This is a case of 1 year old post-burn contracture of right hand with flexion contracture of index and middle fingers at PIP and DIP joints and Boutonniere deformity of ring finger and little finger with hypopigmented patches with stiff joints.

Questions

Q1. What is your plan?
- X-ray of the affected hand in both anteroposterior and lateral view to rule out bony deformities.
- Complete blood count including Hb, TLC, DLC, PT/INR.
- Serum electrolytes.
- Serum urea and creatinine.
- Viral markers.
- List the stages in which the surgery is planned and explain to the patient accordingly.
- Plan is to release the contracture and cover with appropriate tissue (**Fig. 13.3**).

Important questions to be kept in mind before doing surgery:
- What is the nature of the contracture or the limiting scarring? (detailed assessment of every every structure including skin, tendon, joint, nerve - motor and sensory and vascular testing must be done)
- Are there any underlying joint problems (e.g., contracture of the ligaments or capsule, cartilage destruction)?
- Will soft tissue procedures be sufficient?

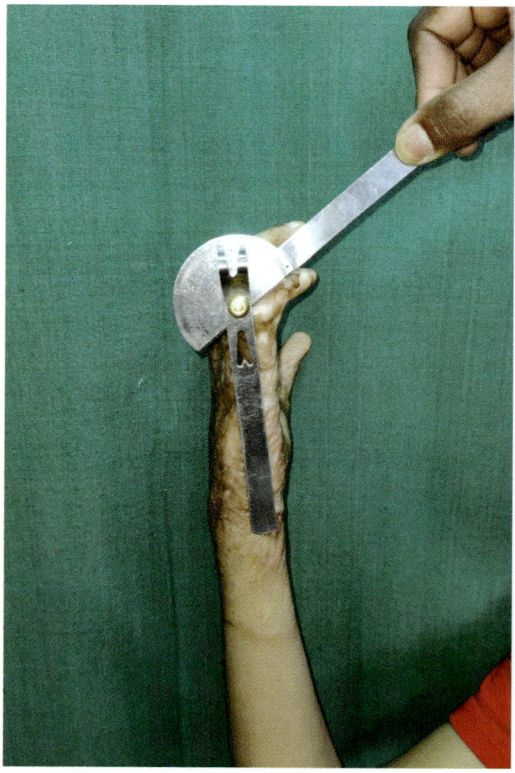

Fig. 13.2 Measurement of angle at proximal interphalangeal (PIP) joint.

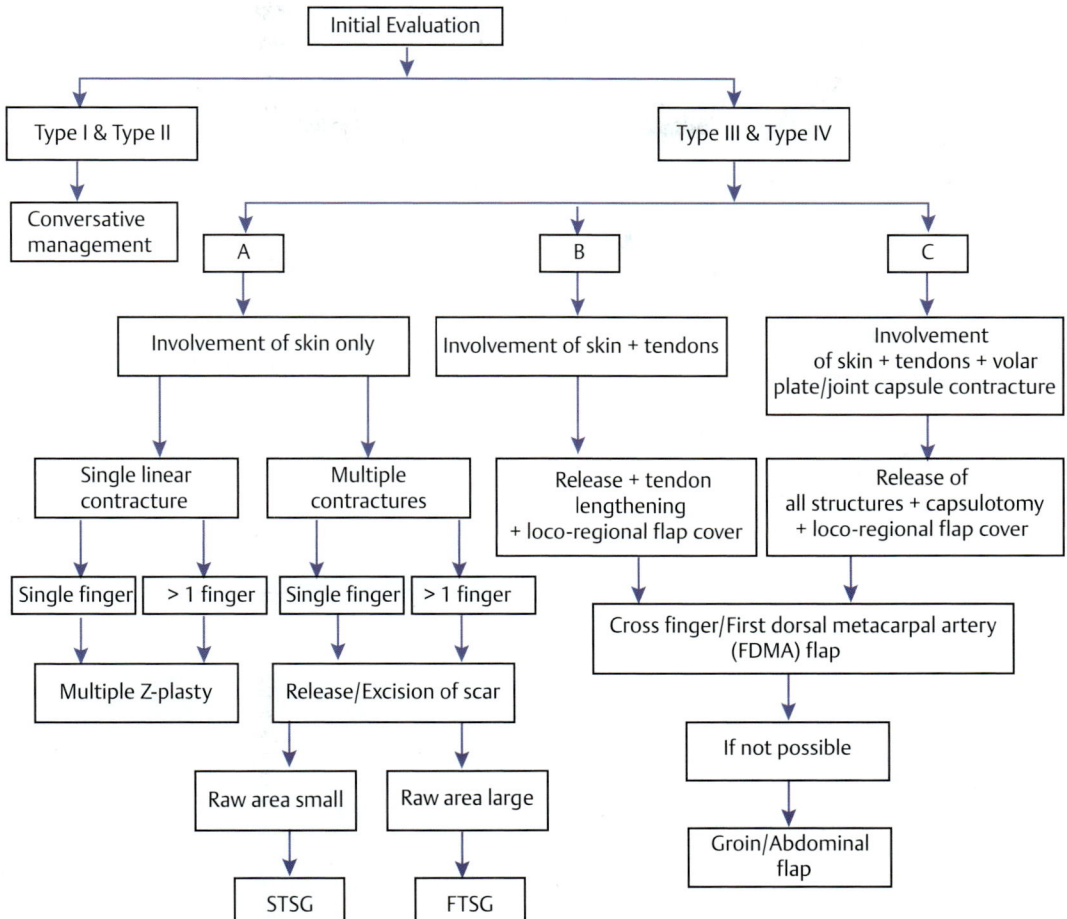

Fig. 13.3 Algorithm for decision making in management of post-burn deformities.

- Which type of coverage is adequate after contracture release?
- From which donor site should skin grafts or flaps be harvested?

Q2. What is the difference between contraction and contracture?

In wound contraction the surrounding skin is pulled circumferentially toward an open wound, while contracture is due to tissue shortening and distortion that causes decrease in joint mobility and function. Contraction is a usual phenomenon in normal wound healing but contracture is the end result of abnormal wound healing.

Q3. What actually happens in contracture formation? What is the composition of contracture tissue?

Refer Q.no. 5 in Chapter 2 Post Burn Contracture (PBC) Neck.

Q4. What is Lai's line? How to mark and what is its importance?

Midlateral line in finger is Lai's line (**Fig. 13.4a, b**). Flex the finger and mark the point at each joint where the flexion crease ends. Then connect these points which identifies the midaxial line or Lai's line. It is important because digital nerve

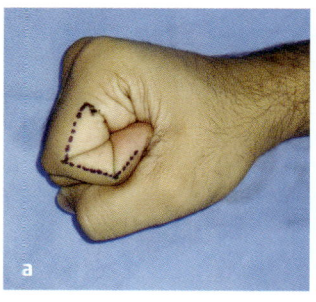 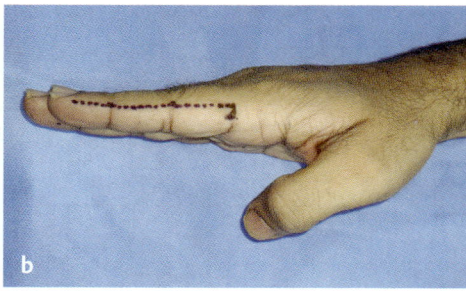

Fig. 13.4 (a, b) Marking of Lai's line (midaxial line).

and artery lie approximately 2 mm volar to this line. So it helps in marking the incision for finger.

Q5. What is the mechanism of syndactyly formation in burns?

There are two mechanisms:
- Skin of the adjacent burned digits fuse together during the healing process (**Fig. 13.5**).
- Granulation or contractures of the digital skin allow distal migration of the web.

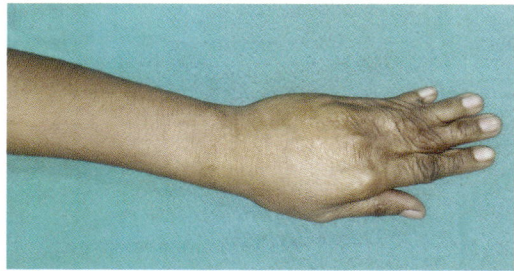

Fig. 13.5 Partial syndactyly after burn injury.

Q6. What is the difference between palmar and dorsal aspect of hand and why is it important in burn injury?

A few attributes differentiate burns at the back and palm of the hands. Burns of palmar skin can totally heal. The reason being the difference in the thickness, palmar skin being more glabrous than the volar aspect of fingers, thickly keratinized, and ready to bear major brunt. This is unique in relation to the result of dorsal burns.

Skin on the dorsum is thin and pliable and can be easily damaged by burns. In addition, the extensor tendons are more superficial and prone to higher possibility of injury from burn. Therefore, burns on the dorsum of hand often requires reconstruction of soft tissue either by graft or flaps than burns on palmar aspect as it heals better (**Fig. 13.6** and **Fig. 13.7**).

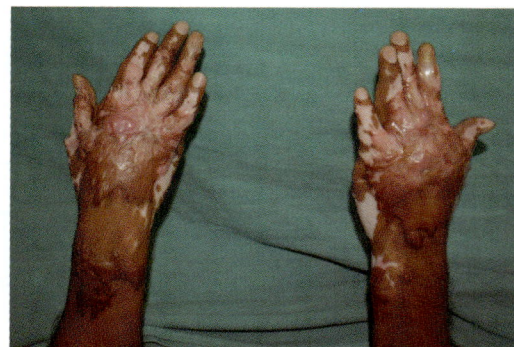

Fig. 13.6 Photograph of a patient showing hypertrophic scars over dorsum of bilateral hands.

Q7. What is the pathophysiology of first web space contracture? (Fig. 13.8 and Fig. 13.9)
- It is due to hypertrophic scarring or skin deficiency in the web space.
- There may be associated contracture of the adductor muscle, fascia, and possibly the basal joint capsule.

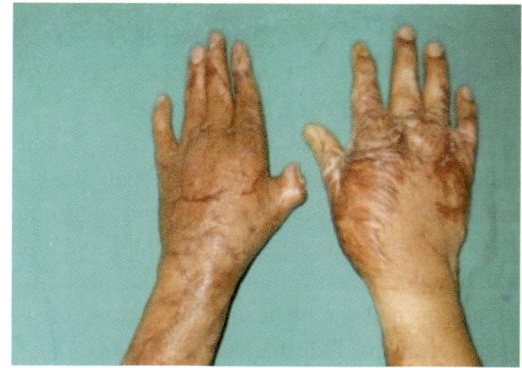

Fig. 13.7 Hypertrophic scars excised and resurfaced with split thickness skin graft (STSG).

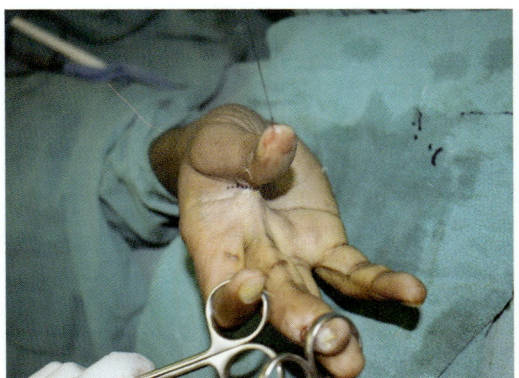

Fig. 13.8 Photograph showing first web space contracture.

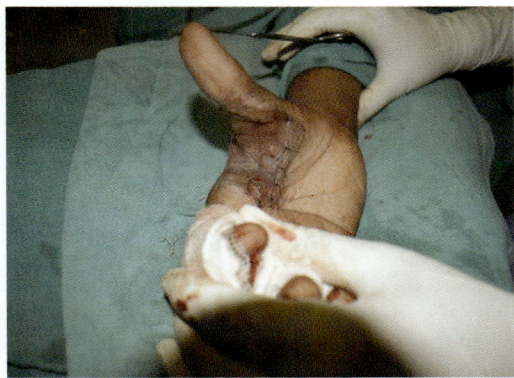

Fig. 13.9 Photograph after release and skin graft.

Q8. What is the cause of scar hypertrophy in burn?

When healing occurs secondarily, there is a significant development of granulation tissue during the healing phase. This granulation tissue is the precursor of scar hypertrophy. Granulation tissue with its high collagen content is responsible for scar hypertrophy and all of its unfavorable sequelae. The tendency of the burn wound to heal with hypertrophy increases directly in relation to the time required for wound healing.

Q9. What are the types of scar hypertrophy?

There are two types:

- Early scar hypertrophy: It occurs in the active phase of burn wound healing. It is usually within 6 months of injury. The scar at this stage is hyperemic, often symptomatic and amenable to conservative measures.
- Late scar hypertrophy: It is static, mature phase of burn wound healing. Mature contracted hypertrophic scars do not respond to conservative measures.

Q10. What is the pathophysiology of post-burn contracture hand?

The untreated severely burned hands usually develop contractures. In most patients, the initial thermal injury is limited to the skin, with sparing of the underlying tendons, joints, and joint capsules. These structures usually affect later on by prolonged healing. The position of the wrist

is one of the key factors in the development of deformity in the burned hand.

After burn, patients' hands assume a position—
the position of comfort

$\downarrow$

Due to synergistic effects of extrinsic extensors and wrist flexion

$\downarrow$

MCP results in extension

$\downarrow$

Laxity of the collateral ligaments in early stage

$\downarrow$

Collateral ligaments become shortened and contracted producing extension deformity that cannot be overcome by the flexor muscles

$\downarrow$

Transverse intermetacarpal ligaments become shortened and thickened, resulting in loss of the arch. PIP joints assume a position of moderate flexion immediately after burning, and if uninhibited, this progresses to extreme flexion.

Q11. Describe the position of comfort and why is it the position of contracture formation?

The position is volar flexion at the wrist, hyperextension at the MCP joints, and variable degrees of flexion at the IP joints with adduction and extension of the thumb. It is called position of comfort as it is least painful. In burns, there is edema formation in the hand so it has a tendency to go into position of comfort and leads to contracture if early splintage in functional position is not done (**Fig. 13.10**).

Q12. How will you differentiate whether contracture is due to skin or tendon or bone?

In cases of flexion deformity of the fingers, when the wrist is brought in flexion and fingers are able to extend then it is due to contracture/shortening of the tendons. But even after flexion at the wrist, fingers are still in flexion, then it is due to skin involvement. In case it is due to involvement of the bone, joints would be totally fixed irrespective of the position.

Q13. List the grading of MCP joint extension contracture.[1]

Type I: • With wrist flexion, passive MP flexion is <30 degrees.
• With wrist extension, passive MP flexion is >30 degrees and scarring is limited to the skin.

Type II: • With wrist flexion, MP flexion is severely limited.
• With wrist extension, MP passive flexion is <30 degrees.
• In addition to dermal contracture deeper structures such as the MP joint capsule are scarred.

Type III: • MP joint is fixed regardless of wrist position.
• MP joint is dislocated and often has articular incongruity.

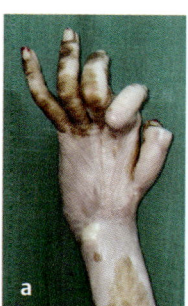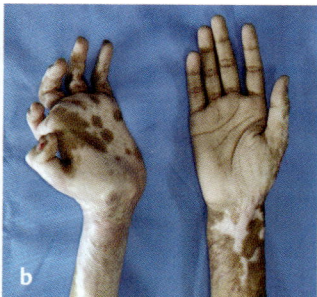

Fig. 13.10 (a, b) Contracture formation in position of comfort.

Q14. List the grading of post-burn flexion contractures of the fingers.

Classified by Kurtzman and Stern:
Type I: Skin only; MCP in passive flexion, PIP can be fully extended.
Type II: Palmar capsular contractures; MCP in passive flexion; no passive extension of PIP possible.
Type III: Soft tissue, joint contractures; fixed PIP regardless of MCP position.

Treatment:
Type I: Release contracture and replace the palmar skin deficiency with z-plasties or full-thickness skin grafts.
Type II: Release of volar plate and division of the checkreins to free the joint. Flap coverage is required if the joint capsule or flexor tendons are exposed.
Type III: These patients often require joint fusion, despite complex soft tissue reconstruction procedures.

Q15. Describe the surgical management of metacarpophalangeal joint deformities.

Type I: Surgical management of Type I includes simple release of scarred skin and resurfacing with thick SSG or FTG because the joint is preserved.
Type II: It requires release of the skin on the dorsum of the hand, release of deeper tissues with capsulotomy. Flap cover is required when the wound bed is unsuitable for skin grafting. K-wire fixation may be required.
Type III: Joint is severely affected, so arthrodesis is the best option.

Q16. What are the recommended ranges of angle of fusion in arthrodesis?

Finger	MCP	PIP/IP	DIP
Thumb	10–20	10–20	N/A
Index	20–30	25–35	5–15
Middle	25–35	30–40	5–15
Ring	30–40	35–45	5–15
Little	35–45	40–50	5–15

Q17. Describe Boutonniere deformity and its management.

Deep dorsal burns damage the central slip of the extensor apparatus over the PIP joint initially or during healing phase.

↓

Lateral bands slide below the axis of rotation of the PIP joints.

↓

Lateral bands become PIP joint flexors rather than extensors and the PIP joint is flexed up to 90 degree and is unable to actively extend.

Treatment

- In acute cases; K-wire fixation and splinting is required.

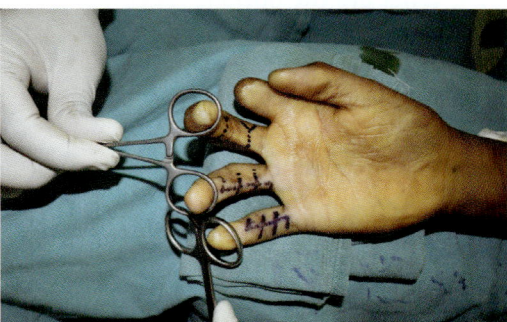

Fig. 13.11 Photograph showing marking of z-plasty for contracture of ring and little fingers.

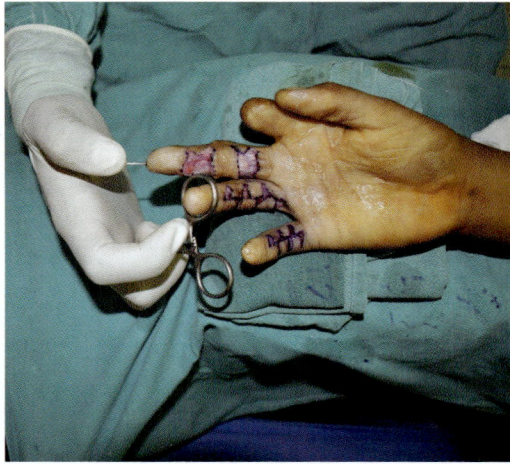

Fig. 13.12 Photograph after release of contracture by z-plasty.

- In chronic cases, surgical treatment is required.
  - Transpose the lateral bands to the dorsum of finger and suture them together.
  - Figure-of-eight tendoplasty.
  - Simple transection of the lateral bands can be done.
  - Tendon graft can be used to repair the central slip.

Q18. How will you manage DIP joint deformity?

Deep dorsal burns at DIP joint can lead to rupture or weakening of the extensor tendon at its insertion into the base of distal phalanx. This causes flexion at the DIP Joint and leads to mallet deformity. If it is associated with hyperextension at the PIP joint it results in swan-neck deformity.

Treatment

- Surgical correction by wedge excision arthrodesis in a functional position is often the only option for functional rehabilitation.

Q19. What are the options of surgery in post burn contracture (PBC) hand?

- Release of contracture by giving incision or z-plasty (**Fig. 13.11** and **Fig. 13.12**).
- Split-thickness skin graft or full-thickness skin graft (**Fig. 13.13**).
- Local flap: Dorsolateral flap, cross finger flap (**Fig. 13.14**).

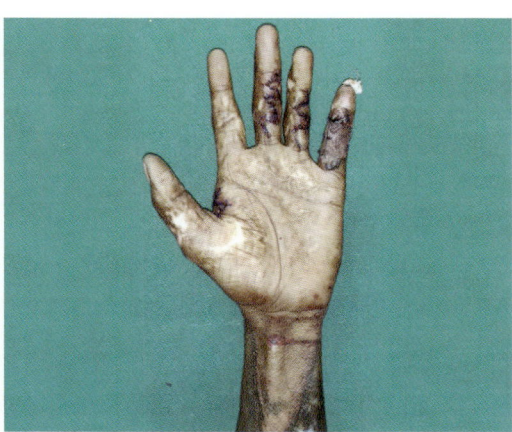

Fig. 13.13 Release of finger contracture and resurfacing with split skin graft (SSG).

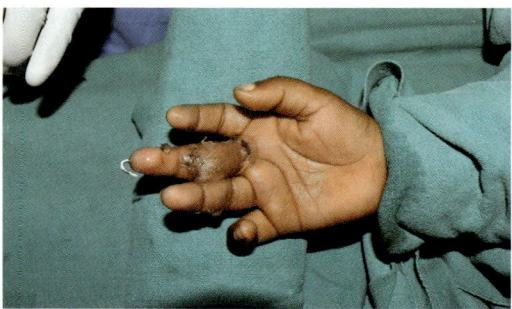

Fig. 13.14 Cross-finger flap in situ after release of contracture.

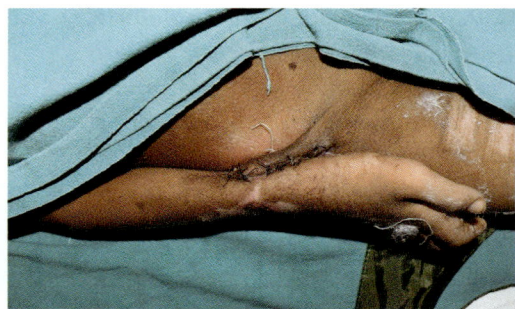

Fig. 13.15 Groin flap for post-burn contracture release at wrist.

- If large then pedicle flap: groin flap, abdominal flap (**Fig. 13.15**).
- K-wire fixation of the joint to keep the joints in the desired position.

Q20. What are the advantages of early skin grafting?
- Minimizes wound edema.
- decreases pain.
- Promotes earlier functional rehabilitation.
- Decreases the possibility of joint contractures and tendon adhesions.

Q21. What are the postoperative problems?
- Vascularity of finger may compromise. If the color of the finger is doubtful then remove K-wire, loosen dressing, and remove tight sutures.
- Graft loss may be there.
- Infection may be there.
- Recurrence of contracture.

Q22. Which graft is preferred for resurfacing of finger contractures?
Full-thickness skin graft is preferred as it is more similar to normal skin in texture, color, and resilience than SSG.

Q23. In which cases do you apply grafts harvested from palm or sole and what are the advantages?
In cases where contracture is present over palmar aspect of fingers in an adult patient, we can take SSG harvested from the ulnar aspect of hypothenar eminence or instep area of the sole. The amount of graft is sufficient to cover contracture of one to two fingers and the most important advantage is the color matching of the graft.

Q24. What are the options for correction of first web space contracture?
- Z-plasties.
- Four-flap z-plasty.
- Five-flap z-plasty.
- Local rotation flaps (first or second dorsal metacarpal artery).
- FTG or SSG.

Q25. What are the surgical options in cases where there is fixed bony deformity or destruction of joint?
In case there is fixed bony deformity or destruction of the joint is present then arthrodesis is the best option.

Q26. What is the postoperative position of the hand? (Fig. 13.16)
It is known as the safe position of the hand:
- The MCP joints should be placed at 40 to 70 degrees of flexion to prevent the collateral ligament from shortening and contracting.
- The IP joints should be maintained in extension.
- The thumb should be abducted and rotated toward the palm to prevent the contraction and fibrosis of its muscles.
- The wrist should be at 35 degrees of extension.

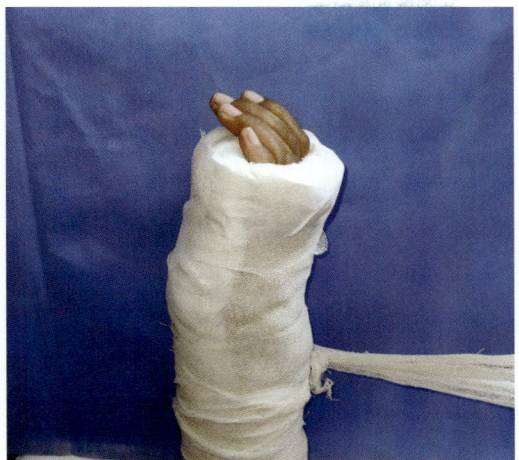

Fig. 13.16 Postoperative position of hand.

Q27. Is there any role of skin substitutes in reconstruction of hand burns?

Skin substitutes are used in cases of both acute burns and late presentations, especially for resurfacing the skin over the palmar and dorsal aspects. Advantage is that skin substitutes heal with less scarring than conventional skin grafts. For optimum function to be obtained, a skin substitute requires a bilaminate system to incorporate the desirable properties of the dermis and epidermis, particularly with respect to pore size. The outer membrane requires a small pore size to allow water vapor permeability and to act as a barrier to microorganisms. The inner layer requires a larger pore size to permit ingrowth of fibrovascular tissues from the wound bed.

Q28. What is Integra?

Integra was designed by Yannas and Burke. It is a bilaminar acellular matrix which consists of an outer Silastic sheet and an inner layer of highly porous structure composed of cross-linked coprecipitate of bovine collagen and chondroitin 6-sulfate derived from shark cartilage. After application, the recipient fibroblasts infiltrate the matrix network and synthesize a neodermis that is very close to the normal human dermis while the artificial dermis undergoes biodegradation. Adequate revascularization requires 2 to 3 weeks, by which time the Silastic membrane, an epidermis-like structure which controls water loss and prevents invasion of microbes, is removed and replaced by an ultrathin (usually less than 0.01 inch) epidermal overlay. The resulting coverage is pliable and nonadherent to deeper structures and it shows no meshed pattern. The donor site heals satisfactorily within 1 week.

Q29. What is AlloDerm?

AlloDerm is an acellular allogeneic dermal matrix processed from human allograft skin with preservation of the type IV collagen of the basement membrane. The final product is devoid of type I and type II major histocompatibility antigens. It is intended to provide a permanent nonimmunogenic template to augment the dermal component of a meshed or sheet split-thickness skin graft when it is used on a full-thickness wound.

Q30. What is biotemporizing matrix (BTM)?

BTM is composed of three layers including biodegrading foam, bonding layer, and sealing membrane which acts as an interface for deep burns down to the muscle. The wound-facing foam is biodegradable, synthetic, nonbiological, polyurethane temporizing dermal substitute intended for use in replacement of tissue loss due to burns or trauma.

Advantages:

- It is nonallergic as it does not contain any sensitizing proteins.
- As it contains synthetic material, it offers a higher resistance to infection.
- Can also be applied on surgically debrided wounds.

Contraindications:

- Severely discharging wounds.

Suggested Readings

1. Robert LM, Malachy EA. Mathes text book of plastic surgery. Elsevier; 2006:186, 605–645
2. Germann G, Philipp K. Green operative. Hand Surgery;61:1–99
3. Singh V, Haq A, Sharma S, et al. Pre-operative scrutiny of late burned hand presentations: crucial step for the improvement of results. Burns Open 2021;5:104–112

Post-Burn Contracture (PBC) Axilla and Knee

Rimpi Jain

Learning Objectives

At the end of this chapter, the students will be able to:

1. Summarize the clinical presentation of PBC axilla and knee.
2. Demonstrate the examination in these patients.
3. Understand the types of contracture and relevant plan of management.
4. Demonstrate the markings of various flaps used for coverage in PBC axilla and knee.

Introduction

Contracture of axilla and knee as a sequela to burns involves reconstructive challenges owing to the restriction in day-to-day activities due to the involved functional impairment. The goal of surgical correction should be to provide the maximum release so as to facilitate the complete range of motion (ROM). The most common treatment methods are incisional contracture release and cover with skin graft or local flaps. A detailed examination of the extent of restrictions in movement and assessment of the severity and type of contracture will help in choosing the most appropriate surgical procedure and affect the outcomes.

PBC Axilla

History

Particulars of the patient (name, age, sex, occupation, residence, etc.).

Chief Complaints

- Difficulty in lifting the arm overhead.
- Difficulty in movements of the shoulder.
- Difficulty in straightening the arm.
- Thickened scar in armpit.
- Itching over the scar.

History of Present Illness

- Patient was apparently well before she/he sustained burn injury.
- Duration and mode of burn—accidental, suicidal or homicidal
- Write in details about the cause of burn—whether flame, scalds, or chemical burn and the exact description of the event.
- Enquire about the temperature and duration in cases of contact burns.
- Whether immediate cooling with water after injury done or not and for how long.
- Whether first aid received and where—local clinic or burn center, details of treatment received, whether required admission, any history of blisters.
- Whether open dressings or close dressings done—at home or by a doctor.
- If admitted, then for how long and what was the condition of the burn wound at the time of discharge.
- Ask about the progression of contracture and duration.
- Any surgical intervention for the wound or contracture.

- Any physiotherapy or splintage provided or not.

Negative History

- Difficulty in combing the hair.
- Difficulty in performing routine household activities.
- Any discharge from the scar.
- History of itching over scar.

Past History

History of diabetes mellitus, hypertension, tuberculosis, or any other medical illness. Any surgery done in the past for the current problems.

Personal History

History of addiction including alcoholism, smoking, marital status, number of kids, employment status. In case of females, ask for the date of last menstrual period (LMP).

Family History

Number of family members dependent on the patient.

Treatment History

History of allergy to food or medications.

General Physical Examination

General survey: Apart from general examination, examine bilateral thighs for graft donor site.

Local Examination of Shoulder and Axillary Region

Inspection

1. Look for attitude of arm at shoulder joint.

2. Look for extent of scar and contracture in terms of definitive landmarks like:
   - Acromion process.
   - Midpoint of arm.
   - Midaxillary line.
   - Anterior axillary line.
   - Nipple.
3. Whether only anterior fold or posterior or both involved.
4. Involvement of axillary pit or not.
5. Examine Scar
   - Whether raised or not.
   - Color of the scar.
   - Margin of the scar.
   - Surface of the scar.
   - Pigmentation.
   - Vancouver scar scale.
   - Any pits or sinuses in the scar.

Palpation

1. Temperature and tenderness over the scar.
2. Measure the extent of scar in both vertical and transverse dimensions.
3. In vertical dimensions how far away it is from the midpoint of inner side of arm?
4. Similarly, in downward direction for how far it extends in the midaxillary line.
5. Similarly, measure the transverse extent of the scar.
6. Palpate the armpit whether there is involvement of the armpit or not.
7. Surface of scar.
8. Margins of scar.
9. Consistency.
10. Blanching or not.
11. Able to pinch the scar or not.
12. Sensations over scar to assess the depth of burn.

Movements

Examine movements at shoulder joint.
1. Abduction: It begins with the arm in a position parallel to the torso and hand in an

inferior position, continues with the movement of the arm to a position perpendicular to the torso, and ends with the movement of the arm so that the humerus is raised above the shoulder joint and hand points straight upward.

2. Adduction: Sometimes hypertrophic scar resists complete adduction due to its thickness.
3. Flexion: The movement of humerus straight anteriorly.
4. Extension: The movement of humerus straight posteriorly.
5. External rotation: The movement of humerus laterally around its long axis away from the midline.
6. Internal rotation: The movement of humerus laterally around its long axis away from the midline.
7. Circumduction.

Measurement of Defect

- The principles of measurement of apparent and true defect remains the same as in PBC neck.
- Measure the apparent defect: The extent of scar in both vertical and transverse dimensions.
- Measure the true defect.
  - On arm: Measure the distance of the farthest point of scar from the midpoint of inner side of arm.
  - On chest: Measure the distance of the farthest point of scar from the midaxillary line.
  - Similarly, measure the transverse extent of the scar from the highest point of axillary pit.
  - Measure the same distance between same landmarks in normal opposite side of axilla. This will be the true defect.

Systemic Examination

As done elsewhere.

Provisional Diagnosis

This is a case of a 35-year-old male patient with 6 months old post flame burn contracture left axilla type 1A with hypertrophic scar and multiple hypopigmented patches.

- Give a complete diagnosis mentioning:
  - Side and site of contracture.
  - Duration.
  - Grading of contracture.
  - Any associated scar anomalies like hypertrophic, hypopigmentation, etc., also need to be mentioned.

Questions

Q1. How will you proceed?

I will plan for contracture release and appropriate skin cover after obtaining preanesthetic fitness for which I will get baseline investigations:

- Blood for Hb, total leukocyte count (TLC), differential leukocyte count (DLC), erythrocyte sedimentation rate (ESR).
- Blood for sugar, urea, creatinine, electrolytes.
- Chest X-ray.
- Electrocardiography (ECG).
- Viral markers.

Q2. What is the grading of axillary contracture?

- Grading of Axillary contractures was given by Kurtzman and Stern.
- Three grades:
  - Type 1A: Contracture involving anterior axillary fold (**Fig. 14.1a, b**).
  - Type 1B: Contracture involving posterior axillary fold (**Fig. 14.2**).
  - Type 2: Contracture involving both anterior and posterior axillary folds (sparing axillary dome) (**Fig. 14.3**).
  - Type 3: Contracture involving both anterior and posterior axillary folds plus axillary dome (**Fig. 14.4a, b**).

Q3. What is the goal of surgical corrections?

The goal is to do the maximum release of the contracture so as to provide the complete ROM

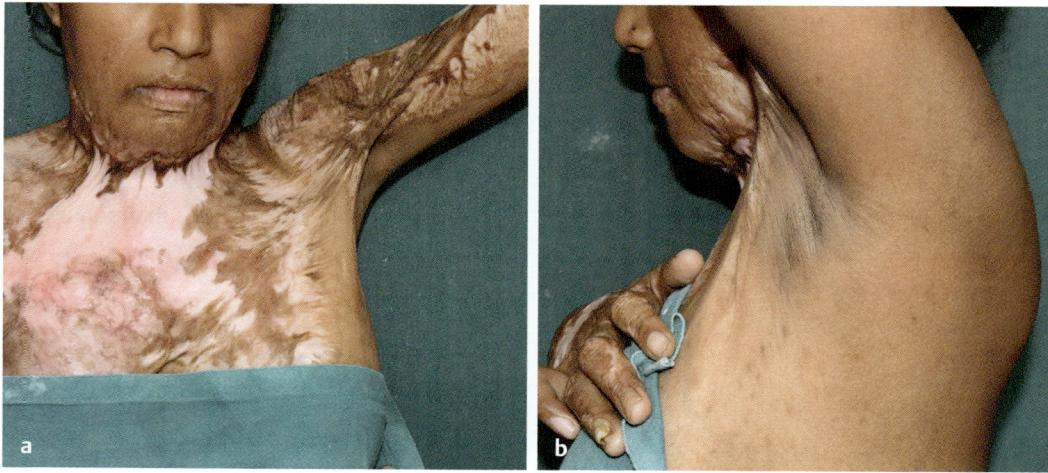

Fig. 14.1 **(a, b)** Grade 1A post burn contracture of axilla.

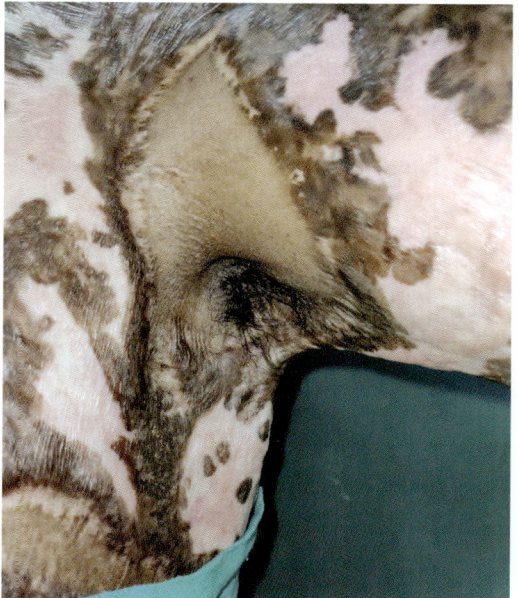

Fig. 14.2 Grade 1B post burn contracture of axilla.

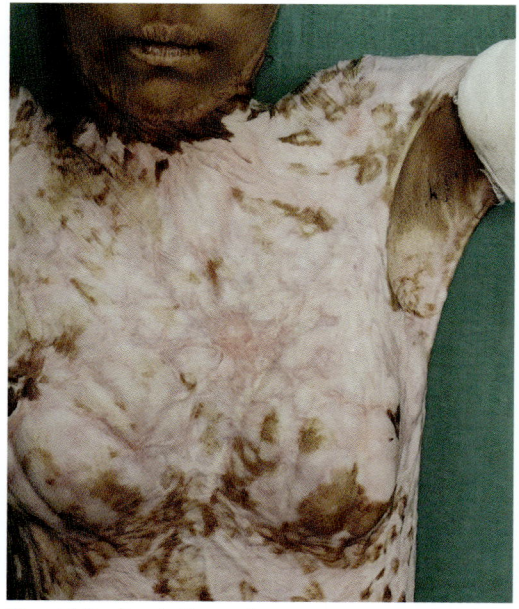

Fig. 14.3 Grade 2 post burn contracture of axilla.

at the shoulder joint with little or no anatomic distortion.

Q4. What are the principles of release of axillary contracture?

- Contracture should be released completely up to normal tissue.
- Incision should begin across the point of maximum tension.
- Avoid damage to underlying vessels and nerves.
- Fish tailing of the incision should be done on either side.
- Ideal material for coverage should be thin, supple, and large well-vascularized healthy tissue.

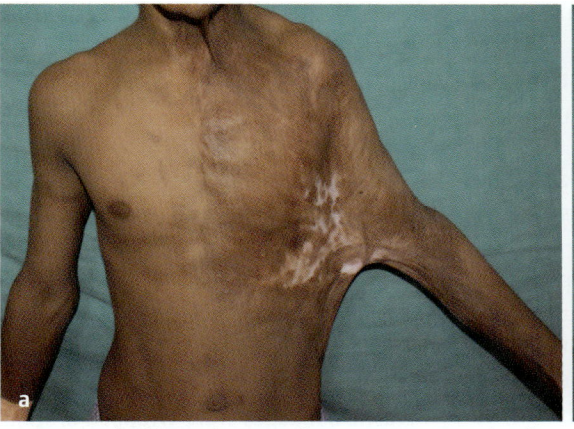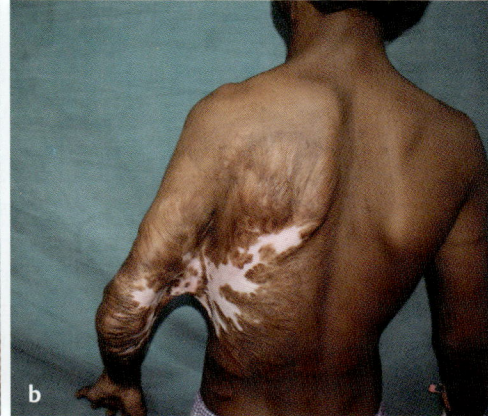

Fig. 14.4 (a, b) Grade 3 post burn contracture of axilla.

Q5. What are the normal ROMs at shoulder joint?

- Flexion:
  - Move your arm from palms against the side of your body to the highest point you can raise your arms over your head.
  - Normal range for shoulder flexion is 180 degrees.
- Extension:
  - Move your hands behind you in straight position.
  - It is between 45 and 60 degrees.
- Abduction:
  - It occurs when the movement of the arm is away from the middle of your body.
  - Normal range is 150 degrees.
- Adduction:
  - When the movement of the arm is toward the middle of the body.
  - Normal range is 30 to 50 degrees.
- Medial rotations:
  - With arms at sides, palm is turned toward body and elbow is bent.
  - Normal range is 70 to 90 degrees.
- Lateral rotation:
  - With arms at sides, palms facing the body and elbow is bent at 90 degrees.
  - Normal range is 90 degrees.

Q6. What is the sequence of contracture release in case of contracture involving axilla, elbow, and hand?

- The sequence of contracture release is always proximal to distal.
- First release the contracture of axilla in the first stage, then elbow in the second stage, and then hand in the next stage.

Q7. What is the surgical approach for different grading of axillary contracture?

- Type 1 and 2 contractures:
  - Z-plasty.
  - V-Y plasty.
  - Contracture release and local flaps.
  - Skin graft.
- Type 3 contracture:
  - Release of contracture and skins grafting.
  - Release of contracture and cover with flaps.

Q8. What are the different procedures for axillary contracture and what are their indications?

- Single Z-plasty: It is indicated when the contracture is linear involving the anterior or posterior axillary fold and the surrounding skin is healthy.

- Multiple Z-plasties: It is indicated for long linear scars.
- V-Y plasty: It is used when sufficient laxity is present perpendicular to the scar contracture axis.
- Five-flap plasty: It is indicated in linear scars having short web where wide release is required.
- Local fasciocutaneous flaps: Local flaps from arm, anterior chest, or back are required in cases of localized moderate bands of contractures of anterior or posterior axillary folds. Donor site should not be scarred.
- Skin grafting: Release of contracture and cover with skin grafting is done when the surrounding skin is scarred and no local flaps are available.
- Parascapular flaps: This is the flap of choice to cover the defect after release of axilla contracture if the width of defect is less than 8 cm. If the width of the defect is more than 8 cm then donor site is covered by split-thickness skin graft.
- Square flap: It was proposed by Hyakusoku et al in 1985.
  - It is a modification of Limberg flap.
  - Also known as three-flap Z-plasty.
  - It is an advancement transposition technique which consists of two triangular flaps which are transposed and a square flap which is advanced.
- Propeller flap: It is used in cases where axillary dome has been spared.

Q9. What is the protocol for postoperative splinting in PBC axilla?

- When splinting is done after Z-plasty and five-flap plasty, then it is required for 2 to 3 weeks.
- When splinting is done after release of contracture and skin grafting then continuous splinting is required for a period of 6 weeks and then night splinting is required for up to 6 months.

Q10. What are the types of splints used in PBC axilla?

- Aeroplane splint:
  - It is made of thermoplastic material or aluminum.
  - The name is given because it is like the aeroplane wing, keeps the shoulder in maximum abduction. The shoulder is in 80 to 120 degrees of abduction after release of axillary contracture.
- Figure-of-8 compression dressing:
  - It was used in the past.
  - Elastic bandages were wrapped around the shoulder joint in a "figure-of-8" to keep the shoulder abducted.

Q11. Describe markings of scapular and parascapular flaps.

- Vascular basis and landmarks (**Fig. 14.5a, b**):
  - The scapular and parascapular flap is based on the circumflex scapular artery (CSA), which is a branch of the subscapular artery.
  - The CSA emerges through the triangular space which is bounded by the teres major inferiorly, teres minor and subscapularis superiorly, and long head of triceps laterally.
  - The CSA is situated two-fifths of the distance from scapular spine to the scapular tip along the lateral border.
- **Axis of scapular flap** extends from triangular space to midline, superior boundary is scapular spine, and inferior boundary is scapular tip.
- **Axis of parascapular flap** extends from triangular space along the lateral border of the scapula to the posterior superior iliac spine.
- The cutaneous branches of the CSA are fairly consistent, and give rise to the transverse and descending branches supplying the scapular and parascapular flaps, respectively.

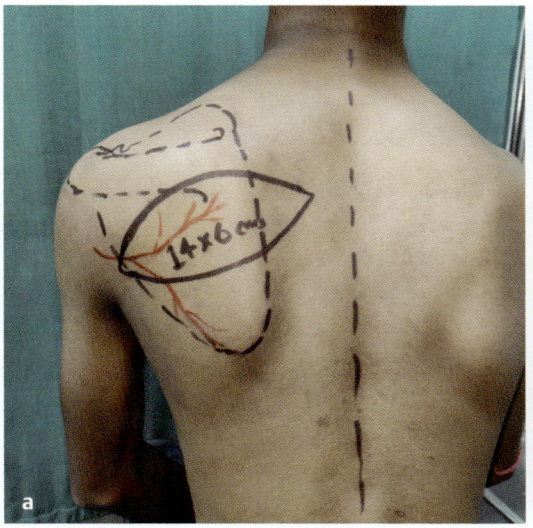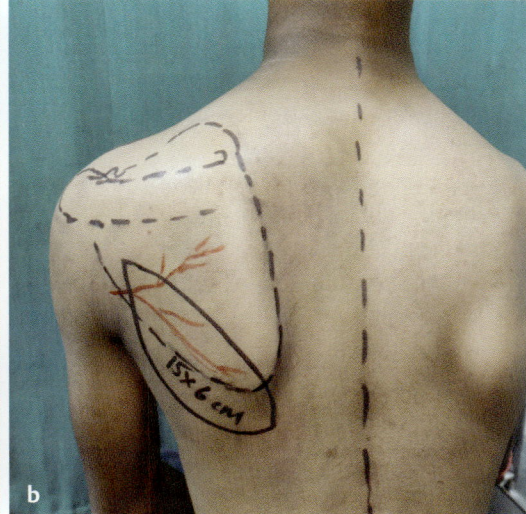

Fig. 14.5 (a, b) Markings of scapular and parascapular flaps.

- Flap harvest:
  - The patient is placed in the lateral decubitus position, with the respective arm extended.
  - The borders of the scapula and triangular space are marked.
  - Preoperative design of the skin flap is based on either the use of the scapular or parascapular flap.
  - A skin island of up to 10 cm × 30 cm in dimension can be harvested. If the width of the skin is more than 10 cm, skin grafting is required.
  - The flap is raised superficial to the deep fascia overlying the muscles of shoulder.
    - In the case of the scapular flap, the medial portion is raised first and dissection proceeds laterally.
    - In case of parascapular orientation, the flap is raised from inferior to superior.
  - Once the superior border of the teres major muscle is reached, care must be taken as the main pedicle emerges immediately superior.
  - The vessels are dissected as they emerge from the triangular space back to its subscapular artery origins.
  - A typical pedicle length of 6 to 10 cm can be achieved.

PBC Knee

History

Particulars of the patient (name, age, sex, occupation, residence, etc.).

Chief Complaints

Usual chief complaints are:
- Inability to straighten the knee (right or left) completely.
- Restricted rotational movements at knee.
- Difficulty in walking.
- Difficulty in sitting, squatting.
- Thickened scar over back of knee.
- Itching over scar.

History of Present Illness

- Patient was apparently well before he/she sustained burn months/years back.
- Whether accidental/suicidal/homicidal (includes acid burn attacks).

- Write about the cause of burn—whether flame burn, scald burn, chemical burn.
- Write in details about the temperature (hot/very hot/extremely hot) and duration of contact.
- Ask about history of facial burn, inhalation injury, difficulty in breathing.
- Ask about the history of blisters.
- After sustaining burns, whether immediate cooling with water done or not and for how long.
- Enquire about the treatment received after burns: About medication.
- Whether open or closed dressing done.
- Whether dressing done by patient at home or by doctor/paramedics.
- Ask about the history of progression of contracture, and time taken in developing contracture.
- History of any surgical intervention.
- Any physiotherapy or splintage provided or not.
- Ask about the condition of the wound at the time of discharge.

Negative History

- Any difficulty in mouth opening and closing.
- Difficulty in eating and drinking.
- Drooling of saliva, if any.
- Difficulty in speech.
- Ask about the range of vision and presence of restriction, if any.
- History of itching over scar --how severe, frequency, any self-medication for the relief.
- Any discharge from the scar or history of recurrent wound breakdown and healing.
- History of pain.

Past History

- History of diabetes mellitus, hypertension, tuberculosis, or any other medical illness.

- Any surgery done in the past for the current problems.

Personal History

History of addiction including alcoholism, smoking, marital status, number of kids, employment status. In case of females, ask for the date of last menstrual period (LMP).

Family History

Number of family members dependent on the patient.

Treatment History

History of allergy to food or medications.

General Physical Examination

- Apart from other general examination, examine bilateral thighs for graft donor site.
- Examine the gait or difficulty in walking.

Local Examination of Knee Region

Exposure
Proper exposure of both the lower limbs up to gluteal region should be done in adequate light and with informed consent.

Inspection

Knee

- Look for attitude of knee joint. Knee joint will be in flexion in case of PBC.
- Look for extent of scar and contracture in terms of definitive landmarks like:
  - Popliteal fossa.
  - Ankle joint.
  - Midpoint of thigh.

Scar

- Whether raised or not.
- Color of scar.
- Margin of scar.
- Surface of scar.
- Pigmentation.
- Vancouver scar scale.
- Any pits or sinuses in the scar.

Palpation

- Temperature and tenderness over the scar.
- Extent of the scar-size measurement in both vertical and transverse dimensions from a definitive landmark.
- Popliteal fossa: How far does the scar/contracture extend from the popliteal fossa in both upward and downward direction.
- Ankle joint: How far away is the contracture from the ankle joint?
- Midpoint of thigh: How far away is the contracture from the midpoint of thigh?
- Also measure contracture in transverse dimension.
- Surface of scar.
- Margin of scar.
- Consistency.
- Blanching or not.
- Able to pinch the scar or not.
- Vancouver burn scar scale.
- Sensations over scar to assess the depth of burn.

Movements

- Look for flexion.
- Look for extension.
- Rotational movements at knee joint.
- Range of movements.

Measurement of Defect

Apparent and True Defect

- The principles of measurement of apparent and true defects remain the same as in PBC neck.

- Apparent defect.
  - Measure the extent of scar both in vertical and horizontal dimensions. This represents the defect occupied by the scar, and therefore, it is "apparent."
  - Then, measure the distance of scar margins from the appropriate landmarks. In knee contracture four landmarks can be chosen, such as:
    - For longitudinal measurements:
      - Above—ASIS/PSIS.
      - Below—medial/lateral malleolus.
    - For transverse measurements:
      - Medial and lateral—tibial tuberosity.
- True defect.
  - Mark the landmarks on the opposite leg and measure the distance from same landmarks on the normal side if the burn is unilateral.
  - You will get four points which can be joined to form the area of defect after contracture release. This is the "true" defect which represents the exact size of flap or graft required.
  - Mark the true defect only after assessing whether you are going to excise/incise the contracture.
  - If contracture is present in bilateral knees, then measure those distances with same landmarks in a normal individual of same age, sex, and build to get the extent of true defect.

Systemic Examination

Same as others.

Provisional Diagnosis

This is a case of a 12-year-old child with 8 months old post flame burn linear contracture of left knee with hypertrophic scar and multiple hypopigmented patches.

- Give a complete diagnosis mentioning:
  - Side and site of contracture.
  - Duration.

– Grading of contracture.
– Any associated scar anomalies like hypertrophic, hypopigmentation, etc., also need to be mentioned.

Questions

Q1. How will you proceed?
I will plan for contracture release and appropriate skin cover after obtaining preanesthetic fitness for which I will get baseline investigations done.

Q2. What is the classification of post burn knee contracture?
- Post burn knee contracture is classified in three groups by Ogawa and Pribaz.
  - Linear (**Fig. 14.6**).
  - Broad band (**Fig. 14.7**).
  - Circumference (**Fig. 14.8**).
- Another classification of knee contracture is given by Dougherty et al. Two forms of knee contractures.
  - Medially or laterally with unburned skin posteriorly.
  - Contracture of the entire popliteal fossa.

- Hudson et al divided into two types:
  - Mild: restriction of <50% ROM of any joint of extremity.
  - Severe: restriction of >50% ROM of any joint of extremity.

Q3. What is the timing of surgery in post burn contracture knee?
- If less than 6 months then release the whole scar by excise as it is immature and cover the entire defect with graft/flap.
- If more than 6 months then release by incision of the contracture.

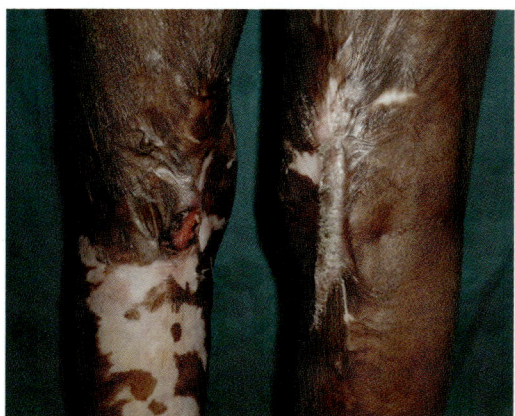

Fig. 14.6 Linear contracture of knee.

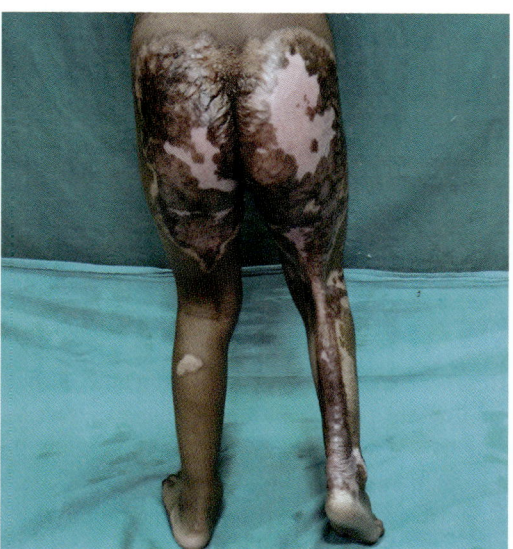

Fig. 14.7 Broad contracture of knee.

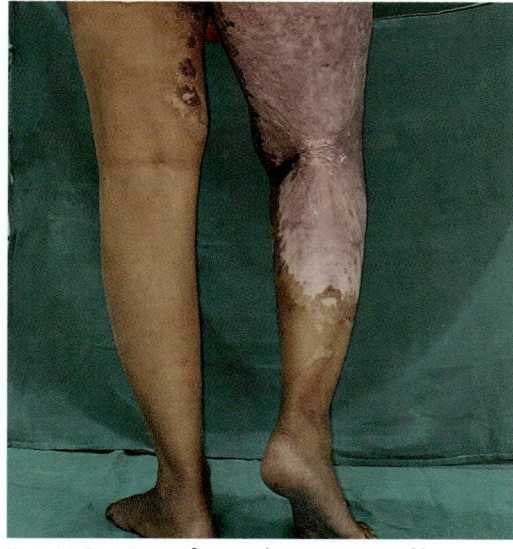

Fig. 14.8 Circumferential contracture of knee.

Q4. What are the principles of release of contracture knee?

Following are the principles:

- Contracture should be released completely up to normal tissue.
- Avoid damage to important underlying structures: artery, vein, and nerves.
- Incision should begin across the point of maximum tension, (i.e., where the contracture is most tight).
- Fish tailing of the incision on either side should be done to avoid linear scar contracture.
- Circulation of the distal part of the limb should be checked constantly during release of knee contracture and release of contracture should be stopped before the appearance of solid structures.
- Ideal material for coverage should be thin, supple, and large well-vascularized healthy tissue.
- Intermediate thickness graft is appropriate as compared to split-thickness skin graft.

Q5. What are the options to cover the defect created after release of knee contracture?

Following are the options:

- Skin grafting.
- Z-plasty, Y-V plasty.
- Flap cover.
- Artificial skin substitutes.
- Tissue expansion with or without flap cover.

Q6. What is the normal ROM of knee joint?

- Knee flexion is 145 to 155 degrees.
  - Slightly more in females: 151.2 to 154 degrees.
  - Slightly less in male: 146 to 149 degrees.

Q7. What are the possible movement at knee joint?

Following are the movements:

- Flexion (blending).
- Extension (straightening).

- Adduction (movement toward middle of the body).
- Abduction (movement away from middle of the body).
- Rotations (inward and outward).

Q8. What is the normal knee active range of motion (AROM)?

It is between 0 degrees of knee extension (a fully straightened knee) and 135 degrees of knee flexion.

Q9. What is the anatomy of popliteal fossa?

- Popliteal fossa is bounded by:
  - Superomedially: Semitendinosus, semimembranosus, gracilis, and sartorius tendons.
  - Superolaterally: Biceps femoris tendon.
  - Inferomedially: Medial head of gastrocnemius.
- Popliteal vessels and tibial nerve and common peroneal nerve cross the fossa deep to the popliteal fascia.
- Short saphenous vein, posterior cutaneous nerve of thigh, posterior division of medially cutaneous nerve of thigh, and peroneal communicating nerve pass through the fat layer superficial to the popliteal fascia.
- The arterial network of genicular arteries supplies the knee joint.

Q10. What are the treatment options?

- Mild contracture can be released by Z-plasty.
- Mild to moderate contracture can be released with Z-plasty, V-Y plasty, or incisional release with skin grafting.
- Severe contracture can be released and covered with skin grafting and local flaps.
  - Bilateral flaps from medial and lateral sides of popliteal area.
  - Gastrocnemius muscle flap.
  - Distally based fasciocutaneous thick flap.
  - Medial sural perforator plus island flap.
  - Proximally based sural flap.
  - Posterior calf fascial flap.

Q11. What are the other treatment options?

- In case of severe contracture and exposed vessels and nerves the defect can be covered with free flap like free anterolateral thigh flap.
- Ilizarov technique can be combined with free flap for severe contracture.

Q12. What is the goal of release of knee contracture?

Goal is to create the normal function and appearance as much as possible.

Q13. What are the postoperative instructions?

- Joint should be immobilized in extension.
- •. Small window should be kept open to look at the flaps vascularity.
- •. Dressing is usually done at 7 to 10 days.

Q14. What are the instructions to be given at the time of discharge?

- Regular dressing should be done.
- Knee should be kept in extension.
- Physiotherapy of knee joint to start after 3 weeks or healing of wound.
- Scar therapy is advised for 6 months.

- Knee joint splint should be advised regularly for 3 months.
- Compression bandages and night splint for 6 months.

Q15. What are the flaps available for cover of defects after PBC knee release?

- Gastrocnemius muscle flap: Refer to chapter 1 on "Lower leg defect."
- Antegrade sural flap: Refer to chapter 1 on "Lower leg defect."
- Proximally based adipofascial flap.
  - It has the same vascular basis as antegrade sural flap but composition is only deep fascia and a thin layer of adipose tissue.
  - It is used as a turnover flap to fill the defect after release of severe knee contractures. Skin graft (SSG) is then placed over the fascial part of the flap and the donor site is closed primarily.
  - **Advantages:**
    - Adipofascial flaps can be used even if surrounding skin is scarred.
    - Does not hinder the complete flexion of knee.
    - Primary closure of donor site.

15 Cleft Lip and Palate

Rimpi Jain and Anupama Kumari

Learning Objectives

At the end of this chapter, the student will be able to:
1. Describe the clinical presentation of a patient with cleft lip and palate.
2. Recall the anatomy and embryological development of face.
3. Understand the stages of repair in cleft lip and palate.
4. Demonstrate the markings of repair in cleft lip and palate.
5. Perform the common surgical procedures.

Introduction

There are several different treatment plans leading to the surgical correction of the cleft lip and palate deformity. Deficiencies of soft tissue, cartilage, and bone in cleft patients are difficult to evaluate accurately. A systematic approach to a cleft child is crucial in deciding the appropriate timeline, choosing the right surgical procedure and, overall, a holistic management.

History Taking

Details of the Patient

- Name, age, gender, whether informant is mother/father.
- Usually, mother is the informant in most cases.

Chief Complaints in Cleft Lip ± Alveolus

- Defect in lip.
- Difficulty in sucking breast milk (in complete cleft lip).
- Abnormal dentition (in grown-up child).

Chief Complaints in Cleft Palate

- Defect in palate.
- Nasal regurgitation of feeds.
- Repeated cold and cough.
- Ear discharge.
- Difficulty in speech—in a slightly grown-up child.

History of Present Illness

- Ask in detail about the progression of symptoms.
- Ask in detail about the feeding history—feeding is given via bottle/katori-spoon, whether mother's milk or top-up, how much amount, how frequently, whether burping done after every feed.

Negative History

- History of breathing difficulty even once or any abnormal sound heard from child's throat or chest. Any history of baby turning blue—to rule out Pierre Robin sequence.
- History of recurrent upper respiratory tract infection or ear discharge.

- History of nasal intonation of voice if child has started speaking words or sentences.
- Presence of any other deformity in the body.

Antenatal History

- Ask about the duration of pregnancy—full term or preterm.
- Whether delivered by normal vaginal delivery or cesarean section.
- Whether the child cried immediately after birth.
- History of drug intake for any chronic illness:
  - Phenytoin.
  - Anticonvulsants.
  - Retinoic acid.
  - Steroids.
  - Diazepam.
- History of maternal epilepsy during antenatal period.
- Smoking history.
- Alcohol intake.
- Diabetes.
- Any history of radiation exposure during pregnancy.
- History of any viral infection like Rubella.
- If any of the above history is positive, then ask in which trimester.
- Ask about the birth weight of the baby.

Family History

- Any history of cleft lip and palate in the siblings.
- History of similar deformity on maternal and paternal side—mother, father, uncle, aunt, grandmother, grandfather.
- History of consanguineous marriage.

Immunization History

- Ask about the vaccines that the baby has received till date.
- Received BCG at birth.

History of Allergy

To any drug or food.

General Examination

- In case of child, anthropometry is very important to assess the normal development of the child. Measure the height and weight of the child.
- In case of infant, height = length.
- Look for features of malnourishment—listless child or not so playful, thin or bloated appearance, loss of muscle mass, dry and rough skin, loss of hair pigmentation. On skin pinch, it will be slow to go back.
- Look for any other skin anomaly.

Systemic Examination

It is important to rule out other deformities.
- Abdomen: Look for the feel of the abdomen or any organomegaly.
- Central nervous system (CNS) (cranium & spine): Higher mental functions are difficult to examine in a child, mother can be asked about the normal milestones of the child.
  - Shape of the skull (look for features of hydrocephalus and presence of meningocele).
- Cardio vascular system (CVS): Auscultate for the heart sounds, any murmur (associated congenital anomalies can be there).
- Respiratory system: Auscultate for normal breath sounds and air entry.
- Genitourinary system: Look for any abnormality, (e.g., hypospadias, undescended testis especially in a syndromic child).

Local Examination of Lip and Palate

Inspection

Lip (Fig. 15.1a, b)

1. Look for facial symmetry.

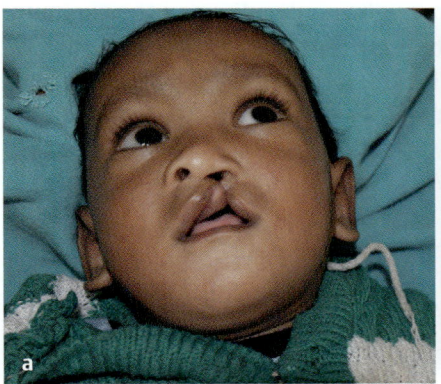
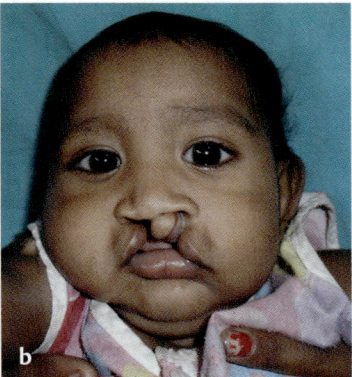

Fig. 15.1 (a, b) U/L and B/L cleft lip.

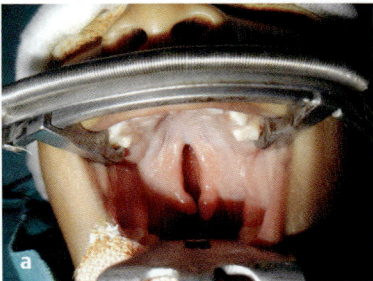
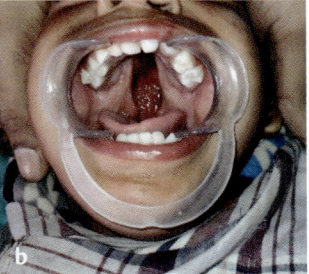
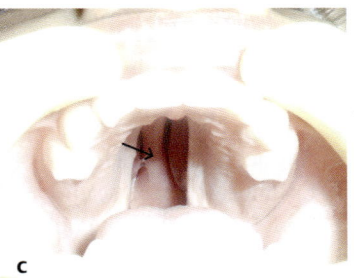

Fig. 15.2 (a, b) Incomplete and complete cleft palate. **(c)** Vomer bone in the midline.

2. Side of cleft whether unilateral or bilateral.
3. Complete or incomplete.
4. Width of cleft.
5. Simonart band.

Alveolus

Look whether cleft in alveolus is present or not.

Palate (Fig. 15.2a, b)

1. Extent of cleft → Complete
   → Incomplete
2. Involvement of hard palate/soft palate/uvula.
3. Width of cleft as compared with the width of palatine shelves.
4. Status of uvula—bifid or not.
5. Look for palatal arch:
   - Whether normal.
   - High arched—in case of Treacher Collin syndrome and Pierre Robin syndrome.
   - Flat.

6. Look for Vomer—whether in midline or deviated, whether one/both sides are visible (**Fig. 15.2c**).
7. Condition of tonsils—whether normal sized or enlarged.
8. Pharyngeal arches—whether inflamed.
9. Posterior pharyngeal wall—any redness present or not.
10. Look for dentition—no. of teeth present, any carious tooth.

Nose (Fig. 15.3)

1. Examine nasal dorsum—may be depressed.
2. Deviation of nasal tip—usually deviated to noncleft side.
3. Look for flaring of ala or alar displacement.
4. Examine nostril—size may be smaller on cleft side.
5. Columella—usually deviated to noncleft side.
6. Septum deviated or not or to which side.
7. Examine nasal sill—intact in incomplete cleft and disrupted in complete cleft lip.

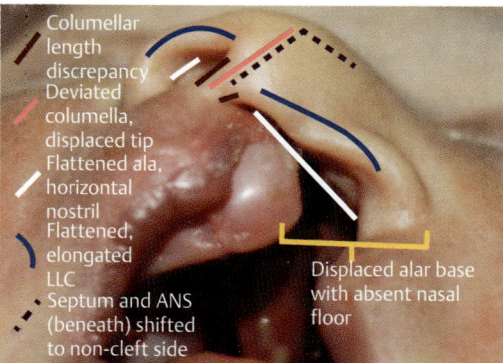

Columellar length discrepancy
Deviated columella, displaced tip
Flattened ala, horizontal nostril
Flattened, elongated LLC
Septum and ANS (beneath) shifted to non-cleft side

Displaced alar base with absent nasal floor

Fig. 15.3 Deformities in the nose.

Ear

1. Rule out chronic suppurative otitis media (CSOM).
2. Any discharge from ear.
3. Any accessory auricle.
4. Examine head and scalp.
5. Look for maxillary hypoplasia or not.
6. Examine mandible for Pierre Robin syndrome.

Provisional Diagnosis

This is a case of a 5-month-old baby with left-sided cleft lip and palate Group III according to Nagpur classification without any associated congenital deformity.

Questions

Q1. How will you proceed?

- I would like to plan the cleft lip repair in this baby. Before surgery, I would go for some investigations for two purposes:
  - Baseline investigations to assess the fitness of the patient for surgery.
    - Blood for hemoglobin (Hb), total leukocyte count (TLC), differential leukocyte count (DLC), erythrocyte sedimentation rate (ESR).
    - Blood urea, serum creatinine.
  - And, a pediatric consultation for ruling out other associated congenital anomalies, if any.
- Preoperative photographs of the patient.
- Dental models.

Q2. How will you decide upon the timing of operation for cleft lip?

According to Millard Rule of 10s, the following criteria must be ensured before embarking upon surgery of cleft lip:

- Weight of baby should be 10 pounds (>4.5 kg).
- Hemoglobin of 10 g/dL.
- Ten weeks of age.
- White blood count (WBC) count should be <10,000/cmm.

Q3. What are the anesthetic considerations and other preoperative precautions to be taken care of during surgery?

- Surgery to be done under general anesthesia.
- Position of patient: Neck should be in extension with pillow under shoulder.
- Throat packing should be done.
- Eye ointment should be applied to protect against corneal injury or eyelid taping is done.
- Once marking of lip repair is done, tattooing should be done and then local anesthetic agent with dilute adrenaline is infiltrated to avoid distortion of markings.

Q4. What are the goals in unilateral cleft lip repair?

- To restore the function of the orbicularis oris muscle.
- To achieve a cosmetically favorable lip.

Q5. What are the goals in bilateral cleft lip repair?

- To bring the lateral parts of the lip together with the middle part of the lip to close the lip.
- To create missing philtral columns.
- To create a Cupid's bow.

Q6. What are the criteria of a good lip repair?

- Steffenson, in 1953 gave criteria for a good lip repair:
  - Skin, muscle, and mucous membrane union should be accurate.

- Nostril floors should be symmetrical.
- Vermilion border should be symmetrical.
- Lip should be slightly everted.
- There should be minimal scar which by its contraction will not interfere with the above requirements.
- Musgrave, in 1963 added two other criteria:
  - Cupid's bow and the vermilion cutaneous ridge should be preserved.
  - Symmetrical nostrils as well as symmetrical nostril floors.

Q6. What are the commonly used classifications of cleft lip and palate?

- Davis and Ritchie:
  - In this classification cleft is divided into three groups according to the position of cleft in relation to alveolar process.
    - Group 1—Cleft is prealveolar which may be unilateral, median, or bilateral.
    - Group 2—Cleft is postalveolar which involves the soft palate only, soft and hard palate or submucous cleft.
    - Group 3—Alveolar clefts which may be unilateral, bilateral, or median.
  - Disadvantages:
    - It does not describe lip deformity.
    - It does not describe cleft of primary palate with intact secondary palate.
- Nagpur classification by Dr. C. Balkrishnan:

Group I	Cleft lip
Group I(a)	Cleft lip with cleft alveolus
Group II	Cleft palate
Group II(S)	Submucous cleft palate
Group III	Cleft lip and palate

- Veau Classification—Four types:
  - Based on morphology.

Type I	Cleft of soft palate only
Type II	Cleft of hard and soft palate extending no further than incisive foramen, thus involving the secondary palate alone
Type III	Complete unilateral cleft
Type IV	Complete bilateral cleft

- Kernahan and Stark:
  - Based on embryology rather than morphology.
    - Incisive foramen divides the primary and secondary palates (**Fig. 15.4**).
    - Elsahy added triangular peaks which indicate nasal floor (**Fig. 15.5**).

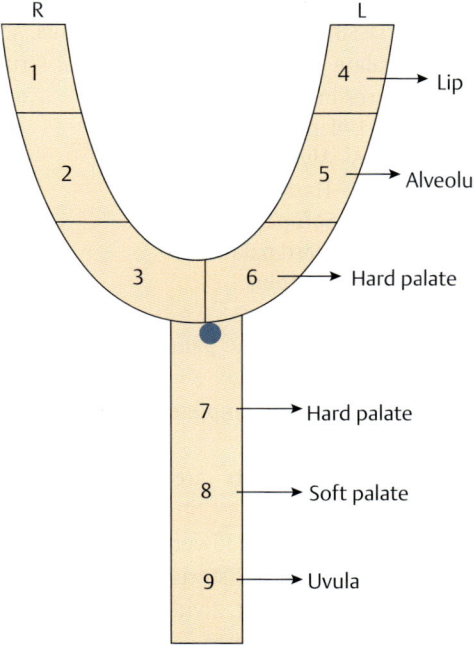

Fig. 15.4 Kernahan and Stark original, striped Y classification.

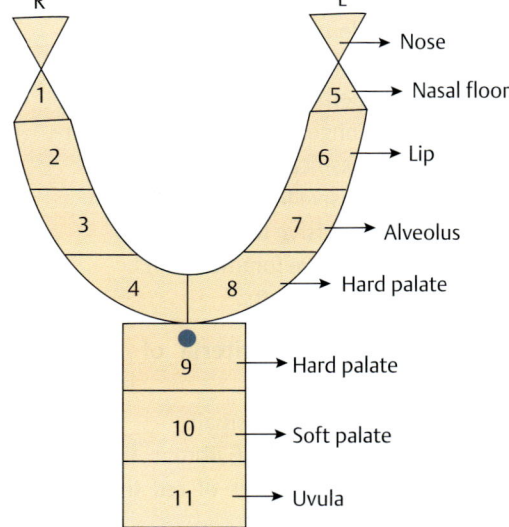

Fig. 15.5 Modified striped Y classification.

- Millard added inverted triangular peaks which indicate nasal deformity.
  - Disadvantage is clefts of the secondary palate cannot be classified into right and left sides.
- Kriens:
  - Kriens proposed the LAHSHAL code for classifying the cleft of lip, alveolus, and palate based on the anatomical structures involved.
    - L—Lip.
    - A—Alveolus.
    - H—Hard palate.
    - S—Soft palate.
    - H—Hard palate.
    - A—Alveolus.
    - L—Lip.
  - Right side of the patient is the left side of the formula.
  - Divides into complete, incomplete, and microform.
  - Complete clefts are represented by capital letters.
  - Partial clefts by lowered letters.
  - Microforms by asterisks.

Disadvantage: Does not divide palate into primary and secondary palates.

- Pruzansky classification:
  - First system to categorize clefts with embryology, physiology, and anatomy.
    I. Cleft lip.
    II. Cleft lip and palate.
    III. Cleft palate only.
    IV. Congenital deficiency of palate.
- Spina classification:
  - Preincisive foramen clefts.
  - Transincisive foramen clefts.
  - Postincisive foramen clefts.
  - Rare facial clefts.

Q7. What are the criteria of microform cleft lip?

- Vermilion notch is small.
- There is a band of fibrous tissue which extends from edges of red lip to nostril floor.
- Ala is irregular on the notched side.

Q8. How does drug produce defect in the lip and palate?

Drug produces anoxia of cells leading to arrest of growth.

Q9. What is the role of nasoendoscopy in cleft lip and palate?

Nasoendoscopy is important in cleft palate patients for the assessment of velopharyngeal function, after palatoplasty.

- In cases where the voice of patients is not normal even after palatoplasty, it is used for assessing the location and gap through which nasal escape of air is present.
- In case of submucous cleft palate, it can examine hypoplastic muscles and thin mucous membrane.

Q10. What is the role of cephalogram in cleft lip and palate?

Helps in identifying how much palate is deficient to posterior pharyngeal wall. Minimum two cephalograms are required. One in static position and second during speaking.

Q11. What is the anatomy of muscles in a cleft lip?

Normal anatomy of orbicularis oris (**Fig. 15.6**):

- The orbicularis oris muscle consists of two parts.
  - The fibers of the superficial portion connect with the maxilla and septum above and with the mandible below.

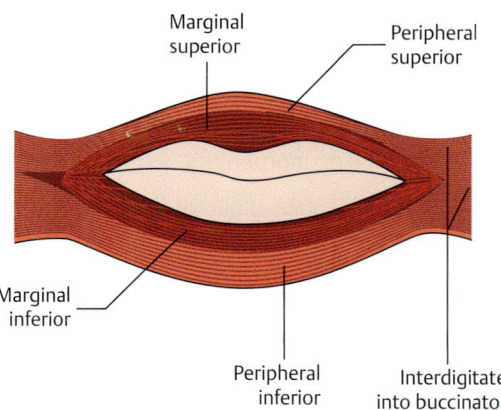

Fig. 15.6 Normal anatomy of orbicularis oris.

- In the upper lip, these consist of:
  - The lateral bands originating from the alveolar border of the maxilla.
  - The medial bands connecting the upper lip to the septum.
  - Between the two medial bands is the philtrum.
- In the lower lip:
  - The superficial layer is composed of slips arising from either side on the midline and inserts into the mandible.
  - The deep fibers encircle the orifice of mouth.

Unilateral cleft lip soft tissue dysmorphology may be summarized as follows:

- In a complete unilateral cleft:
  - The fibers of the orbicularis muscle proceed horizontally from the corner of the mouth toward the midline and turn upward along the margins of the cleft.
  - Laterally, they terminate beneath the base of the ala of the nose.
  - Medially beneath the base of the columella, where most of them attach themselves to the periosteum of the maxilla.
- In incomplete cleft in which the cleft does not exceed two-thirds of the lip height:
  - The muscle fibers reach over the tip of the cleft and pass from the lateral to the medial lip segments.

Q12. What is the difference between incomplete and microform cleft lip?

- In incomplete cleft lip, there is cleft of mucosa, muscle, and skin while in microform cleft lip, muscles and mucosa are generally intact.
- Microform cleft lip has three components:
  - A small vermilion notch.
  - A visible band of fibrous tissue which extends from the edges of the cleft lip to the nostril floor.
    - These bands may mimic the normal philtral columns, but on close inspection, they stream cephalad in a lateral direction compared with the normal lip and converge on the midnostril floor.
  - An irregularity of the ala on the side of the notch or band.

Q13. What is the difference between complete and incomplete cleft lip?

- Incomplete cleft lip extends from the vermilion-free border to the nose, sparing only a thin band of soft tissue (Simonart band) at the nasal sill.
- In complete cleft lip, cleft extends to the floor of the nose.

Q14. What is Simonart band?

It is a bridge of tissue connecting the medial and lateral lip elements.

- It contains only mucous membrane, skin, and fibrous connective tissue.
- There is usually a complete diastasis of the orbicularis oris muscle.

Q15. What is Randall-Tennison (RT) lip repair?

Given by Tennison in 1952 and modified by Randall in 1959.

- It is a triangular flap repair.

Indications: Wide clefts.

Advantages:

- Natural Cupid's bow is preserved.
- Flap produces fullness near the vermilion cutaneous ridge.
- Wasting of minimal tissue.

Disadvantages:

- Scar intrudes upon the philtrum thereby noticeable.
- Disproportionate growth tendency is there.

Q16. How do you mark in RT lip repair?

- Castroviejo calipers are used for measurements in RT repair.
- Markings of RT lip repair is more of mathematical calculation.
- Markings of points (**Fig. 15.7a–c**)
  - 1- Centre of cupid's bow
  - 2- Peak of cupid's bow on non-cleft side
  - 3- Peak of cupid's bow on cleft side

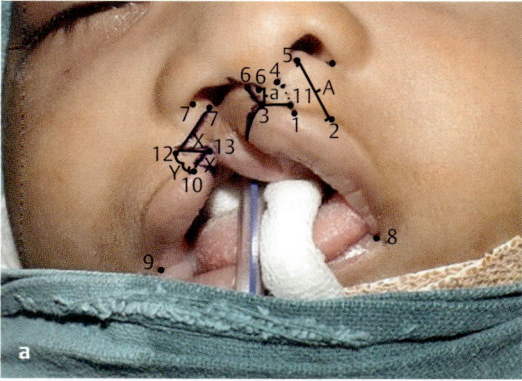 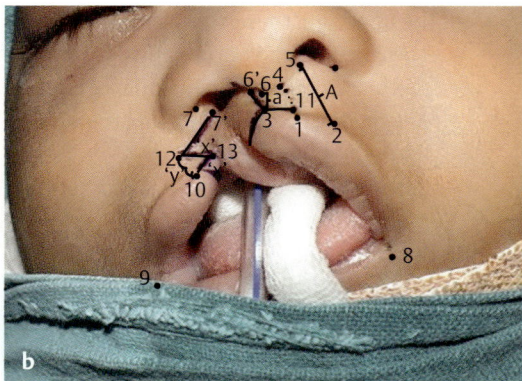

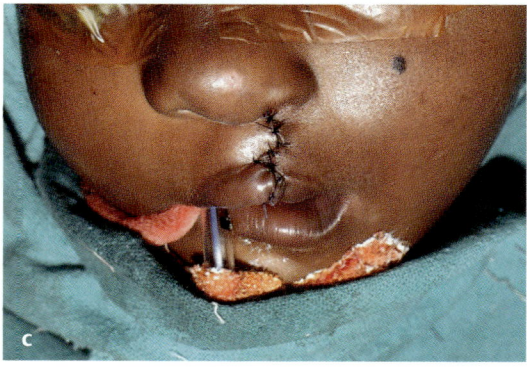

Fig. 15.7 (a–c) Markings of RT lip repair.

4- Mid-point of columellar-labial angle

5- Columellar base on non- cleft side

6- Columellar base on cleft side

6'- Point at 1/3rd of nasal sil length at columellar base on cleft side

7- Alar base on cleft side

7'- Point at 2/3rd of nasal sil length at alar base on cleft side

8- Oral commissure on non-cleft side

9- Oral commissure on cleft side

10- New peak of cupid's bow on cleft side (Noordoff's point or point at which white roll is thinned out); distance 9-10 = 8-2

- Markings of lines (in sequence):
  - An isosceles triangle with base away from the cleft margin needs to be drawn.
  - For drawing the triangle, two measurements are important: "x" and "y" (in mm).
  - Join points 1–4 to get the midline (incision must not cross the midline

otherwise there will be lengthening of lip on noncleft side).

- Draw a perpendicular line from point 3 to get point 11.
- Measure the distance 3–11 to get distance "x" (in mm) (the sides of the triangle).
- Measure the length of philtral column on noncleft side 2–5 to get "A" (in mm).
- Measure the distance 3–6' to get "a" (in mm).
- "A" – "a" = "y" (in mm) is the base of the triangle (the difference in the length of philtral columns on noncleft and cleft side).
- From point 7', draw an arc at distance "a" mm on the cleft side, away from cleft margin.
- From point 10, draw another arc at distance "y" mm on cleft side to cut the previous arc and get point 12.
- From point 10, draw an arc at distance "x" toward the cleft margin.

– From point 12, draw another arc at distance "x" to cut the previous arc to get point 13.
– Incision line on cleft side: Join points 7′, 12, 13, 10 and extend vertically from point 10 down on mucosa till sulcus.
– Incision line on noncleft side: Join points 6′, 3, 11 and extend vertically from point 3 down on mucosa till sulcus.
– points 6′ and 7′ are placed to match the nasal sil width.

Q17. What is Millard I lip repair?

Also known as rotation advancement repair.
Indications: Mild-to-moderate degree of clefts.
Contraindications: Wide cleft.
Advantages:
- This method is a highly flexible one so that you can do constant modification throughout surgery.
- Flap margins follow natural lines (the philtral pillar and the nostril sill).

- Preserves Cupid's bow and philtral dimple.
- Outward pout of lip is preserved.
- Secondary revisions can be done.
- Disproportionate growth is rarely a problem.
- Good access to nose and supplies tissue for deficiency of nose, alar base, and nasal floor.

Disadvantages:
- Not used in wide clefts.
- Frequent contracture of vertical scar, resulting in notching of vermilion or shortening of entire lip in vertical dimension.

Q18. How do you mark in Millard's lip repair?

- Markings of Millard lip repair (**Fig. 15.8a–c**):
  1- Centre of cupid's bow
  2- Peak of cupid's bow on non-cleft side
  3- Peak of cupid's bow on cleft side
  4- Alar base on non-cleft side
  5- Mid-point of collumelar-labial angle

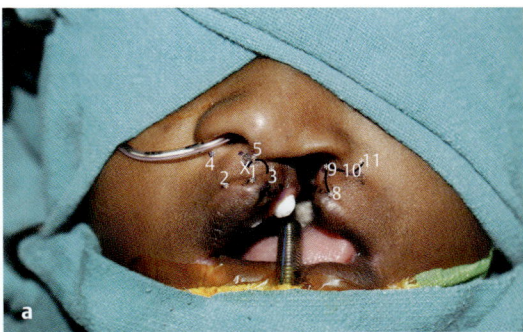

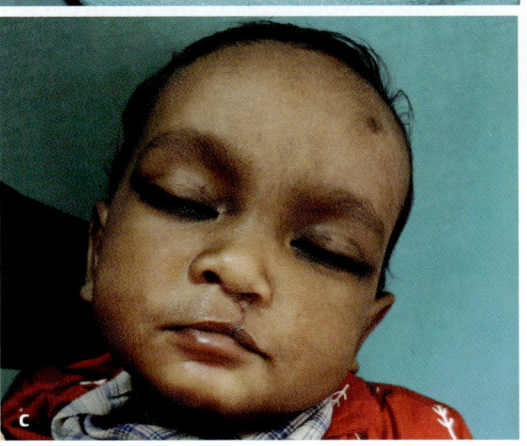

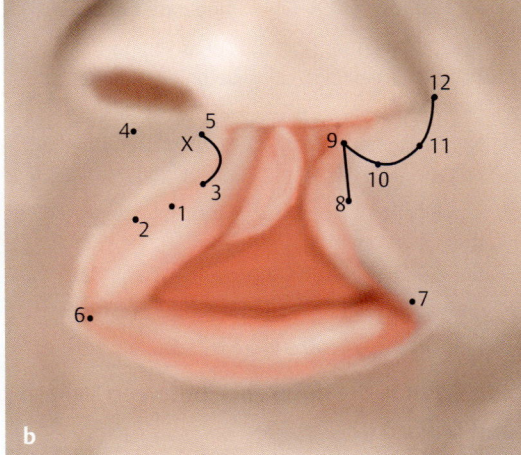

Fig. 15.8 (**a–c**) Markings of Millard's lip repair.

6- Oral commissure on non-cleft side
7- Oral commissure on cleft side
8- New peak of cupid's bow on cleft side
9- Superior tip of advancement flap
10- Mid-point of alar base on cleft side

- Incision is made along line 3–5 as traction is maintained on the tubercle.
- The incision is continued until the Cupid's bow is rotated downward into the normal position.
- A lateral flap is made so that 3–5 equals 8–9.
- Flap X lies between 3–5 and freshened margins of cleft and it forms the sill of the nostril.

Q19. What are the differences between Randall-Tennison and Millard repair?

Differences between RT and Millard.

RT lip repair	Millard lip repair
1. Lower triangular repair	1. Upper triangular repair
2. For wide clefts	2. For mild and moderate clefts
3. Preoperative planning (marking) important	3. Cut as you go technique
4. No management for columella	4. Columella lengthening can be done
5. Tendency to disproportionate growth	5. No such tendency
6. Secondary revisions not easy	6. Secondary revisions easy

Q20. What is the difference between Millard I and Millard II?

The medial flap which is used in Millard I procedure to reconstruct the nasal sill is used to lengthen the columella in Millard II procedure.

Q21. What are the types of ink used in marking?

- Methylene blue.
- Bonney's blue.

Q22. What is Bonney's blue?

Bonney's blue contains 10 g of gentian violet and 10 g of brilliant green in 950 mL of 95% alcohol.

Q23. What dilution of adrenaline will you use and how will you prepare?

- 1:2,00,000 dilution of adrenaline is used in a child less than 1 year of age.
- It means 1 mg of adrenaline is to be diluted in 200 mL of saline (1 mL of ampoule contains 1 mg of adrenaline).
- It is prepared as:
- 1 mg of adrenaline to be mixed in 200 mL of saline.
- 1 mg adrenaline in 200 mL saline means 10^{-3} g adrenaline in 200 mL saline.
- So, the final dilution prepared is 1 in 200,000.

Q24. What are the advantages and disadvantages of adrenaline solution and where do we actually infiltrate?

- Adrenaline is infiltrated in:
  – Planned dissection planes of the lip.
  – Supraperiosteal plane of the cleft-side maxilla.
  – Between the skin and cartilage of the planned nasal dissection.
- Advantages: It helps in decreasing the bleeding and thereby maintains hemostasis.
- Disadvantages: It distorts the marking points of lip repair.

Q25. How do you measure the width of cleft and nasal sill? When do you say it is a wide cleft?

- Castroviejo caliper is used to measure the width of cleft and nasal sill.
- Width of nasal sill—distance between medialmost point of alar base and base of medial crus of columella.
- Width of cleft—distance between the marked highest point of Cupid's bow on cleft side and point at which white roll disappears.

- Wide cleft is when width of cleft is >10 mm.

Q26. What are the indications of secondary lip procedures?

- Long lip.
- Short lip.
- Tight lip.
- Whistle deformity.

Q27. What is whistle deformity and how do you correct it?

- In whistle deformity, there is central vermilion notching and deficiency of visible mucosa and vermilion.
- The underlying cause is the tissue deficiency of orbicularis oris muscle in the prolabium.
- It is corrected by z-plasty and V-Y advancement flap.

Q28. Describe the cleft lip nasal deformities?

Nasal deformities are divided into the following categories:

- **Nasal tip:**
  - Displacement of medial crus medially and downward which causes shortening of columella and decreased projection of the dome of alar cartilage on the affected side.
  - Displacement of dome of ala toward lateral side which causes widening of nasal floor.
  - Angle between medial and lateral crura is more obtuse.
  - Displacement of lateral crura in downward position.
- Lateral bony platform:
  - Hypoplasia of the maxilla in the region of the pyriform aperture is usually present.
- Midline supporting structures:
  - Distortion of columella is due to the deviation of the caudal edge of the cartilaginous septum toward the noncleft side.

Q29. What is tripod theory of cleft lip?

- The tripod consists of the dorsal portion of the septum and nasal bones and the two alar arms (**Fig. 15.9**).
- In cleft lip nasal deformity, tilted tripod is present.
- Tilting effect is due to maxillary hypoplasia and secondary deformity of the septum and cleft ala, so it is considered as a tilted tripod.

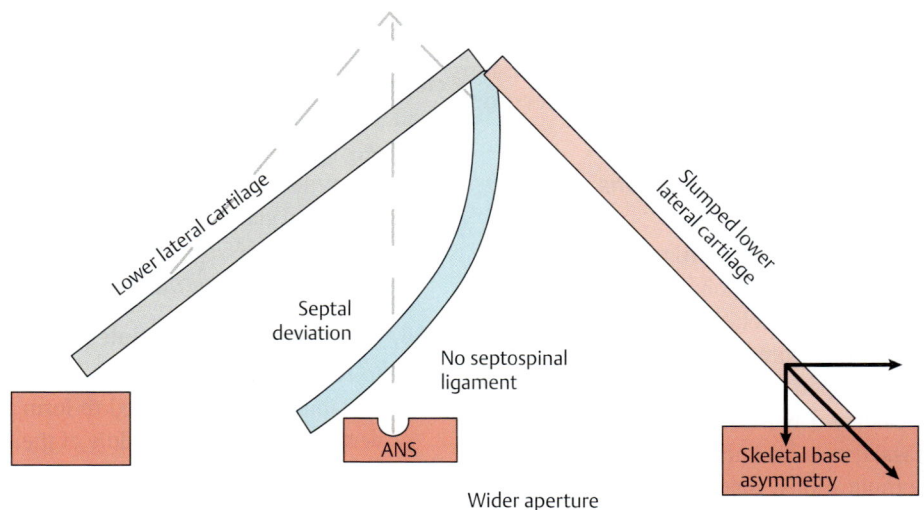

Fig. 15.9 Schematic representation of tripod theory of cleft lip.

Q30. What are the different nasal corrections that can be done at the time of lip repair?
- Repositioning of the flared ala.
- Augmentation of ala with bone grafts.

Q31. What is the postoperative care in a cleft lip repair child?
- Early care:
  - Airway monitoring is very important in early postoperative period as there are chances of accumulation of blood and secretions in the airway from endotracheal intubation and alterations in the lip and nose anatomy.
  - Pain control is an important aspect of postoperative care; nerve blocks often decrease the need for analgesic medication.
  - Arm restraints of the child.
  - Antibiotics.
- Late care:
  - Scar taping.
  - Scar massage.
  - Nasal stenting.
    - It is used to maintain the reconstructed nasal shape and prevent damages that result from wound scarring, cartilage memory, and nasal scar contracture.
    - Silicone nostril conformers are placed at the time of primary rhinoplasty to maintain the form and position of the reconstructed nasal deformity and are used for weeks to months.

Q32. What are the complications of a cleft lip repair?
- Early complications: Airway obstruction, hematoma, infection, anesthesia-related problems, and dehiscence.
- Long-term complications: Stitch granuloma, hypertrophic scarring, nostril floor breakdown with use of nasal stents, oronasal fistula, and notching.
- Complications specific to nasal stenting include infections, pressure necrosis, or soft tissue loss.

Q33. What are the other techniques of lip repair?
- Randall–Graham lip adhesion.
  - Advantages:
    - Indicated in very wide clefts.
    - Molds underlying distortions of maxilla and premaxilla.
    - It causes stretching of attenuated and displaced adjacent soft tissues.
  - Disadvantages: Wastage of tissue which occurs when scar resulting from lip adhesion is excised.
- Rose Thompson straight line repair.
  - Advantages:
    - Scar lies in a satisfactory direction.
    - Easy procedure.
    - No future disproportionate growth.
  - Disadvantage: Sacrifice large amount of tissue.
- Lemesurier rectangular flap repair.
  - Advantages:
    - It produces normal natural fullness at vermilion-cutaneous ridge.
    - Markings are easier.
    - Conserves lateral vermilion which is desirable in wide clefts.
  - Disadvantages:
    - Produces scar over the philtrum.
    - It causes disproportionate growth so that repaired side becomes long.
    - Revision of lip is difficult.

Q34. In bilateral cleft lip repair which side is closed first?
In bilateral cleft lip repair wide side is closed first because:
- Asymmetric bilateral cleft is converted to unilateral cleft.
- And narrower or incomplete cleft is left to be closed at the second stage.

Q35. What are the principles of bilateral cleft lip repair?
- Prolabium should be used to form the full vertical length of the middle of the lip.
- Preservation of vermilion ridge of the inferior border of the prolabium.

- Vermilion muscle flaps from lateral lip segments are used to reconstruct thin prolabial vermilion but no lateral lip skin should be brought beneath the prolabium.
- Protruded premaxilla should be repositioned.
- Expansion of the collapse of maxillary process behind the protruding premaxilla.
- Bone grafting is required to stabilize the premaxilla when it is not united on both sides. Not required if one side is fused with maxilla.
  - Simultaneous repair of both sides of lip can be done:
    - When premaxilla is within the alveolar arch.
    - Size of prolabium is adequate.
      - If there is a protruding premaxilla and a small prolabium, two-stage repair is done.
      - Closure of one side of bilateral cleft lip results in increase in blood supply to prolabium which leads to increase in the size of prolabium.
      - After 6 to 8 weeks of first operation, there is sufficient tissue in the prolabium to reconstruct the lip.

Q36. What are the indications of lip adhesion?

- Indications of lip adhesion are:
  - Cleft >10 mm wide with an associated discrepancy of 4 to 5 mm or more in the vertical cleft length between SBAR-CPHR and SBAL-CPHL'.
  - Complete cleft of the primary palate in which there is a prominent protruding premaxilla resulting in a long vertical discrepancy between the premaxilla alveolus and maxilla.
  - Older children with wide clefts and no presurgical orthodontics.
- Cleft tissue deficiencies are more important than cleft width as a criterion in decision making for an adhesion cheiloplasty.

- Advantages:
  - It causes narrowing of the cleft by decreasing tension across the maxilla.
  - Easier correction of the nasal deformity because of a better bony framework on which the nose can be reconstructed.
  - Development of more muscle or elongation of a short lip before definitive cheiloplasty.
- Disadvantage:
  - The disadvantage is that even with no dissection of the muscle, the operative area is firm with scar tissue, secondary to the healing process.

Q37. What are the anthropometric points and measurements in a cleft lip?

- The anthropometric markings for measurements in a unilateral cleft lip are (**Fig. 15.10a, b**):
  - CHR—Commissure right side.
  - CHL—Commissure left side.
  - HR—Right horizontal length.
  - HL—Left horizontal length.
  - VR—Right vertical length.
  - VL—Left vertical length.
  - CPHR—Base of noncleft side philtral column/noncleft side Cupid's bow.
  - CPHL—Cleft side Cupid's bow.
  - IS—Central Cupid's bow.
  - CPHL'—Base of cleft side philtral column.
  - SBAR—Right base of ala.
  - SBAL—Left base of ala.
  - SN—Midpoint of columella base.
  - CPHSR—Highest point of philtral column on right side.
  - CPHSL—Highest point of philtral column on left side.
  - CPHSL'—Highest point of the philtral column on the cleft side.
- Cupid's bow, vermilion, commissure, columellar base, and alar base.
  - The points of the Cupid's bow (CPHR, IS, CPHL) are marked on the epidermis–vermilion junction line along with the

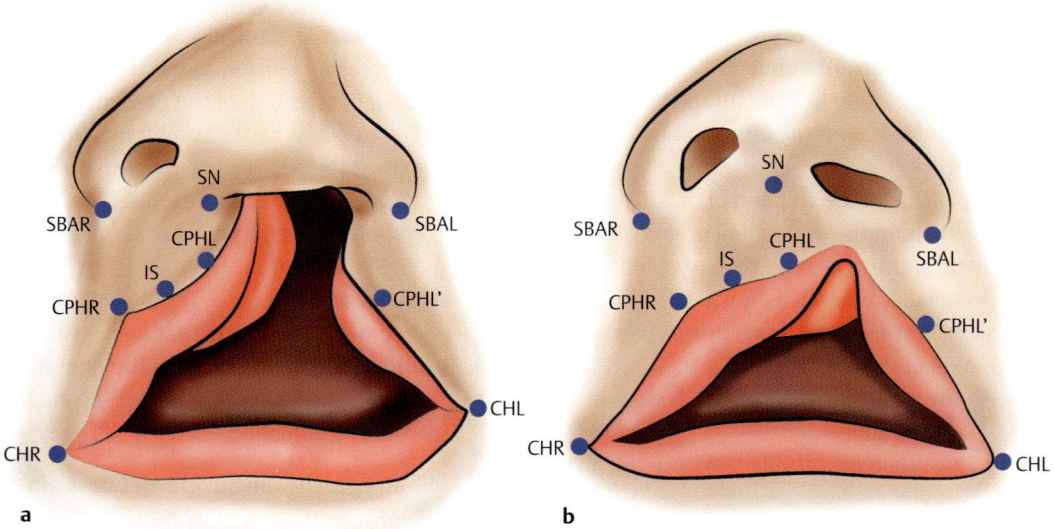

Fig. 15.10 (a, b) Anthropometric in a cleft lip.

white skin roll (WSR). Gentle upward lift on the nasal tip with a finger helps to define point IS.

– The distance between IS and CPHL should be equal to the distance between CPHR and IS.

– If the point IS is toward the cleft margin then the point CPHL will be moved higher and it will be more difficult to level the Cupid's bow.

– The vermilion–mucosa junction line, the red line, is also marked.

– Then mark the midpoint of columella base (SN), highest points of the philtral columns (CPHSR, CPHSL), bilateral base of the ala (SBAR, SBAL) and commissure (CHR, CHL).

– Lastly, the width of the WSR at point CPHR is marked out. The width of the WSR is usually around 2 mm at the age of 3 to 6 months old.

• Base of philtral column on the cleft side.

– The base of the philtral column on the cleft side (CPHL') is a definite anatomic point.

– Point CHPL' is where the WSR changes direction and the vermilion first becomes widest which is usually 3 to 4 mm lateral to the converging point of red line and WSR.

– The width of the WSR flap corresponds to the measurement on the noncleft side.

– The split point of the nasolabial groove (the point where the skin-mucosal junction changes its direction at the deepest point of the nasal vestibulum on the cleft side) is also marked.

• Proposed point of medial nasal sill.

– Gentle inward pressure on the cleft side ala base helps to define the position and direction of the cleft side nasal sill.

– The proposed point of the medial nasal sill, which is usually the highest point of the philtral column on the cleft side (CPHSL'), is the point where the nasal sill ends medially and meets the base of columella during skin closure.

– This point is marked ~8 mm from a tangential line on the ala–facial groove in a 3- to 6-month-old baby.

– This distance helps in achieving an over-corrected nostril width on the cleft side.

Measurements:
- Peaking of Cupid's bow:
  - The discrepancy between the heights from the central columella base (SN) to the two peaks of the Cupid's bow (CPHR and CPHL) is critical for leveling the Cupid's bow.
  - A shorter rotation incision from CPHL to CPSHL is performed if the discrepancy is less than 2 mm.
- Lateral lip height and length: Vertical length is more important aesthetically compared with the horizontal length.
- Vermilion width:
  - The vermilion width beneath point CPHL is always deficient compared with the counterpart vermilion at point CPHR or CPHL'.
  - Inadequate reconstruction of this vermilion deficiency will result in free border deformities like exposed mucosa, color mismatching, and dry crusting as seen in a straight-line vermilion closure.
  - Therefore, the vermilion medial to point CPHL' should be used to correct the vermilion deficiency beneath the Cupid's bow.
- White skin roll:
  - The width of the WSR is usually widest above point CPHR.
  - The WSR remains quite prominent between points CPHR and LS but becomes narrower toward point CPHL.
  - Measurement of the width of WSR at point CPHR is done and transferred to the cleft side.
  - The measured WSR at point CPHR is always wider (e.g., 2 mm wide at the age of 3–6 months old) than the observed WSR at point CPHL'.
  - A triangular WSR flap is designed above point CPHL'. This 2-mm WSR flap helps to level Cupid's bow and correct the WSR deficiency at point CPHL.

Q38. How does presurgical alveolar or nasoalveolar molding help?
- Nasoalveolar molding (NAM) is a passive form of presurgical infant orthopedics (PSIO).
- It is mostly indicated in cases of wide unilateral clefts and for all complete bilateral clefts.
- It helps in narrowing the cleft gap by aligning the maxillary arch which subsequently brings the edges of the clefted lips together.
- NAM helps in correcting the cleft lip nasal deformity, particularly with the bilateral cleft where it extends the columella through tissue expansion and improves sagittal projection, as well as the size, shape, and symmetry of the nasal apertures.

Q39. What are the types of alveolar and nasoalveolar molding available?
- Presurgical nasoalveolar molding (NAM, for complete cleft lips) or nasal molding (for incomplete cleft lips) is started soon after the first visit.
- Usually it takes 3 to 4 months for the completion of the molding process. There are several techniques including:
  - Sleeping in prone position.
  - Lip taping.
  - Presurgical orthopaedics with an acrylic plate with lip taping.
- NAM techniques:
  - Modified Grayson's: A passive orthopaedic appliance is used together with taping of the lip.
  - Liou's (modified Figueroa's): This device is composed of a dental plate, nasal molding components, and adhesive tape (Micropore).
    - Both molding techniques require outpatient adjustments every 1 to 2 weeks.
  - Nasoalveolar molding with a spring device.

– Nasal molding with silicone nasal conformer: used for incomplete cleft lips.

Q40. What is Latham device?

- The device is a form of active PSIO used to align cleft tissues.
- The Latham device requires an additional surgery for placement and is secured with surgical pins.
- This device requires the child's guardian to turn the screw daily and weekly visits to the orthodontist.

Q41. What are the goals of palate repair?

The goals are:

- To repair the palatal defect.
- To reconstruct the palatal muscle.
- To provide adequate palatal movement.
- To provide good speech.
- To isolate the oral cavity from nasal cavity.

Q42. What are the muscles of palate?

- Levator veli palatine (**Fig. 15.11a, b**):
  – Cylindrical muscle.
  – Origin: From posteromedian Eustachian tube.
  – Insertion: Into palatal midline.
  – Function Elevates velum, Eustachian tube dilatation.
  – Forms the posterior three-fourth of the velum.
- Tensor veli palatine:
  – Triangular muscle with fleshy belly and tendinous at each end.
  – Origin: Greater wing of sphenoid (scaphoid fossa):
    - Superolateral aspect of cartilaginous and membranous part of entire length of Eustachian tube.
    - Angle between the axis of tensor veli palatine and the Eustachian tube is 30 to 40 degrees.
  – Insertion: Tendon of tensor veli palatine hooks around the anterior aspect of the hamulus, forming a 90-degree turn as it enters the soft palate.
  – Function: It pulls the tube inferiorly, laterally, and anteriorly.

– Tendon spreads to form aponeurosis which occupy the anterior quarter of the velar length.

- Salpingopharyngeus:
  – It is a vestigial muscle.
  – Origin: Posteroinferior tip of Eustachian tube.
  – Insertion: In the palatapharyngeus.
- Musculus uvulae:
  – It is a paired muscle.
  – Origin: Anteriorly to the aponeurosis in midline.
  – Insertion: Posterior connective tissue of the midline velum.
  – Function: It forms the knee in velopharyngeal closure.
- Palatapharyngeus:
  – This muscle occupies the central 50% of velar length. It consists of two heads separated by levator veli palatine.
  – Origin: Posterior border of aponeurosis and levator.
  – Insertion: Lateral pharynx and larynx.
  – Function: It forms the cleft muscles of Veau along with the fibers of levator.
- Palatoglossus:
  – It arises from transverse muscle fibers of tongue.
  – It inserts into muscles of palate.
- Superior constrictor:
  – Quadrangular muscle.
  – Origin: Medial pterygoid plate.
  – Insertion: Pharyngeal ligament.
    - It is deepest of pharyngeal constrictors.
    - It causes medial excursion of lateral pharyngeal walls, and anterior displacement of posterior pharyngeal wall.
    - Main component of Passavant ridge.

Q43. What is Passavant's ridge?

- It is formed by some fibers of palatopharyngeus which pass circularly deep into the mucous membrane of pharynx and forms a sphincter internal to superior constrictor.

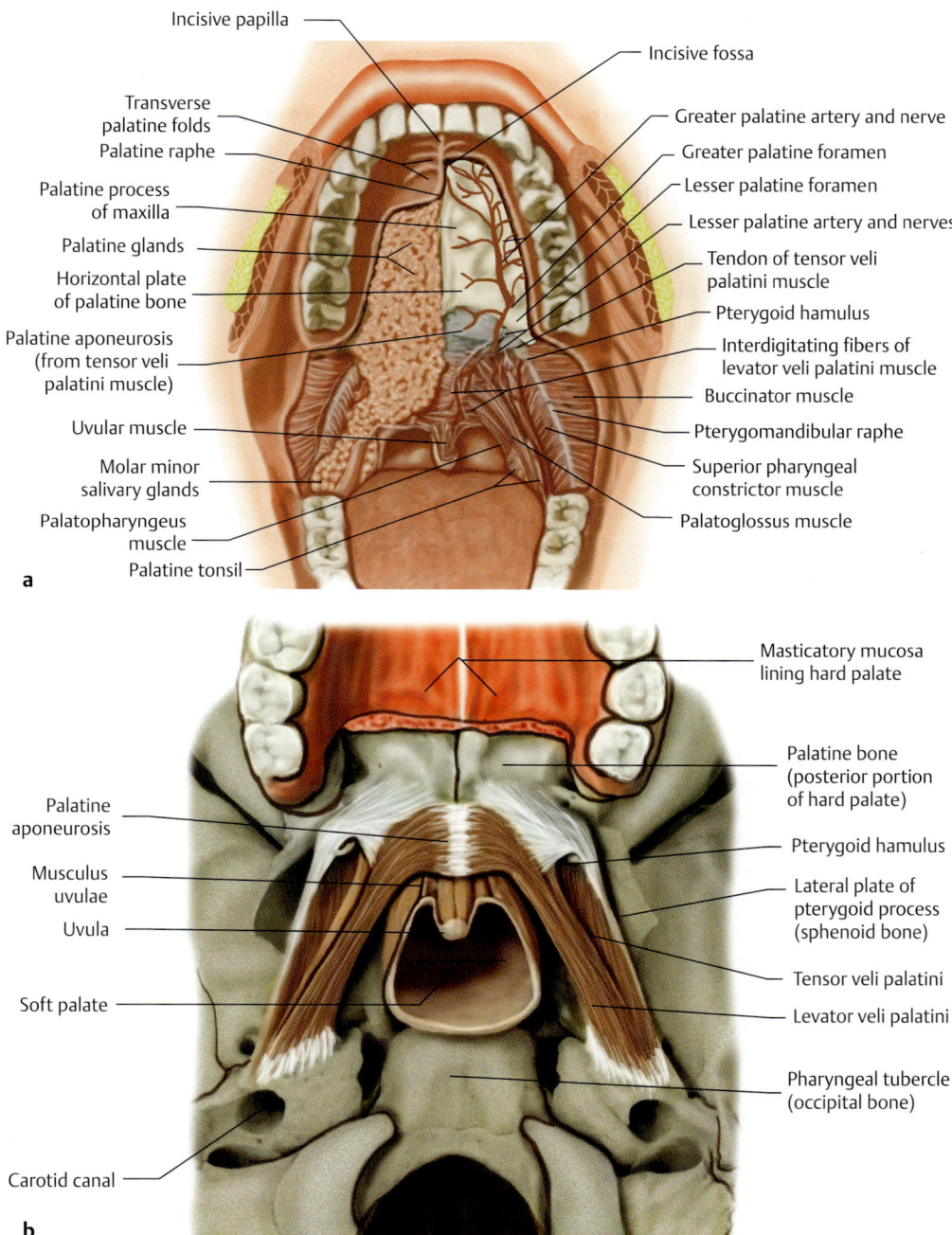

Incisive papilla

Incisive fossa

Transverse palatine folds

Palatine raphe

Greater palatine artery and nerve

Greater palatine foramen

Palatine process of maxilla

Lesser palatine foramen

Palatine glands

Lesser palatine artery and nerves

Horizontal plate of palatine bone

Tendon of tensor veli palatini muscle

Pterygoid hamulus

Palatine aponeurosis (from tensor veli palatini muscle)

Interdigitating fibers of levator veli palatini muscle

Buccinator muscle

Uvular muscle

Pterygomandibular raphe

Molar minor salivary glands

Superior pharyngeal constrictor muscle

Palatopharyngeus muscle

Palatoglossus muscle

Palatine tonsil

a

Masticatory mucosa lining hard palate

Palatine bone (posterior portion of hard palate)

Palatine aponeurosis

Pterygoid hamulus

Musculus uvulae

Lateral plate of pterygoid process (sphenoid bone)

Uvula

Tensor veli palatini

Soft palate

Levator veli palatini

Pharyngeal tubercle (occipital bone)

Carotid canal

b

Fig. 15.11 **(a, b)** Anatomy and muscles of palate.

- These fibers constitute Passavant's muscle which on contraction produces ridge on posterior pharyngeal wall.
- Soft palate comes in contact with this ridge.

Q44. How to do preoperative feeding of the baby?

- Hold the baby at 45- to 60-degree angle.
- Nipple should be with enlarged hole—Preemie and Duckbill nipples.
- Small and frequent feeds
- Burping to be done after each feeding.

Q45. Which muscles form the levator sling?

- Levator veli palatine.
- Palatapharyngeus.

Q46. What are the cleft muscles of Veau?

- Musculus uvulae.
- Levator veli palatine.
- Palatopharyngeus.

Q47. What is the optimum age for palatoplasty?

Nine to 12 months. Development of babbling is an indication to reconstruct the palate.

Q48. What are the principles of palatoplasty?

- Anatomical closure of the defect should be done.
- Abnormal position of the muscles of the soft palate should be corrected especially levator veli palatine.
- Muscle sling should be reconstructed.
- Soft palate should be retropositioned so much that during speech the posterior part of the soft palate comes in contact with the posterior pharyngeal wall during speech.
- There should be no minimal or no raw area on the nasal side or the oral surface.
- Suturing should be done tension free.
- There should be two-layer closure in the hard palate region and three-layer closure in the soft palate.

Q49. Which endotracheal tube is used for anesthesia in cleft lip and palate?

- For cleft lip: Normal endotracheal tube, size should be appropriate for the age.
- For cleft palate:
  - Ring–Adair–Elwyn (RAE) tube: This tube is named after the inventors Ring, Adair, and Elwyn, who described the use of their novel oral preformed tube in pediatric patients in 1975 (**Fig. 15.12**).
    - Distinguishing feature of this tube in comparison to normal ET tubes is that there is a preformed bend which reduces the risk of kinking and obstruction.
    - There is a black marker bar on the tube at the point of maximum angle of the bend.
  - South pole tube.
  - Flexometallic tube or armored tube.
  - Normal tube with a metallic mount.

Q50. What are the different techniques of palatoplasty?

- Von-Langenbeck bipedicle flap technique (**Fig. 15.13a, b**):
  - Incision is given along the oral side of cleft edges and along the posterior alveolar ridge.
  - The bipedicle mucoperiosteal flaps are raised.

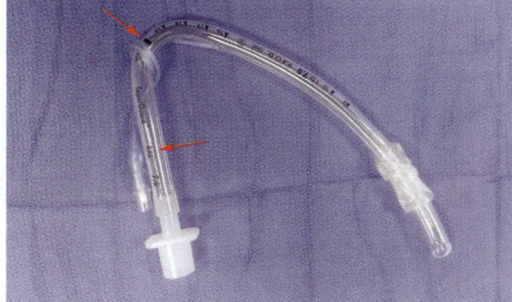

Fig. 15.12 Ring–Adair–Elwyn (RAE) endotracheal tube.

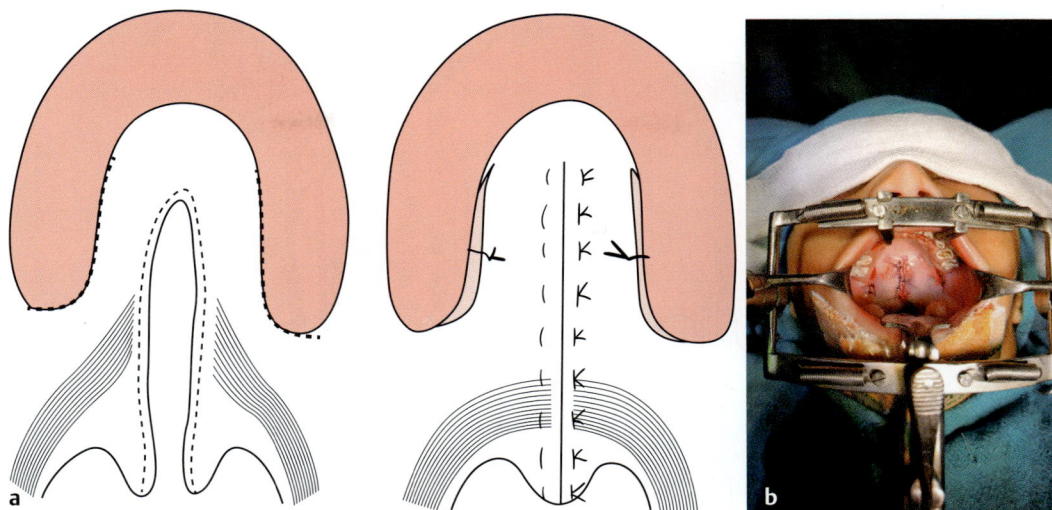

Fig. 15.13 **(a, b)** Von Langenbeck technique.

- Flaps are mobilized medially with preservation of the greater palatine arteries and closed in layers.
- The hamulus may need to be fractured for easy closure of the defect.
- Veau-Wardill-Kilner pushback technique (**Fig. 15.14a, b**):
  - In this technique V to Y incision is given and the hard palate closure is done.
  - The hamulus is fractured, and the muscle closure is done as a separate layer.
  - Advantages: It causes increase in palatal length which improves velopharyngeal function.
  - Disadvantages:
    - This technique creates a larger area of denuded palatal bone anterolaterally.
    - Associated with a higher incidence of fistula formation.
  - Victor Veau:
    - Known as father of cleft lip and palate.
    - Born in a small village of Burgundy.
    - He advocated Ganzer V-incision and nasal mucoperiosteal closure of hard palate including vomerine flap.
    - Coined the term "Suture musculaire".

- William Edward Mandall Wardill:
  - He fractured the hamulus, divided posterior palatine vessels, and modified Ganzer's V-Y by transecting mucoperiosteal flaps in their middle to ensure adequate blood supply.
  - He used three-flap method for incomplete clefts.
  - For complete cleft, four-flap method.
- Thomas Kilner:
  - He dissected the nasal mucosa from medial pterygoid plate and along posterior border and free edge of hard palate.
  - This freeing of soft tissue called filleting revealed gain in length of 1 cm.
  - He used French Reverdin needle for suturing, which is well adapted for awkward closure of nasal and oral palatal mucosa.
- Bardach's two-flap palatoplasty (**Fig. 15.15a, b**):
  - The main goal of this technique is complete closure of the entire cleft without tension, with minimal exposure of raw bony surfaces.
  - Most applicable in relatively narrow clefts. It is a modification of the

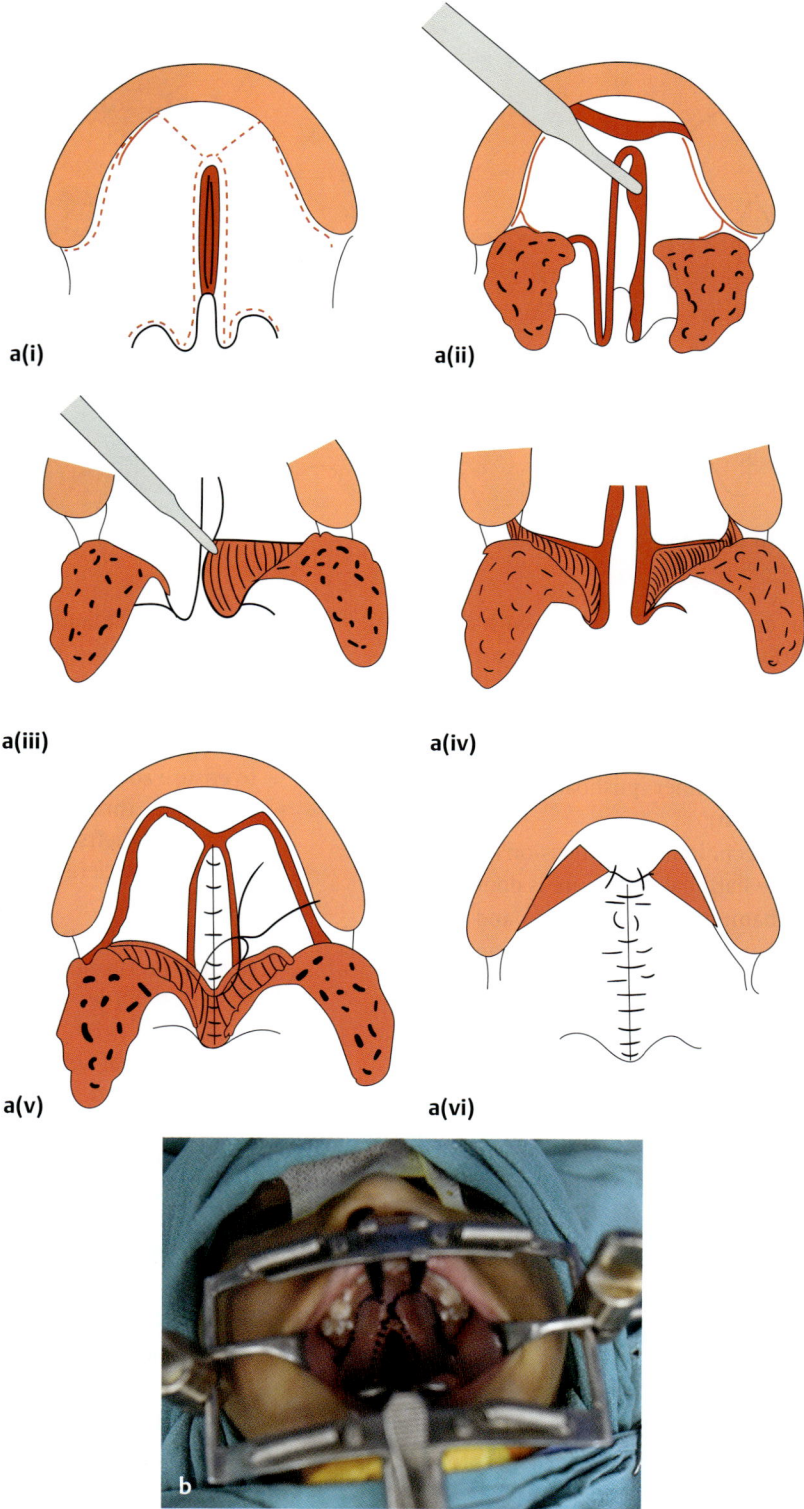

a(i)

a(ii)

a(iii)

a(iv)

a(v)

a(vi)

b

Fig. 15.14 **(a, b)** V-W-K palatoplasty.

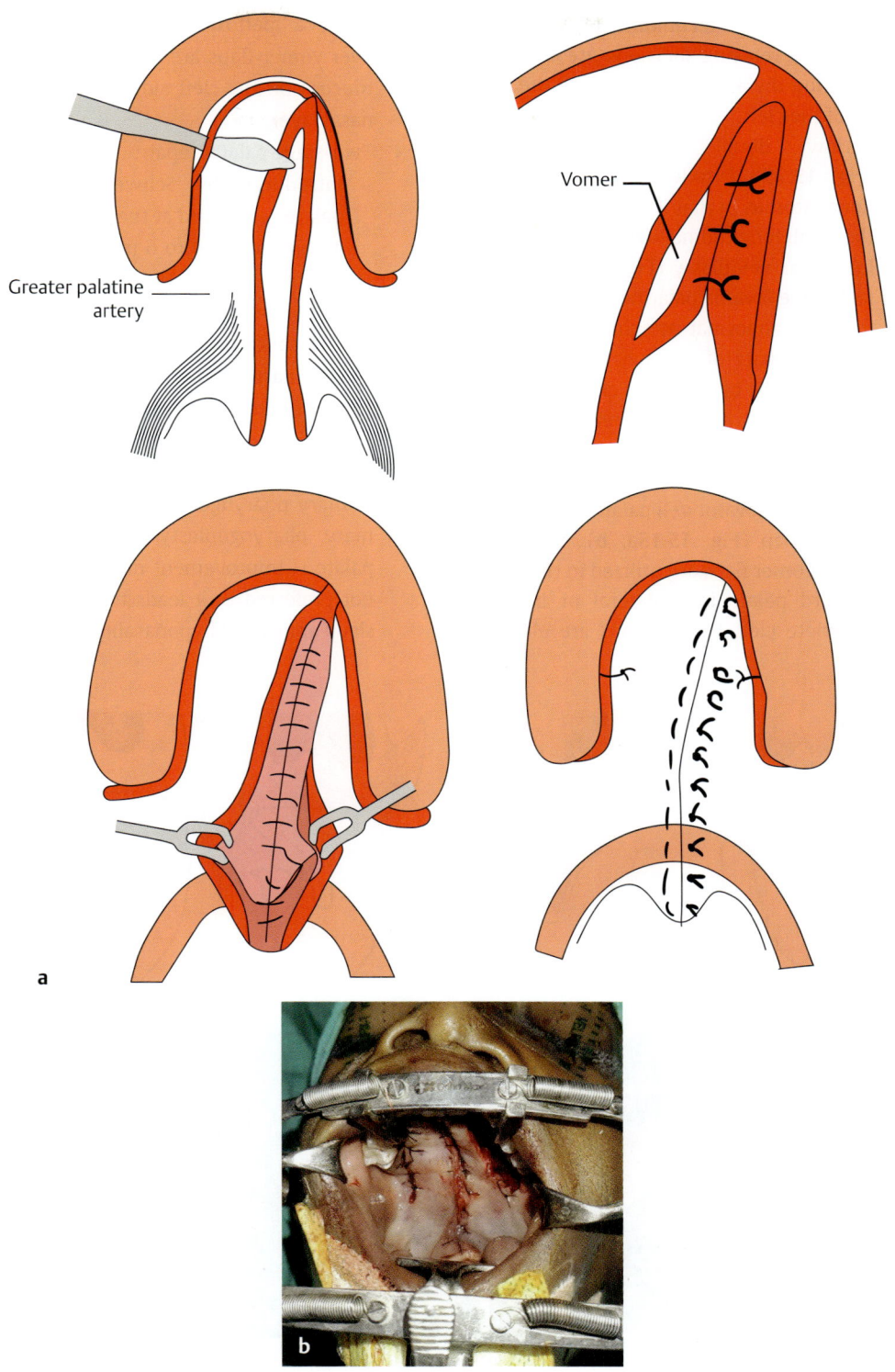

Fig. 15.15 (a, b) Bardach's two-flap palatoplasty.

Langenbeck technique. In this technique relaxing incisions are extended along the alveolar margins to the edge of the cleft.

- Furlow double opposing z-plasty (**Fig. 15.16**): Disadvantage is that it is nonanatomic, in that it completely ignores the small longitudinal uvular muscle.
- Intravelar veloplasty (**Fig. 15.17**): In this technique levator palatine muscle is freed from its abnormal attachment from the posterior part of the palatine bone and also from the aponeurosis and rarely from the hamulus and then reapproximated in midline. In addition, it lengthens the palate and restores the normal muscular sling of the levator veli palatini.
- Vomer flap (**Fig. 15.18a, b**): Superiorly based vomer flaps are utilized in the repair of hard palate in unilateral or bilateral complete cleft palate. Flaps are elevated using a periosteal elevator and turnover vomer flaps are sutured to the nasal mucosa on the cleft side to complete the nasal layer.

- Two-stage palatal repair:
  - Introduced by Schweckendiek. Soft palate is repaired at the time of cleft lip repair around 4 to 6 months. The hard palate was obturated and repaired at ~4 to 5 years of age.
  - The rationale is that the hard palate cleft narrows during the time between procedures, requiring less dissection and thus resulting in less maxillary growth disturbance.
- Primary pharyngeal flap: The goal of primary pharyngoplasty in cases of cleft palate is improvement of speech but it is not preferred as it leads to problems like sleep apnea and hyponasality.

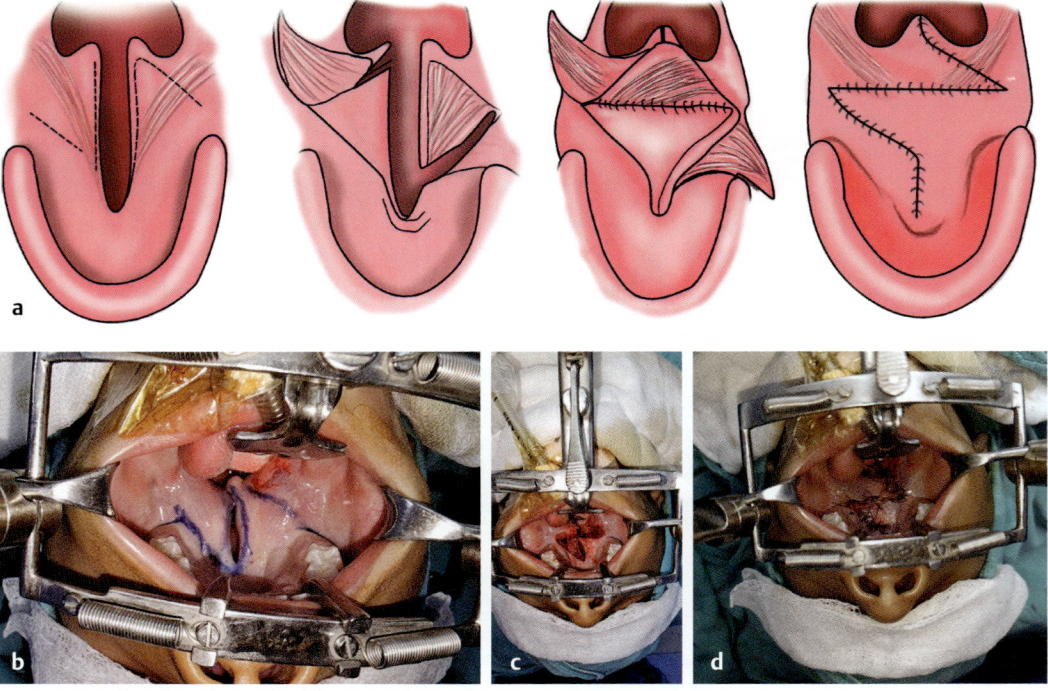

Fig. 15.16 **(a–d)** Furlow's double opposing z-plasty.

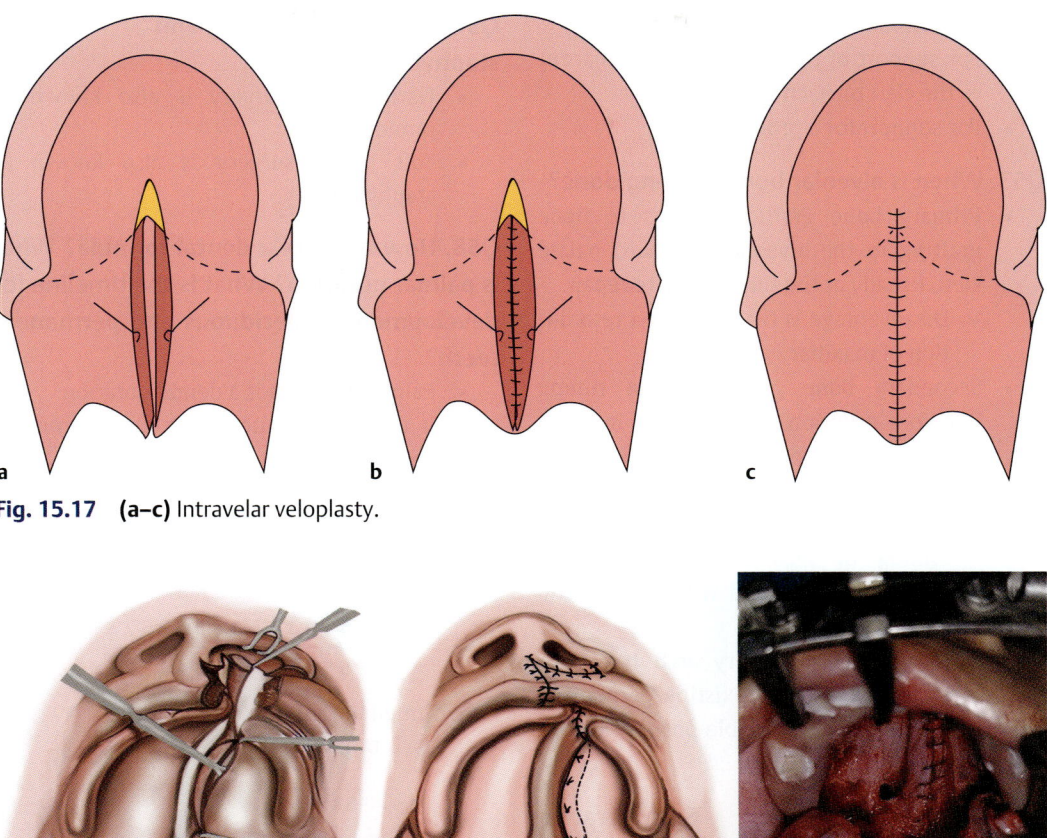

Fig. 15.17 **(a–c)** Intravelar veloplasty.

Fig. 15.18 **(a, b)** Vomer flap.

- Raw area free palatoplasty: Back cut is given in nasal mucosa and palatal lengthening is done and raw area is covered with local flaps like vomer flap and buccal mucosal flap. On oral side, all lateral incisions are sutured so as to leave no raw area anywhere.
- Hole in one-repair technique: In one stage cleft lip and palate repair is done.
- Alveolar extension palatoplasty: When there is large gap, incision is extended up to the alveolus and flaps are large.

Q51. What is the Calnan's triad and where is it found?

It is a triad used for diagnosis of submucous cleft palate.
- Midline clear zone (zona pellucida).
- Bifid uvula.
- There is a palpable notch in posterior hard palate.

Q52. What are the indications of alveolar bone grafting?

- For closure of nasoalveolar fistula.

- For stabilization of the maxillary arch.
- For support of the roots of teeth adjacent to the cleft on each side.
- For support for a prosthesis.

Q53. When is alveolar bone grafting done?

- Primary bone grafting: Refers to bone grafting in the alveolar and hard palate cleft, usually at the time of palate repair.
  – Disadvantage is that there is a retardation of maxillary growth.
- Secondary bone grafting: Ideal timing is before eruption of the canine into the cleft. If the grafting is done after eruption of the canine, there is a chance of late root resorption.
  – Timing of secondary bone grafting must be coordinated with orthodontic treatment.
  – Ideally, the maxillary arch has been expanded and the existing permanent teeth are in reasonable position before the procedure.

Q54. What are the postoperative instructions?

- Baby should be nursed in lateral position.
- Remove tongue stitch in the evening.
- Allow clear liquids in evening.
- Arms should be restraint.
- Adequate postoperative analgesia should be given.
- Give mouth wash correctly.
- In summer months beware of hyperpyrexia.

Q55. At what age child should be sent to speech therapy?

Two-and-half years.

Q56. Which part of soft palate touches the pharynx?

The junction of anterior two-third and posterior one-third of the soft palate touches the posterior pharynx at the level of C1 vertebra.

Q57. What is uranoplasty and staphyloplasty?

- Hard palate surgery is also known as uranoplasty.
- Soft palate surgery is also known as staphyloplasty.

Q58. How to write a dental formula? What is palmar notation? What is the timeline for development of deciduous and permanent teeth?

- Palmer notation is a dental notation.
- It is used for numbering and naming of teeth.
- It consists of a symbol designating in which quadrant the tooth is found and a number indicating the position from the midline.

$$87654321 | 12345678$$
$$87654321 | 12345678$$

- Timeline for tooth development:
  – Temporary:

Central incisor	6–7 mo
Lateral incisor	7–9 mo
First molar	12–14 mo
Canine	16–18 mo
Second molar	20–24 mo

  – Permanent:

First molar	6 y
Lower central incisor	6 y
Lower lateral incisor	7 y
Upper central incisor	7 y
Lower lateral incisor	8 y
First premolar	10 y
Lower canine	10 y
Second premolar	11 y
Upper canine	11 y
Second molar	12 y
Third molar	17 y

Q59. What are the different types of syllables?

- **Fricatives:** They are consonants which are made when the air is squeezed through a small hole in the mouth like the gap between the teeth, (e.g., v, f, z, s, h).
- **Plosives:** They are consonants which are produced by forming a complete obstruction to the flow of air out of the mouth, (e.g., p, t, k, b, d).
- **Affricates:** Also called semiplosive, a consonant sound that begins as a plosive (sound with complete obstruction of the breath stream) and concludes with a fricative (sound with incomplete closure and a sound of friction). For example, "t" followed by "s."

Q60. What is wide cleft palate? What are the surgical techniques used in a wide cleft?

- Wide cleft palate is defined as when the palatal defect is >60% of the width of the entire palate or in which the width of both palatal shelves is less than the width of the palatal defect.
- Techniques used to repair wide cleft palate are:
  - Primary pharyngeal flap with palatoplasty.
  - Double transposition flap.
  - Buccal musculomucosal flaps.
  - Mucoperiosteal hinge flap with pushback palatoplasty.
  - Free-tissue transfer flaps.

Q61. Why noncuffed endotracheal tube is used in children?

Noncuffed tube is used because for the same external diameter, lumen is smaller in cuffed tubes, which results in decreased air flow and increased resistance.

Q62. What are the historical developments in cleft palate?

- Johann Friedrich Dieffenbach (1826): Closure of hard palate by giving relaxing incisions bilaterally within the alveolus and around maxillary tuberosity and elevated bipedicle flaps.
- Bernhard von Langenbeck (1861): He was the first to describe the mucoperiosteal plane of dissection and to use its advantage in mobility to cleft palate closure.
- Dieffenbach (1845): Extended his relaxing mucoperiosteal incisions through bone.
- Ganzer (1917): Developed various retrodisplacement procedures.
- Dorrance(1925): Developed variation in retrodisplacement. He made a relaxing incision within the alveolar ridge from one maxillary tuberosity to the contralateral one, thereby producing a transverse flap (posteriorly based) which was mobilized toward the posterior pharyngeal wall.

Q63. What are the postoperative complications?

- Immediate complications:
  - Hemorrhage:
    - From bare membranous bony palate and from edges of mucoperiosteal flap.
    - Bleeding is common after palate repair.
    - There are inevitably raw surfaces, which may ooze for 12 to 24 hours.
    - Light pressure on the hard palate repair at the conclusion of the procedure often controls bleeding.
  - Respiratory obstruction.
  - Hanging palate.
  - Dehiscence of the repair.
  - Oronasal fistula.
- Late complications:
  - Bifid uvula.
  - Velopharyngeal incompetence.
  - Abnormal speech.
  - Maxillary hypoplasia.
  - Dental malpositioning and malalignment.
  - Otitis media.

Q64. Does type of cleft palate repair have any relation to the site of fistula formation?
- The pushback palatoplasty causes greater degrees and duration of hypoxemia than the von Langenbeck technique, so chances of fistula formation are more.
- Furlow repair was shown to markedly reduce fistulas relative to the V-Y pushback or von Langenbeck technique.

Q65. What is the algorithm of treatment in a cleft lip and palate child?
The algorithm is as shown in **Fig. 15.19a, b**.

Q66. What are rings of Delaire?
It is formed by the following muscles:
- Nasolabial muscles:
  - Transverse nasalis.
  - Levator labii superioris alaeque nasi.
  - Levator labii superioris.
- Bilateral:
  - Orbicularis oris upper lip (oblique head).
  - Orbicularis oris upper lip (horizontal head).
  - Orbicularis oris lower lip.
- Labiomental:
  - Depressor anguli oris.
  - Depressor labii inferioris.
  - Mentalis.

Q67. What is the incidence of cleft lip and palate?
- Cleft lip and palate: 46%.
- Isolated cleft palate: 33%.
- Isolated cleft lip: 21%.
  - Side: Left:Right:Bilateral = 6:3:1.
  - Sex:
    Cleft lip and palate: Male:Female = 2:1.
    Isolated cleft palate (M:F) = 1:2.

Q68. What are the syndromes associated with cleft lip and palate?
- Syndromes associated with cleft lip:
  - Van der Woude syndrome:
    - Autosomal dominant.

- Associated lower lip pits or blind sinuses.
- Syndactyly.
- Waardenburg syndrome.
- Down syndrome (Trisomy 21).
- Trisomy 13.
- Stickler syndrome:
  - Autosomal dominant.
  - Caused by connective tissue dysplasia.
  - Cardiac anomalies.
- Pierre Robin sequence:
  - It is a sequence because a group of anomaly that results from a single disrupted event.
    - Micrognathia and retrognathia prevent the normal descent of tongue.

    - Tongue interferes in upward rotation of palatal shelves.

    - Paired palatal shelves do not fuse, which results in horseshoe-shaped cleft palate.

    - Tongue fall-back in pharynx causes airway obstruction.
  - Treatment:
    - Prone positioning.
    - Nasopharyngeal airway protection.
    - Gavage feeding.
    - Apnea monitoring.
    - Supplemental oxygen.
    - Temporary endotracheal intubation.
    - Tongue lip adhesion.
    - Tracheostomy (severe cases).
    - Early distraction lengthening of mandible.
    - Palatoplasty (may be delayed for several months).
- Syndromes associated with cleft palate:
  - Velocardiofacial syndrome:
    - Also known as DiGeorge syndrome.
    - CATCH 22 syndrome.

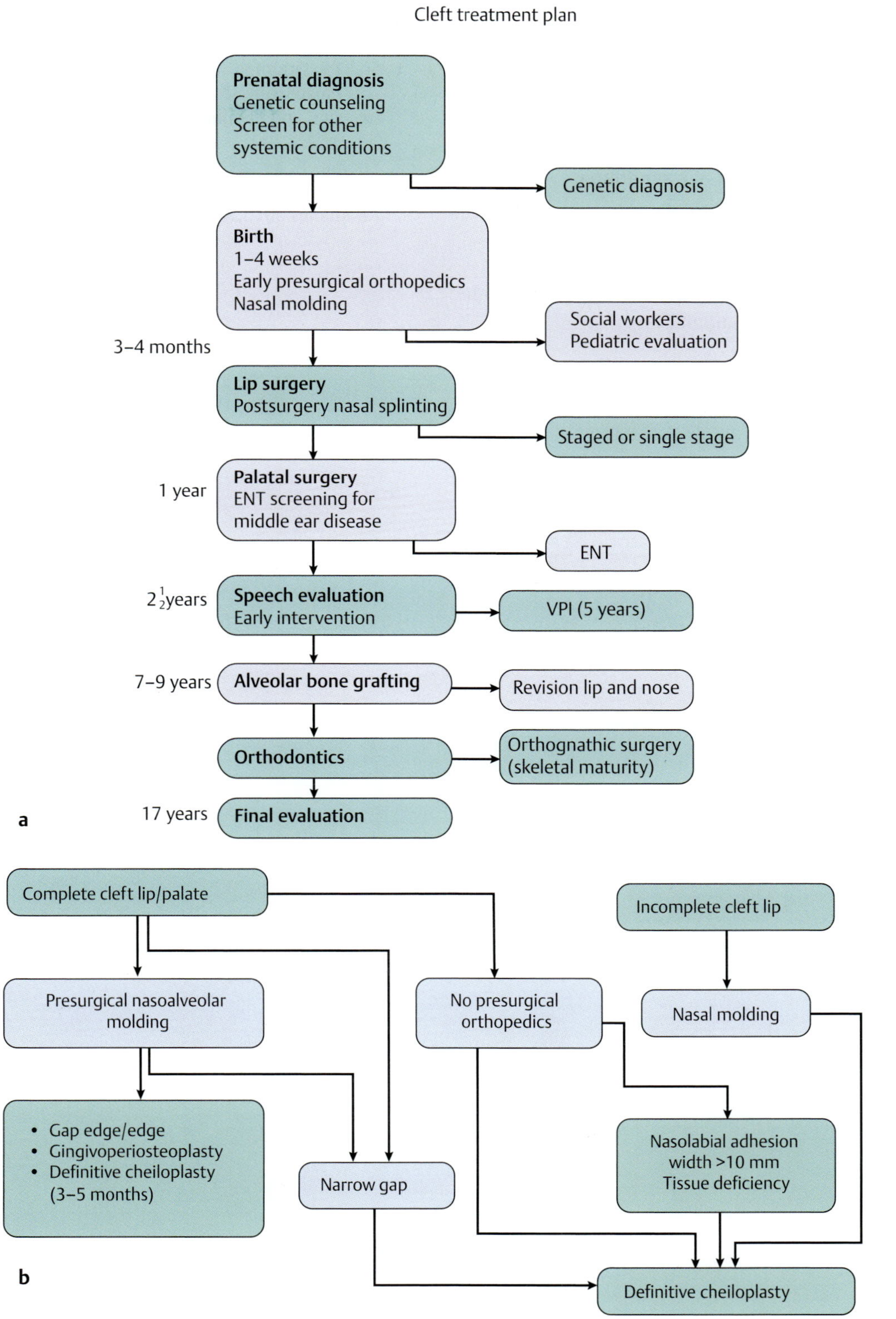

Cleft treatment plan

Fig. 15.19 **(a, b)** Algorithm of treatment in a cleft lip and palate child.

- C—Cardiac anomaly.
- A—Abnormal face.
- T—Thymic aplasia.
- C—Cleft palate.
- H—Hypocalcemia.
- 22—Long arm of chromosome 22.
- Treacher Colin syndrome.
- Apert syndrome.
- Crouzon's syndrome.
- Klipple Feil syndrome.
- Shprintzen syndrome: Associated cardiac anomalies.

Suggested Readings

1. Stål PS, Lindman R. Characterisation of human soft palate muscles with respect to fibre types, myosins and capillary supply. J Anat 2000;197 (Pt 2):275–290
2. Thomas C. Repair of cleft palate: Evolution and current trends. J Cleft Lip Palate Craniofacial Anomalies 2015;2(1):6

16 Vascular Anomalies

Saurabh K. Gupta and Veena K. Singh

Learning Objectives

At the end of this chapter, the student will be able to:
1. Understand the difference between the pathogenesis of vascular tumors and malformations.
2. Demonstrate the examination of a vascular swelling and make a proper diagnosis.
3. Distinguish between the various presentations of vascular anomalies.
4. Interpret the radiological findings of vascular anomalies.
5. Understand the management of different types of vascular anomalies at various stages of presentation.

Introduction

Vascular anomalies are broadly classified into vascular tumors and vascular malformations (VMs). Vascular tumors are basically due to endothelial cell hyperplasia and comprise hemangioma and other proliferative lesions. VMs are due to defect in vascular morphogenesis and remodeling. VMs are classified into slow-flow and fast-flow lesions. Identification of the lesion on the basis of its history, clinical presentation, and radiological findings is the most crucial step in choosing the correct management.

History

Particulars of the patient (name, age, sex, occupation, residence, etc.).

Chief Complaints

- Swelling over the affected area.
- Discoloration of the affected area.
- Bleeding episodes.
- Ulceration of affected area.
- Visible pulsations over the affected area.
- Pain associated with the lesion.

History of Present Illness

- **Location** of swelling:
  - Head and neck region.
  - Trunk and abdomen.
  - Extremities.
- **Duration** of swelling (mode of onset):
  - Noticed at birth.
  - Few days/months after birth.
  - Or, later on when the child grew up.
  - Noticed after any trauma to that area.
- **Progression** of the swelling:
  - Noticed at birth but swelling is stable.
  - Noticed at birth but increasing since then.
  - Noticed later in life and swelling subsiding in due course of time.
- Whether swelling is solitary in body or there are multiple similar lesions.
- Whether swelling is associated with increase in the volume of affected part, (e.g., in extremities).
- Any feeling of heaviness over the affected area.
- Any aggravating or relieving factors, (e.g., if the swelling subsides while lying down or it increases in size when the affected part is in dependent position).

- **Discoloration of the affected area:**
  - Any discoloration like crimson red, bright red, violet, or pale blue color associated with the swelling (suggestive of VMs).
  - Any change in color during the course.
  - Ask whether swelling becomes pale on applying pressure.
  - Whether the discoloration is solitary or similar lesions are present elsewhere in the body.
- **Bleeding episodes:**
  - To enquire about any bleeding episodes associated with the swelling.
  - Whether bleeding was spontaneous in occurrence or associated with any trauma.
  - Whether the blood loss was bright in color or slightly dark in color.
  - How much amount of blood was lost during the episode, (e.g., a single handkerchief or a towel, etc.).
  - How did the bleeding stop—whether by itself or after applying pressure or the patient needed hospitalization for bleeding.
  - Any history of visible clots in the swelling (may be due to past bleeding episode over the affected area).
- **Ulceration:**
  - Whether swelling is associated with ulceration of the affected area.
  - How did the ulcer occur—spontaneously or associated with trauma or due to friction of the swelling with surrounding area.
  - *Enquire for:*
    - Any discharge from the ulcer, either fresh blood or serosanguinous discharge or pus.
    - Any foul smell originating from the ulcer (due to secondary infection).
    - Progression of the ulcer—whether increasing with time or on treatment.

- **Visible pulsations:**
  - To enquire about any visible pulsations noted by the patient/informant (visible pulsations indicate the communication of the lesion with underlying arterial vessels).
- **Pain associated with swelling:**
  - Whether the swelling is associated with pain.
  - Whether pain is continuous or intermittent or occasional.
  - If pain subsides by any postural change, (e.g., lying down on bed).
    - Nature of pain: Dull aching, throbbing, sharp shooting, burning (irritation of a local nerve by the swelling).
    - Whether patient needs medication to relieve the pain (oral or injectable).
    - Pain relieved after how much duration of medication.

Past History

- Any history suggestive of diabetes mellitus, hypertension, tuberculosis.
- Any other medical illness.
- History of any surgical intervention in the past.

Personal History (in Grown-up Patients)

- History of smoking, drinking, any other addictions.
- Patient's occupation and social obligations.
- Marital status.

Family History

- Number of members in the family.
- Any family member suffering from the same problem and has taken treatment for the same.

Treatment History

- Whether any treatment taken for the current problem, both medical and surgical.

History of Allergy

- Any allergy to drugs.
- Any food allergy, etc.

General Physical Examination

- It remains same as for other cases but the area affected is to be examined in detail.

Systemic Examination

- Abdomen   ⎤ Refer chapter 3 on
- Respiratory system ⎥ "Carcinoma oral
- CNS   ⎥ cavity".
- CVS   ⎦

Local Examination of Lesion

Inspection

1. **Location** of the swelling:
   - Midline over scalp, trunk.
   - Extremities.
2. **Color** of the swelling:
   - Red—Bright red, dark red.
   - Cherry colored.
   - Blinds in appearance like red blemishes.
3. **Shape:** Whether
   - Ovoid.
   - Pear-shaped.
   - Kidney-shaped.
   - Spherical.
   - Irregular.
   - Bosselated.
   Generally, the vascular malformations are spherical swellings.
4. **Size:** Approximate size of the swelling should be mentioned in both vertical and horizontal dimensions.

5. **Surface:** In some swellings, surface depicts a lot about its character, (e.g., irregular bosselated surface is characteristic of vascular swellings).
6. **Margins:** Margin of the swelling may be clearly defined or indistinct. They may be either pedunculated or sessile.
7. **Number:** To notice whether the swelling is single or multiple. Whether swellings are in vicinity of each other or scattered over a large area.
8. **Skin over the swelling**:
   - Whether red and edematous, any venous prominence, any pigmentation.
   - Whether tense or glossy.
   - Presence of any scar over the swelling suggests previous surgical intervention.
   - Sometimes, appearance is of peau d' orange (because of blockage of small lymphatic drainage in the skin).
9. **Any visible pulsations:**
   - Look carefully for any pulsations over the swelling.
   - It suggests communication with underlying arterial system.

Palpation

The findings on inspection must be corroborated with palpation.

1. **Temperature:**
   - Felt by the back of fingers and compared with normal areas.
   - Local temperature may be raised due to excessive vascularity of swelling.
2. **Tenderness:** Presence of tenderness indicates infection.
3. **Size, shape, and extent:**
   - By gently palpating the swelling, try to get an idea about the deeper dimensions of the swelling.
   - Both vertical and horizontal dimensions should be measured and mentioned.
   - Extent of the swelling should also be noted.

4. **Surface:**
   - Palmar surface of fingers should be used to palpate surface of swelling.
   - Swelling surface can be smooth or associated with irregular bumps.
5. **Edges/Margins:**
   - Edges or margins of the swelling should be palpated carefully. May be well defined or indistinct merging into the surrounding structures.
   - Margins should be felt by the tip of fingers. **"Slip sign"** is elicited—It can be used to differentiate swellings. For example lipoma slips away from the palpating finger, but a cystic lesion or VM yields to the palpating fingers and cannot slip away from the examining finger.
6. **Consistency of the swelling:**
   - Soft, (e.g., lipoma, cysts).
   - Firm, (e.g., lipoma).
   - Hard, (e.g., chondroma).
   - Bony hard, (e.g., osteoma).
   - Stony hard, (e.g., carcinoma).
   - Check whether swelling is getting molded or not. Sometimes, the swelling pits on pressure in case there is associated edema.
7. **Fluctuation:**
   - One finger of both hands is used simultaneously.
   - Pressure is applied on one pole of swelling. This increases pressure within the cavity of the swelling and transmits equally at right angles to all parts of its wall.
   - The other finger can feel the increased pressure within the swelling.
8. **Translucency:**
   - For this test darkness is required. A drill of paper is held on one side of swelling while a torch is held on the other side of the swelling.
   - Swelling will be seen to transmit the light in case it is a translucent swelling.
   - This test is positive if the swelling contains clear fluid, (e.g., water, serum, lymph, plasma, or highly liquefied fat).

9. **Impulse on coughing:**
   - The swellings which are in continuity with visceral cavities show impulse or coughing.
   - Look for impulse on coughing in suspected vascular swellings over abdominal regions or near groin.
10. **Reducibility:**
    - Swelling reduces and ultimately disappears when it is pressed upon.
    - This characteristic differentiates the vascular swellings from hernia, lymphavarix, varicocele, meningocele, etc.
11. **Compressibility:**
    - This means swelling can be compressed to an extent but will not disappear completely. Those swellings may not have connections with the adnominal, pleural, spinal, or cranial cavity.
    - These swellings are liquid filled and mostly VMs, (e.g., arterial capillary or venous hemangiomas).
    - The swelling immediately appears when the pressure is taken off.
12. **Pulsatility:** A swelling may be pulsatile if:
    - It arises from an artery (expansile pulsation)—both fingers are raised and separated with each beat of the artery.
    - If it lies very close to an artery (transmitted pulsation)— both fingers are raised but not separated with each beat of the artery.
13. **Thrill:** In cases of high-flow VMs, a sound like purring of a cat will be heard on palpation.
14. **Attachment to the overlying skin:**
    - Look whether the skin over the swelling can be pinched or not by trying to hold the skin between the thumb and index finger and lift it.
    - It is not possible in the swellings that arise from skin.
    - This is known as "PINCH TEST."
15. **Relation to the structures in vicinity:**
    - To examine whether the skin is attached to the nearby structures.

- If a swelling is present over the muscle, make the muscle taut and check the movement of swelling over the muscle. The swelling would not move if it is attached to the underlying muscle.
16. **Peripheral pulses and vascularity:**
    - Arterial pulses distal to the swelling must be examined.
    - Capillary refill time must be seen if swelling is in palm or any finger.
17. **Motor and sensory examination:**
    - Important in lesions over face and extremities for documentation of findings before surgery and comparison of any deficit after surgery.
18. **Regional lymph node examination:** It is necessary to examine the regional lymph nodes. The fair knowledge of the areas draining to a particular group of lymph nodes is necessary to generally rule out any infection or malignant pathology.

Percussion

- This examination is not of much use in case of a swelling.
- Generally done to get a vague idea about the contents of a swelling.

Auscultation

- In auscultation, bruit may be heard in case of arterial malformations (AM). arterio-venous malformations (AVMs), etc.

Movements

- Movements of nearby joints should be examined for normal activity or any impairment.

Provisional Diagnosis

This is a case of slow-flow VM likely to be of venous origin over the left forearm in a 16-year-old female without any functional and neurovascular deficit.

Questions

Q1. What are your differential diagnoses?
- It can be any other swelling like lipoma, neurofibroma.
- It can be any other vascular anomaly like lymphatic malformation.
- Pyogenic granuloma.
- Kaposiform hemangioepithelioma.

Q2. How will you proceed?
I will go for certain investigations to get the details of the lesion. Once my diagnosis is confirmed, I would plan for surgical excision for which I would like to get the baseline investigations for anesthetic fitness.
- If facilities are available, I would go for MR angiography (**Fig. 16.1a–c**).
- Magnetic resonance (MR) imaging:
  – The best imaging in vascular anomalies as it is noninvasive and provides the details of the lesion and also the surrounding structures.
  – MR angiography can also distinguish the slow-flow lesions from the high-flow ones.
  – In smaller children, MRI is a problem as it requires sedation or general anesthesia.

Q3. If MRI facility is not available, then how are you going to investigate this case?
There are other investigations which can be done to confirm the diagnosis.
- X-ray: For any skeletal abnormality or phleboliths (seen in venous malformations).
- Color Doppler ultrasound: For assessing the blood flow velocity and is helpful in differentiation of high-flow and slow-flow lesions.
- CT scan: Only for intraosseous VMs or secondary changes in the underlying bone due to long-standing lesion.

Q4. How will you classify vascular anomalies?
Vascular anomalies are broadly classified into tumors and malformations (**Table 16.1**).

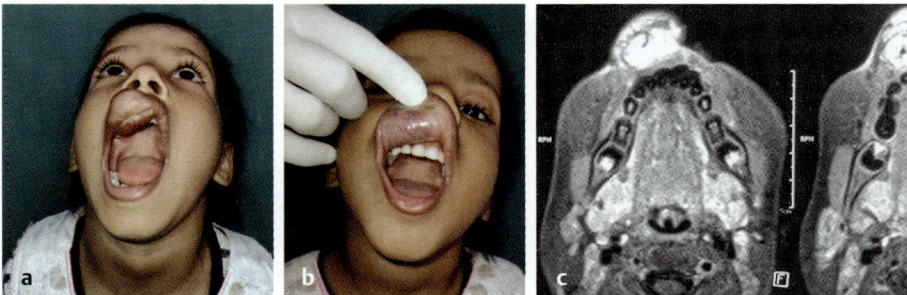

Fig. 16.1 (a–c) Vascular malformation upper lip and increased uptake in the magnetic resonance (MR) angiography.

Table 16.1 International Society for the Study of Vascular Anomalies Classification of Vascular Anomalies

Vascular tumors	Vascular malformations
Infantile hemangioma	Simple
Congenital hemangioma	Capillary malformations
Tufted angioma	Venous malformations
Hemangiopericytoma	Lymphatic malformations
Progenic granuloma	Arterial malformation
Kaposiform hemangioendothelioma	Combined
Spindle cell hemangioendochelioma	Capillary-lymphatic-venous malformation
Rare hemangioendotheliomas (epithelioid, composite, retiform, polymorphous, Dabska tumor, etc.)	Capillary-venous malformation
Dermatologic-acquired vascular tumors (targetoid hemangioma, glomeruloid hemangioma, microvenular hemangioma, etc.)	Capillary-lymphatic malformation
	Lymphatic-venous malformation
	Arteriovenous malformation
	Capillary-arteriovenous malformation
	Lymphatic-arteriovenous malformation
	Arteriovenous fistula

Q5. What is the difference between vascular tumors and vascular malformations?

- **Vascular tumors** are characterized by endothelial cell hyperplasia as seen in infantile hemangioma.
  - It increases in size during infancy and regresses in childhood.
- **Vascular malformations** are characterized by defective vascular development leading to abnormal blood vessels.
  - They never regress but persist or continue growing in size with time.

Q6. What are the other congenital anomalies associated with hemangioma?

- **PHACES syndrome: P**osterior fossa malformations (Dandy-Walker malformation is the most common), **h**emangiomas of cervicofacial region, **a**rterial anomalies, **c**ardiac anomalies, **e**ye abnormalities, and **s**ternal defects.
- Hemangiomas in lumbosacral region may be associated with occult spinal dysraphism or genitourinary anomalies.

Q7. What is an infantile hemangioma (IH)?

- Infantile hemangioma is benign endothelial tumor characterized by rapid growth and slow regression (**Fig. 16.2**).
- They manifest as single lesion in 80% cases and multiple in 20% cases.
- There are three phases in its life cycle:
  - Proliferating phase (0–1 y of age).
  - Involuting phase (1–4 y).
  - Involuted phase (>4 y).
- Proliferative phase:
  - Marked by clusters of rapidly dividing and plump endothelial cells with less vascular channel, sparse connective tissue, and multilaminated basement membranes.
  - Markers like VEGF (vascular endothelial growth factor), MMP-2 (matrix metalloproteinase-2), bFGF (basic fibroblast growth factor) are seen in increased amounts.
- Involuting phase:
  - Decreased proliferation of endothelial cells.
  - Mature blood vessels are seen with large vascular channels.
  - Fibrosis starts and markers like tissue inhibitors of MMP-2 are seen.

- Involuted phase: Most of IH are replaced by adipocytes and connective tissues containing dense collagen.
- *Clinical course:* IH grows very fast in the first 9 months of child, and by then, the growth reaches a plateau and regression of tumor starts after 12 months.

Q8. How to manage the infantile hemangioma?

- Treatment of infantile hemangioma depends upon the following factors:
  - Location.
  - Size.
  - Growth phase.
  - Age of the patient at the time of presentation.
- There can be various options:
  - Observation and local care.
  - Medical management.
  - LASER.
  - Surgical management.
- **Nonoperative management:**
  - **Observation:**
    - Small IH needs only observation, and close follow-up is required for continuous monitoring of its progression and development of any complication.
    - If during the proliferating phase, lesion becomes large and causes obstruction, destruction, or ulceration of vital structures, then intervention is required.
  - **Local care:**
    - Superficial IH may have ulceration because overlying skin becomes thin and liable to damage by friction.
    - They should be kept lubricated with creams and ointments. Occlusive dressings may be applied to prevent desiccation and crust formation.
    - Pain may be relieved by topical analgesia like viscous lidocaine.
    - Local infections should be prevented.

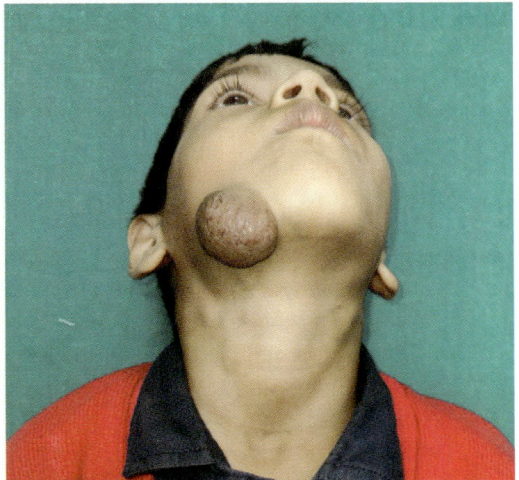

Fig. 16.2 Hemangioma over right lower jaw.

Q9. What are the drugs available for treatment of hemangioma?

Pharmacological treatment: Indicated only in hemangiomas causing complications like ulceration, local tissue deformity, or amblyopia (only in 10% of cases).

- **Steroids:**
  - **Topical corticosteroids:**
    - Are only useful in superficial IH. It may lead to cutaneous atrophy and discoloration.
  - **Intralesional corticosteroids:**
    - If lesion is affecting vital structures or obstructing visual axis or nasal passageway, intralesional steroids can be used.
    - Triamcinolone (3 mg/kg) injection stops the growth of lesion.
    - Generally two to three injections are required at the gap of 2 to 3 weeks.
    - Subcutaneous fat atrophy is a known side effect.
  - **Systemic steroids:**
    - IH >3 to 4 cm in diameter are treated by oral corticosteroid.
      - ○ *Dosage:* Prednisolone 2 to 3mg/kg/d as a single morning dose for 4 to 6 weeks and discontinuation between 10 and 12 months of age.
      - ○ **Response observed is:**
        - ◇ Decreased growth rate.
        - ◇ Fading color.
        - ◇ Softening of lesion.
    - **Side effects:** 20% infants develop cushingoid features which resolve after stopping the therapy. Other side effects can be hypertension, immunosuppression, hirsutism.
- **Propranolol:**
  - **Dosage:** 2 mg/kg/d in three divided doses during the proliferative phase. It should be stopped after weaning for 2 months once the proliferative phase ends.
  - 90% tumors show response and regular monitoring is required.

- **Mechanism of action:** inhibition of hypoxia-induced factor 1 alpha-VEGF pathway which results in inhibition of the angiogenesis mediators.
- **Side effects** like bradycardia and hypotension have been seen in few patients so all patients should have cardiologist consultation and baseline cardiac investigations.
- **Interferon alpha:**
  - Recombinant interferon, IFN-α-2a or IFN-α-2b, is a second-line drug.
  - **Indications:** IH not responding to steroids, contraindications to systemic steroids, complications, and parental refusal of steroids.
  - Simultaneous treatment with IFN and steroids is not recommended.
  - **Dose:** 2 to 3 Mu/m^2 (million units/m^2) as subcutaneous injection daily.
  - Response is >80% in 6 to 10 months of therapy.
  - **Side effects:** Fever for initial 1 to 2 weeks, raised liver enzymes, neutropenia, spastic diplegia.
  - Effective in vascular tumors causing Kasabach-Merritt phenomenon.
- **Vincristine:**
  - It is also a second-line drug used only in cases where steroids and interferons cannot be used.
  - Is administered through central venous line.
  - Side effects are peripheral neuropathy, constipation, sepsis.

Q10. What is the role of LASER in hemangioma?

- Pulsed dye laser (PDL) is generally used but has a very limited role as penetration is very less. It is only indicated in the later stages of involution to fade the residual lesions.
- Other lasers used are Nd:YAG (neodymium: yttrium-aluminum-garnet) and KTP (potassium titanyl phosphate).

Q11. When is surgery done in cases of hemangioma?

Surgical treatment: Surgery is required only in the following cases:

- Infant can't be given pharmacotherapy.
- Small localized tumor.
- Tumor situated at vital areas like eyelids and is supposed to create a problem in vision.

Q12. What is Kasabach-Merritt phenomenon?

- It is a life-threatening event in which a vascular tumor traps the circulating platelets and destroys them, leading to thrombocytopenia and consumptive coagulopathy which finally results in the loss of clotting factors and disseminated intravascular coagulopathy (DIC).
- Mainly associated with kaposiform hemangioepithelioma and tufted angioma.
- Once Kasabach-Merritt phenomenon resulting in DIC takes place, do not give platelet transfusion (only indicated if active bleeding is present or any surgical intervention is required) or heparin (as it stimulates the growth of vascular tumor leading to increased platelet trapping).
- Proper management of DIC must be followed.

Q13. What are the pathological considerations in infantile hemangiomas?

- In infantile hemangiomas, marker CD133 is found positive on immunohistochemistry which represents the proliferation of hemangioma-initiating stem cell population.
- This stem cell population forms blood vessels which express glucose transporter protein (GLUT-1). GLUT-1 is positive on immunohistochemistry in infantile hemangioma.
- The endothelial cells of the blood vessels also show low expression of vascular endothelial growth factor receptor (VEGFR-1).

- Also, there are mutations in genes responsible for expression of VEGFR-2 and tumor endothelial marker (TEM-8).

Q14. What are congenital hemangiomas?

- Congenital hemangiomas are vascular anomalies that arise in fetus, fully developed at birth and do not grow after birth.
- These lesions do not express GLUT-1.
- They are two types of congenital hemangiomas:
  - **RICH (rapidly involuting congenital hemangiomas):**
    - It presents as a single, elevated lesion with telangiectasia in the center with surrounding halo.
    - It might cause high-output cardiac failure due to shunting of blood circulation.
    - It rapidly evolves after birth and approx. 50% of lesions are gone by 7 to 8 months.
    - Rest lesions are gone by 12 months of age.
    - After involution, they do not leave much adipose tissue component.
    - RICH generally do not require surgical resection because it regresses quickly.
    - Complication can occur in few cases like congestive heart failure controlled by corticosteroids or embolization.
    - At later stages, fat grafting may be required for atrophic areas.
  - **Noninvoluting congenital hemangiomas (NICH):**
    - Do not involute as the name suggests.
    - It presents as a flat lesion of pink or blue color with a central telangiectasia.
    - It requires surgical management at some point of time.
    - NICH requires surgery later for remaining lesions.

Q15. What are capillary malformations (CMs) and how are they treated?

- Most common vascular anomalies, and present as pink or red discoloration of the skin (**Fig. 16.3**).
- Also known as "macular stains" and located on the central aspect of face and neck as "salmon patch" or "nevus simplex."
- Comprises of thin-walled capillary to venular sized channels in the dermis.
- Some CMs may be a part of a syndrome: Klippel-Trenaunay syndrome, Parkes-Weber syndrome, Cobb's syndrome, Sturge-Weber syndrome.
- Extensive CM in extremity is often associated with increased circumference and limb length discrepancy.

Management:
- **LASER (light amplification by the stimulated emission of radiation):** Pulsed dye laser (PDL, wavelength 577, 585, or 595 nm) helps by lightening the color.
  - Head and neck region have better response rate.
  - Treatment should be started in infancy for superior results.
  - Other lasers such as long PDL, alexandrite or Nd:YAG, and IPL (intense pulsed light) can also be used.

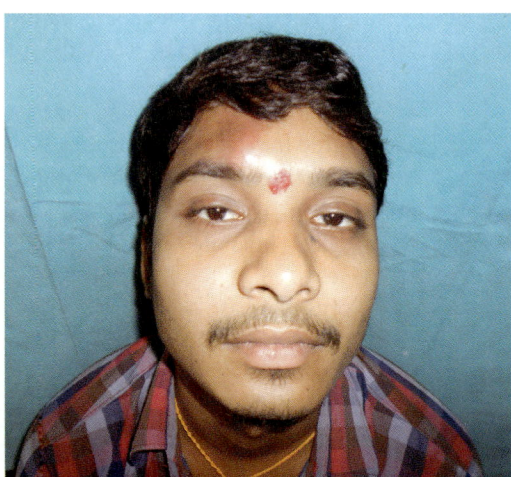

Fig. 16.3 Capillary malformation (port wine stain) over right forehead.

- Trunk or extremities soft tissue overgrowth can be addressed with liposuction, excision and linear closure, skin grafts or flaps.

Q16. What are the syndromic associations of capillary malformations?

- **Klippel-Trenaunay syndrome:**
  - Combined capillary-lymphatic-venous malformations.
  - Manifests as limb hypertrophy.
- **Parkes-Weber syndrome:**
  - Arteriovenous malformations.
  - Cutaneous capillary malformations.
  - Skeletal or soft tissue hypertrophy of the limb.
- **Cobb's syndrome:**
  - Capillary malformation over the back along with AVM of spinal cord.
- **Sturge-Weber syndrome:**
  - Capillary malformation over face in the area of trigeminal nerve.
  - Vascular anomalies of leptomeninges of brain and eye.
  - Seizures.

Q17. What are lymphatic malformations (LM)?

- LM comprises lymphatic fluid-filled anomalous channels, vesicles, or pouches.
- They are formed when small lymphatic sacs are separated off the main lymphatic system.
- Regression is not seen in LMs but depending on the flow of lymphatic fluid, bleeding, and inflammation, they either expand or contract.
- They are categorized into:
  - Microcystic.
  - Macrocystic.
  - Combined.
- **Macrocystic LMs** cause soft tissue and bony hypertrophy like macrocheilia, macrotia, macroglossia, and macromala.
- **Microcystic LMs** are also known as "lymphangioma circumscriptum" and manifest on trunk, axilla, or extremities as an

irregular group of vesicles or hyperkeratotic papules.

- **Combined LMs** may be seen over cheek, forehead, or orbit and cause soft tissue and bony hypertrophy. It may also be seen in cervicofacial region, cervicoaxillary region, extremities, and pelvic area.

Q18. What are the complications associated with LM?

- Lesions leading to overgrowth in mandible may cause class III malocclusion and anterior open bite.
- Bulky tongue causes impaired speech and is affected frequently by infections, swelling, and bleeding.
- In cervicofacial region, LM may cause airway obstruction thereby needing tracheostomy.

Q19. What are the treatment options of lymphatic malformations?

- Asymptomatic lesions are observed.
- **Sclerotherapy:**
  - Sclerotherapy is the first line of management for large or problematic macrocystic/combined LMs.
  - Aspiration is done and inflammatory substance is injected which causes cyst walls to collapse.
  - **Main sclerosants used are:**
    - Doxycycline.
    - Sodium tetradecyl sulfate (STS).
    - Ethanol.
    - Bleomycin.
  - **Side effects of sclerotherapy:**
    - Cutaneous ulceration.
    - Ethanol—central nervous system (CNS) depression.
    - Hemolysis.
    - Pulmonary hypertension.
    - Thromboembolism and arrhythmias.
    - Extravasation in muscle causes atrophy or contracture.
- **Surgical treatment:**
  - Surgical aspiration generally associated with morbidity:
    - Iatrogenic injury.

- Blood loss and deformity.
- Recurrence is generally common.
  - **Surgical resection is the only way to cure LM. It may be done for:**
    - Microcystic LM causing bleeding, infection, distortion of vital structures.
    - Macrocystic/Combined LM not responding to sclerotherapy.

Q20. What are the characteristics of venous malformation (VM)?

- They are present at birth sometimes but not always evident.
- They manifest as bluish discoloration, compressible swelling which increases in size when the extremity is in dependent position. Patient may complain of pain and stiffness in that particular part on getting up in the morning.
- Phleboliths are often found in VMs, and episodic thrombosis occurs.
- VM grows proportionately to child and is usually a solitary lesion (**Fig. 16.4**).
- *Associated problems:*
  - **Craniofacial VMs** are usually unilateral and extend to the underlying

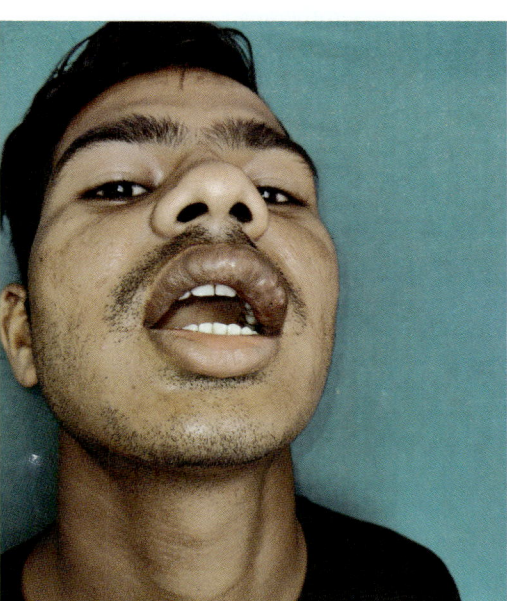

Fig. 16.4   Venous malformation over upper lip.

muscle, bone, salivary glands, leading to epistaxis, hemoptysis, airway problems, abnormal dentition, and speech.

- **Extremities VM** can involve skin only or extend into muscles, joints, and bone, and may cause limb hypertrophy.
- **Blue rubber bleb nevus syndrome** is associated with multiple VMs in the palm, sole, trunk, and gastrointestinal system leading to intestinal bleeding.

Q21. What are the treatment options for VMs?

- Large extensive extremity VMs are treated by pressure garments customized to the extremity to reduce blood stagnation and further progression.
- Coagulation profiles should be done for all large VMs as these patients are at risk for DIC.
  - **Sclerotherapy:**
    - First-line treatment for VMs as percutaneous sclerotherapy.
    - Common sclerosants used are 3% STS, absolute ethanol, or hypertonic saline.
    - Pressure garments are also prescribed for the patients along with sclerotherapy.
  - **Surgical resection:**
    - Complete resection is not possible and surgery is more of debulking.
    - It is not the preferred method as the VMs are associated with multiple smaller channels and there are risks of bleeding and other complications.

- **Indicated only if:**
  - Lesion is small and chances of complete removal are fairly high.
  - Existing deformity after completion of sclerotherapy.

Q22. What are the characteristics of arteriovenous malformations (AVMs)?

- The characteristic features are:
  - AVMs are fast-flow lesions where there is a direct connection between the artery and vein without intervening capillary bed.
  - Pure arterial malformations occur as a solitary lesion or in association with AVMs.
  - The AVM has an epicenter called "nidus" which consists of arterial feeders, micro and macro-AV fistulas and ectatic veins.
  - Intracranial AVMs are more common than extracranial AVMs.
- They have a natural history as described by **Schobinger** (**Table 16.2**).

Q23. What are the treatment options for AVMs?

- **The treatment options are:**
  - **Small, localized AVM:**
    - Surgical excision and reconstruction.
  - **AVM with recurrent bleeding, ulceration, ischemic pain, and increased cardiac output:**
    - Early embolization and surgical resection for stage I/II if this is easily

Table 16.2 Stages of Arterio-Venous malformations (Schobinger)

Stage	Clinical findings
I. (Quiescent phase)	• Usually asymptomatic • This is the duration between birth and adolescence • Appearance of involuting capillary malformation
II. (Progressive phase)	• Starts during adolescence • Presents as enlarged, warm lesion with palpable thrill and bruit on auscultation
III. (Destructive phase)	• Associated complication starts like pain, bleeding, ulceration
IV. (Decompensation phase)	• Cardiac decompensation with congestive heart failure

achievable and reconstruction is not a problem.

- Selective or superselective arterial embolization done through a catheter to temporarily stop blood flow into the AVM nidus.
- Embolization has to be followed by surgical resection within 24 to 48 hours, otherwise collaterals will form and original blood flow will be restored.
- The main aim of the embolization is to reduce the intraoperative bleeding. It does not shrink the boundaries of the AVM.
- The resection must be targeted toward complete excision and not only ligation of the arterial feeders, otherwise there would be rapid recruitment of the arterial feeders to supply the nidus.

Q24. What are the substances used for embolization?

- They are categorized into either:
  - Solid (polyvinyl alcohol [PVA] particles).
  - Liquid (N-butyl cyanoacrylate) (N-BCA).
- Temporary embolization substance is used for the patient planned for definite surgical resection (Gelfoam powder, PVA Embospheres).

Q25. Describe pyogenic granuloma and how they are treated.

- "Pyogenic granuloma" is basically a misnomer. They are generally lobular capillary hemangioma.
- It is generally a single papule with a peduncle, small with a diameter of 5 to 6 mm (**Fig. 16.5**).

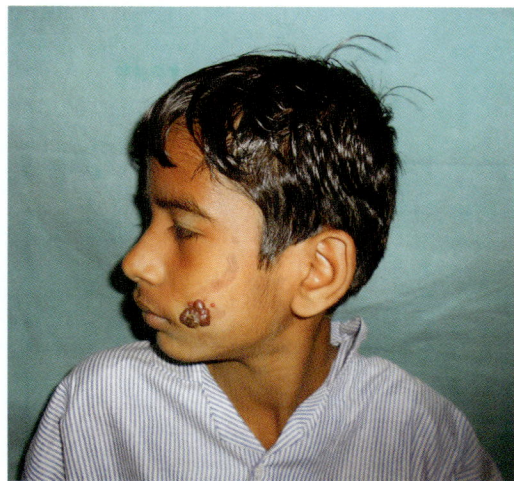

Fig. 16.5 Pyogenic granuloma over left cheek.

- It is found mainly in skin (80%).
- **Treatment:**
  - It rarely involutes and requires intervention.
  - The major associated problem is bleeding.
  - Many treatment modalities are described like curettage, shave excision, Laser therapy, and excision.
  - Lasers are generally not effective.
  - Full-thickness excision is generally more definitive treatment.

Suggested Readings

1. Chim H, Gosain AK. In: Thorne CH, ed. Grabb and Smith's plastic surgery: congenital anomalies and paediatric plastic surgery. 7th ed. Wolters Kluwer; 2014:206–220
2. Greene AK, Muliken JB. In: Neligan PC, ed. Plastic surgery: craniofacial, head and neck surgery, and pediatric plastic surgery. Vol. 3. 4th ed. Canada: Elsevier; 2018:866–887

Learning Objectives

At the end of this chapter, the students will be able to:
1. Understand the anatomy of penis.
2. Describe the clinical presentation of patients with hypospadias.
3. Demonstrate the examination of patients with hypospadias.
4. Understand the pathophysiology of hypospadias.
5. Understand the planning and management of hypospadias.
6. Understand the type of surgery according to the position of penile meatus and grading of chordee.

Introduction

Hypospadias is one of the most common genital anomalies in male newborns, 1 in 250 to 300. The urethral meatus is located at the ventral surface of the penis varying from glans to the perineum proximally. The optimum timing for surgery is at 6 to 18 months. The goal is to give the patient a cosmetically acceptable penis, enabling him to micturate while standing and maintaining his fertility. A good clinical examination and thorough knowledge of the anatomy and available surgical options provides a strong foundation for the surgeon to achieve his/her goals and give quality life to the patient.

History

Details of the patient (name, age, religion, address).

Mention of the informant is important. In most cases, it is usually the mother.

Chief Complaints

- Passage of urine from undersurface of penis.
- Bending of penis.
- Narrowing/Thinning of urinary stream.
- Retention of urine and distension of abdomen.
- Abdominal pain due to retention of urine.

History of Present Illness

- History of child having the above problems since birth, may be few complaints arise later in life.
- Write in details about the progression of symptoms like bending of penis and narrowing of urinary stream, with the age of the patient.
- Enquire about increase in the bending of penis during morning erections.

Negative History

- History of undescended testis—the mother can be asked whether scrotal sac is empty.
- History of inguinal hernia—whether any swelling is seen in the inguinal region when the child cries or cough.
- Any other deformity present in the body since birth like cleft lip and palate, fusion of fingers.

Antenatal History

- Ask about the duration of pregnancy—full term or preterm, as hypospadias is sometimes associated with low birth weight.
- Ask about the maternal age at pregnancy as hypospadias is associated with increased maternal age.
- Whether delivered by normal vaginal delivery or cesarean section.
- History of maternal diabetes and hypertension.
- History of taking any fertility drugs and in vitro fertilization.
- History of taking antiepileptic drugs.
- History of increased blood pressure during antenatal period as it is associated with pre-eclampsia.
- Smoking history of mother.
- Alcohol intake by the mother.
- Ask about the birth weight of the baby.

Past History

- Any history of circumcision done in the past.
- Any other medical illness which the child is suffering from.

Family History

- History of hypospadias in other siblings.
- History of hypospadias on maternal and paternal side.

Immunization History

Ask about the vaccines which the child has received for the age.

History of Allergy

Whether the child is allergic to any medicine or food material.

Examination

General Physical Examination

- In case of child, anthropometry is very important.
- Measure height and weight.
- Observe the build and nutrition.
- Measure temperature/pulse/BP (using child cuff)/respiratory rate.
- Look for pallor/jaundice/cyanosis/edema.
- Look for neck glands/neck veins.
- Any skin abnormalities.
- Look for other congenital anomalies in the body like:
  - Undescended testis, inguinal hernia.
  - Syndactyly.
  - Cleft lip and palate.

Systemic Examination

CNS Examination

Examine general behavior of the child and milestones as child may have mental retardation in cases associated with with WAGR syndrome hypospadias.

CVS Examination

Auscultate for normal heart sounds.

Per Abdomen

- Palpate for kidney as there may be hydronephrosis due to the obstruction.
- Palpate the hernial sites.
- Examine for undescended testis.
- Palpate the scrotum for testis.

May be examined under heading "local examination" also

Respiratory System

Measure the respiratory rate, whether regular, abdominothoracic, or thoracic; also auscultate for normal air entry, breath sounds.

Local Examination of Genital Region

Inspection

1. Ask the patient to hold the penis so that the undersurface can also be inspected.
   - Penis:
     - Curvature—usually curved downwards (**Fig. 17.1**).
     - Size—usually smaller in size than normal for the age.
     - Look for the presence of dorsal hooded prepuce and deficiency of prepuce on the ventral aspect.
     - Flattened and spatulated glans.
     - Look for deviation of median raphe. It is deviated mostly to left side.
     - Look for presence of chordee.
     - Comment on the local condition of skin.
   - Urethral opening:
     - Look for the site of meatus and describe the exact anatomical location.
     - Examine the shape of the urethral opening—whether it is fish mouth opening or pin-hole meatus.
     - Pin-hole meatus usually leads to stasis of urine→ cystitis→ hydroureter→ hydronephrosis.
     - Look for accessory urethral fistula.
   - Examination of scrotum:
     - Look for the presence and location of bilateral testis—whether descended in the scrotal sac.
     - Scrotum well developed or not.
     - Hypoplastic penis may be engulfed in bifid scrotum.
     - Bifid scrotum in scrotal type causes difficulty in sex determination.
   - Examination of hernial sites: Ask the patient to cough or make the baby cry and look for presence of inguinal hernia.

Palpation

1. After proper exposure of the genital region and from umbilicus up to the knees and adequate light with proper explained informed consent (from the parent or the adult patient).
   - All the inspection findings are corroborated on palpation.
   - The penis must be held by pulling the dorsal preputial skin and undersurface of the penis must be examined (**Fig. 17.2**).
     - Examination of chordee by making it stretched by pulling the ventral skin and dorsal hood simultaneously.
     - Presence and degree of ventral curvature.
     - Location and shape of the meatus and the degree of proximal spongiosal hypoplasia.
     - Quality (width and depth) of the urethral plate.
     - Size of the glans and the depth of the navicular fossa.
   - Degree of ventral skin deficiency: Availability of the foreskin.
   - Measure the penile length.

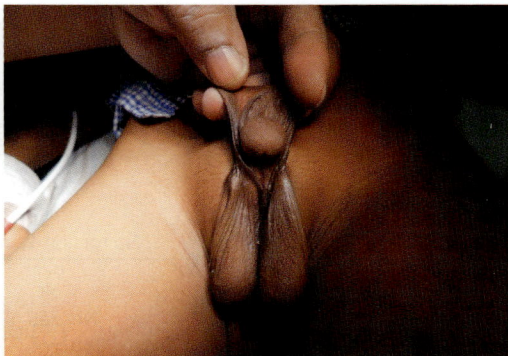

Fig. 17.1 Downward curvature of the penis.   **Fig. 17.2** Dorsal hooding.

2. Scrotal abnormalities:
   - Penoscrotal transposition and bifid scrotum.
   - Palpate the scrotum for testis.
   - Palpate for undescended testis.
3. Palpate the hernial sites.

All the relevant findings can be documented in a tabular format (**Fig. 17.3**).

Provisional Diagnosis

This is a case of a 3-year-old child with proximal penile hypospadias with moderate chordee with no other congenital anomaly.

Questions

Q1. How will you proceed?

I would like to go for some investigations and plan for surgery.

- Investigations:
  - Baseline investigations for surgical fitness of the patient:
    - Blood for CBC, ESR.
    - Blood for renal function tests.
    - Urine routine microscopy.
    - Urine for culture and sensitivity.
    - USG abdomen—to look for urinary tract back pressure changes.
      - Rule out stone in bladder.
      - Look at thickness of bladder wall.
      - Any diverticula or sacculations in bladder wall.
      - Kidneys present or not.
      - Kidneys are in normal position or ectopic position.
      - Fused or horseshoe-shaped kidney.
- After obtaining fitness of the patient for surgery, I would like to proceed in two stages:
  - Chordee correction.
  - Urethroplasty.

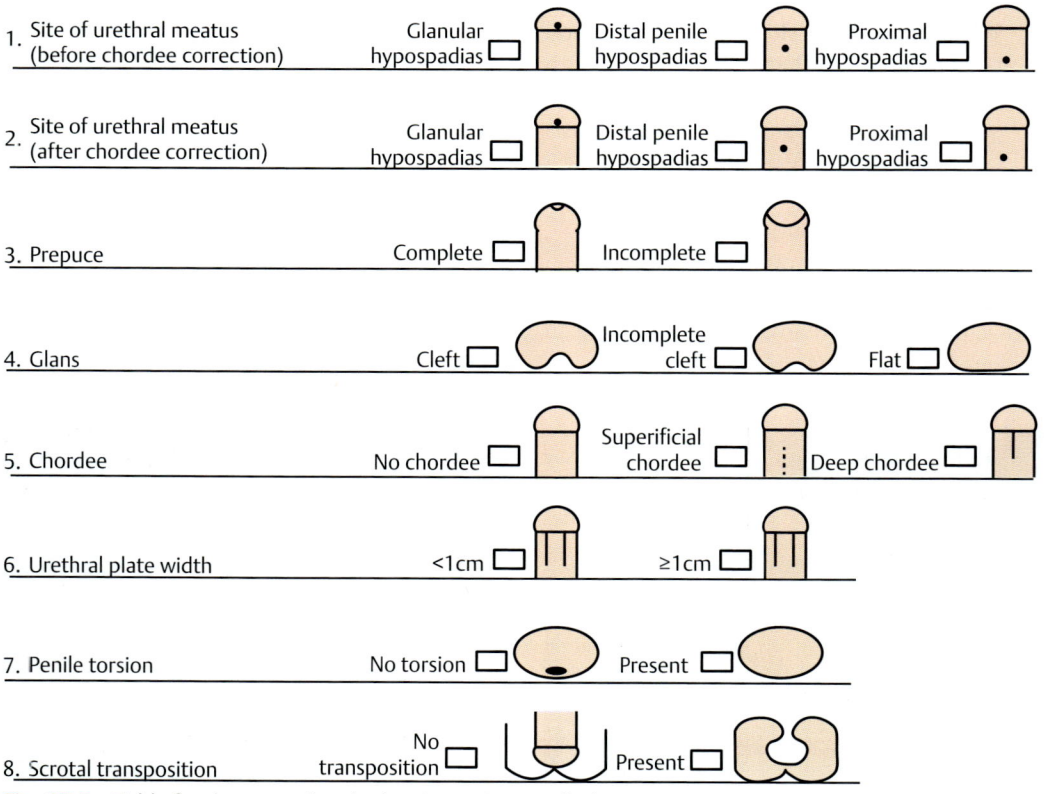

Fig. 17.3 Table for documenting the local examination findings.

Q2. What are the prerequisites of urethroplasty?

- No meatal stenosis should be there.
- No chordee should be there.

Q3. What is the best time for surgery?

Ideal time for surgery is between 6 and 12 months because:

- Genital awareness starts around 18 months of age.
- As the genital awareness begins child becomes uncooperative and it becomes very difficult to hospitalize the child.
- Hence, the best time for surgery is between 6 and 12 months of age.

Q4. What are the treatment goals?

Following are the treatment goals:

- To reconstruct a straight penis.
- Slit-like meatus on the ventrum of the terminal aspect of the glans.
- Micturition in the standing position.
- Normal sexual function.

Q5. What are the components of hypospadias surgery?

Regardless of the technique employed, following are the components of hypospadias surgery:

- Correction of penile curvature (orthoplasty).
- Urethroplasty.
- Meatoplasty.
- Glanuloplasty.
- Scrotoplasty.
- Finally, skin coverage.

Q6. Define hypospadias.

- Hypospadias—Dr. John W. Duckett coined the term "hypospadiology."
  - Hypo = below.
  - Spadon = a fissure or a hole.
- Hypospadias is an anomaly classically defined as an association of three anatomic developmental anomalies of the penis:
  - An abnormal opening of the urethral meatus, which may be located anywhere from the ventral aspect of the glans penis to the perineum.
  - An abnormal ventral curvature of the penis (chordee).
  - An abnormal distribution of foreskin, with a hood present dorsally and deficient foreskin ventrally.

Q7. What is the incidence of hypospadias?

One in 250 to 300 newborn males.

Q8. How do you classify hypospadias?

Sheldon and Duckett (1987) classified hypospadias based on the level of meatus following the treatment of penile curvature (**Fig. 17.4a–e**):

- Anterior → 50 to 70%
  - Glanular.
  - Coronal.
  - Subcoronal.
- Middle → 30%
  - Distal penile.
  - Midshaft.
  - Proximal penile.
- Posterior → 20%
  - Penoscrotal.
  - Scrotal.
  - Perineal.

Q9. What are the syndromes associated with hypospadias?

Nearly 200 syndromes are associated with hypospadias:

- Smith-Lemli-Opitz syndrome.
- WAGR syndrome →
  - W → Wilms tumor.
  - A → Aniridia.
  - G → Genital anomalies.
  - R → Mental retardation.
- Hand-foot-genital syndrome → bilateral thumb and great toe hypoplasia.
- Opitz G syndrome → hypertelorism, tracheoesophageal defects, cleft lip/palate, and mild mental retardation as well as hypospadias.
- Wolf-Hirschhorn syndrome.
- 13q deletion syndrome.

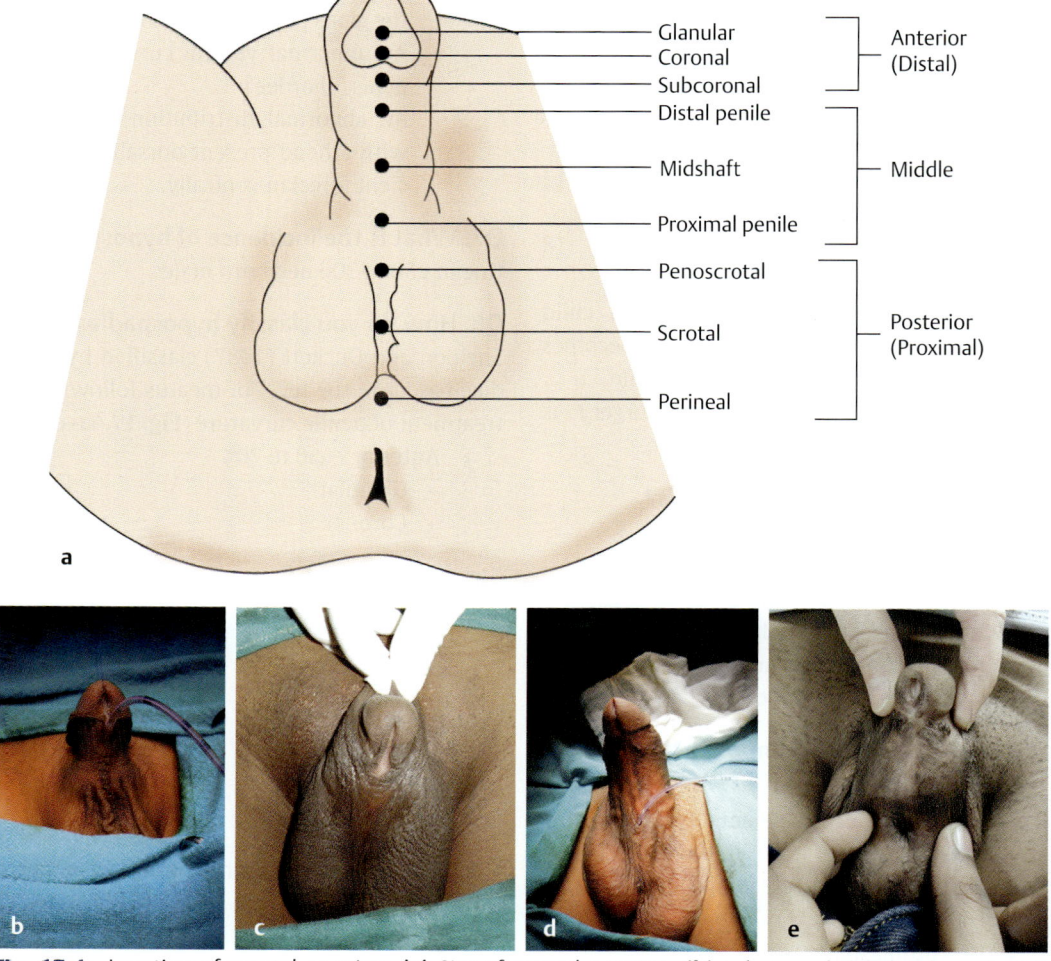

Fig. 17.4 Location of meatal opening. **(a)** Site of meatal opening, **(b)** subcoronal, **(c)** distal penile, **(d)** proximal penile, **(e)** penoscrotal.

Q10. What are the anatomical parts of penis?

- Penis consists of three parts: root (radix), body (shaft), and glans (**Fig. 17.5**).
- The core of the penis contains three erectile tissues, namely, the two corpora cavernosa and the corpus spongiosum.
    - Root:
        - The root of the penis is the most proximal part of the penis.
        - It is fixed to the pubic symphysis via the two suspensory ligaments of the penis.

- It contains three erectile tissues, which include two crura and the bulb of the penis, and two muscles called the ischiocavernosus and bulbospongiosus.
    - Shaft:
        - The body, or shaft, is the free part of the penis between the root and glans.
        - The shaft of the penis contains three erectile tissues: the two corpora cavernosa and the corpus spongiosum.
        - The corpora cavernosa lie one next to another in the dorsal

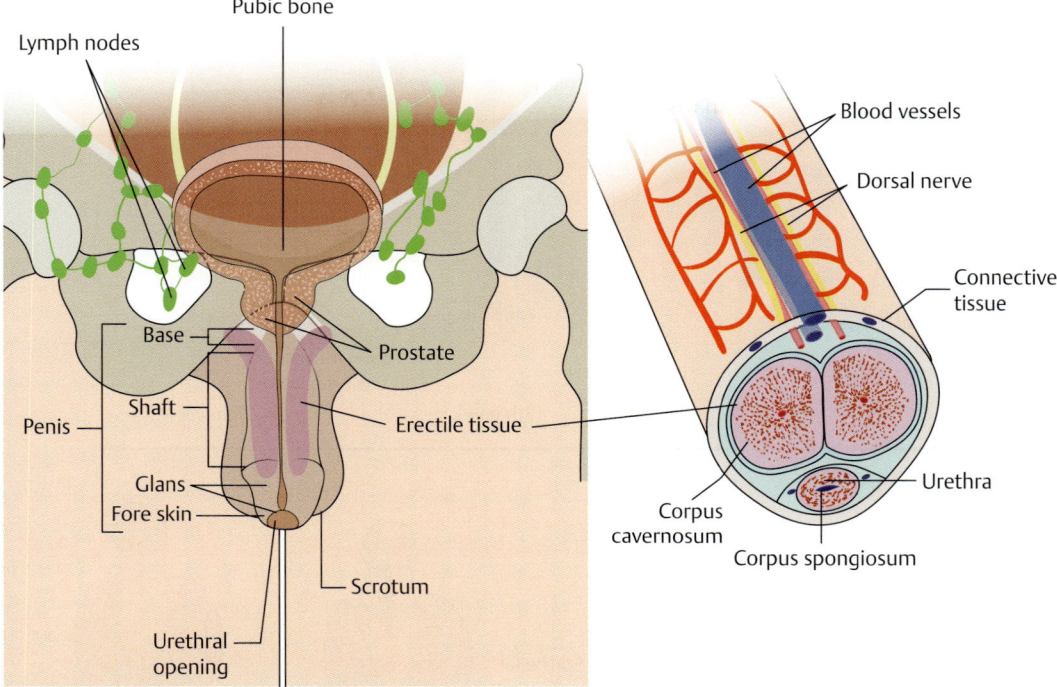

Fig. 17.5 Anatomical parts of penis.

compartment of the penis, while the corpus spongiosum lies in the ventral groove between them.

- The corpora cavernosa are the two erectile masses found within the dorsal part of the penis.
- Each begins within the root of penis as the crus of penis, traverses the shaft, and terminates within the glans.

  – Glans:
  - This is the most distal, or end, part of the penis.
  - It gets its shape from the bulbous expansion of the corpus spongiosum.
  - Urethral opening is present in the glans.

Q11. What are the parts of urethra?

The male urethra is divided into three parts:

- Prostatic urethra:
  - The prostatic urethra originates at the neck of the bladder and is located in the prostate.

  – It is the widest part of the urethra, which then connects to the membranous urethra, found in the urogenital diaphragm.

- Membranous urethra:
  - The membranous urethra is surrounded by the sphincter muscle, which is what holds urine.

- Spongy urethra:
  - Last, the spongy urethra makes up the bottom portion of the urethra which is again divided into bulbous and penile urethra.
  - This is the longest part of the urethra and runs from urogenital diaphragm to the tip of the penis.

Q12. What is the embryological development of male genitalia?

- Development of external genitalia is same in male and female prior to the 11th week of gestation (**Fig. 17.6**).
- At 11th week, the genitalia consists of:
  - Central urethral groove.

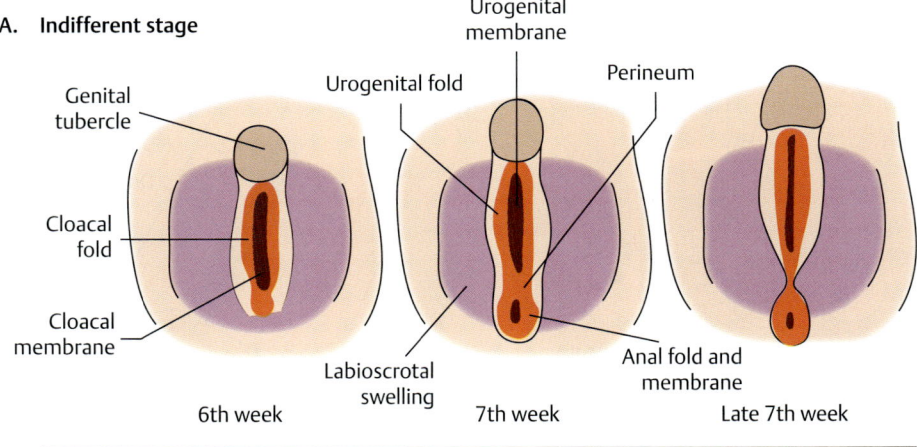

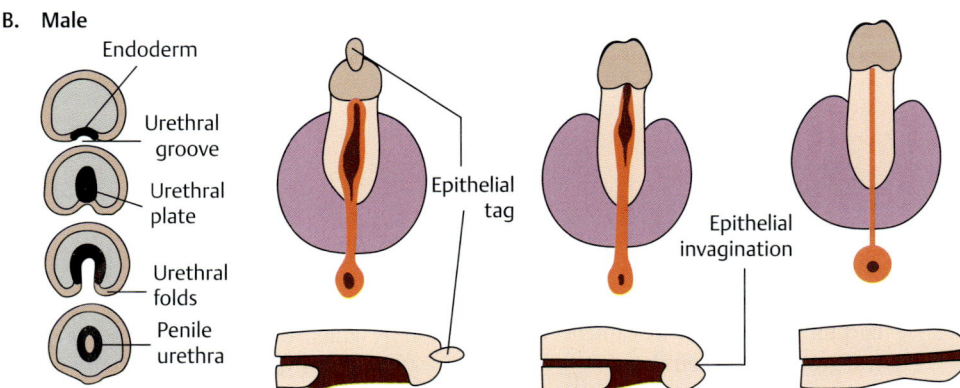

Fig. 17.6 Embryological development of the male genitalia.

- Urethral folds on either side of the urethral groove.
- Labioscrotal swellings on either side of urethral folds.
- Genital tubercle.
- Genital tubercle forms the phallus.
- Urethral folds fuse over the urethral groove forming the penile urethra.
- Labioscrotal swellings form the scrotum.

Q13. What is the difference between normal and hypospadias penile anatomy?

- Normal penile anatomy (**Fig. 17.7**):
  - The penis is made of two corpora cavernosa which are covered by a thick, elastic tunica albuginea.
  - There is a midline septum between the two corpora cavernosa.
  - Corpora spongiosum, which covers the urethra, lies in the ventral position to the paired corpora cavernosa.
- Fascial layers:
  - The buck's fascia surrounds the corpora cavernosa and it splits to encompass the corpus spongiosum.
  - Above the Buck's fascia is the dartos fascia which lies below the skin and this fascia contains the blood supply to the prepuce.
  - The classic dogma is that the neurovascular bundle lies in the 11 o' clock and 10 o' clock positions but recent studies have shown that the neurovascular bundle completely fans out around corpora cavernosa, all the way to the junction of the corpus spongiosum.

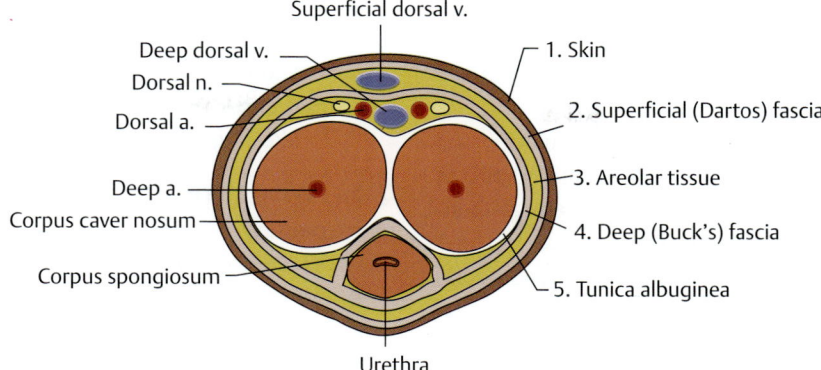

Fig. 17.7 Normal penile anatomy.

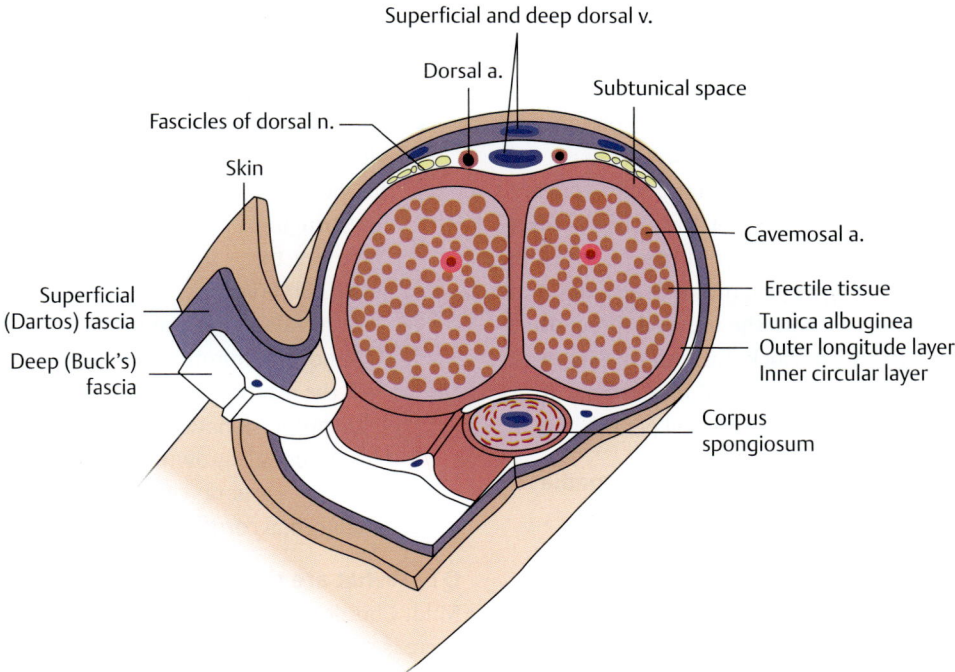

Fig. 17.8 Hypospadias penile anatomy.

- Blood supply:
  - The prepuce is supplied by two branches of the inferior external pudendal arteries and the superficial penile arteries.
  - These arteries divide into the anterolateral and posterolateral branches.
  - In hypospadias surgery, the island flap is typically based on the anterolateral superficial vessels.

  - The onlay island flap, tubularized island flap, and de-epithelialized pedicle flap are dependent on careful preservation of these blood vessels.
  - The outer skin survives from the intrinsic subcutaneous vessels.
- Hypospadias penile anatomy (**Fig. 17.8**):
  - As compared to the normal penis, the anatomy of the hypospadias penis is not different from the normal penis.

- The neuronal innervation, corpora cavernosa, the architecture of the tunica albuginea, and the blood supply are all similar.
- There is variance in vascularity and nerve supply which is limited to the region of the abnormal urethral spongiosum and the glans.
- Difference in vascularity: Hypospadias penis has endothelium-lined vascular channels filled with red blood cells while the normal penis has well-defined, small capillaries around the urethra, fanning into the glans penis.
- Difference in neuronal supply:
  - In both the normal penis and the hypospadias penis, the nerves start as two well-defined bundles superior and slightly lateral to the urethra.
  - Where the two crural bodies converge into the bodies of the corpora cavernosa, the nerves diverge, spreading around the cavernosal bodies up to the junction with the urethral spongiosum.
  - The 12 o' clock position in a hypospadiac penis is spared of neuronal structures unlike the normal penis.

Q14. What is the etiology of hypospadias?
- Genetic background:
  - Familial (4–10%):
    - 6 to 8% fathers of affected boys.
    - 14 to 15% of male siblings.
- Endocrinopathies:
  - Leydig cell dysfunction.
  - Defects in the testosterone biosynthetic pathway-impaired 3β-hydroxysteroid dehydrogenase +/– 17,20-lyase or 17α-hydroxylase activity—proximal hypospadias.
  - SRD5A2 on chromosome 2 mutation (9%).
  - Androgen receptor gene mutation—rare.
- Gene mutations:
  - Fgf8, Fgf10, and Fgfr2.
  - Nuclear estrogen receptors—ER2.

- Estrogen-responsive genes—ACT3, Cyr61, CTGF, and CADD45β.
- Endocrine disruptors—natural or synthetic compounds exerting estrogen-like and/or antiandrogen effects.

Q15. What are the risk factors for hypospadias?
The risk factors can be:
- Placental dysfunction.
- Low birth weight.
- Preterm birth.
- Prepregnancy maternal obesity.
- Extremes of maternal age (<24 and >40).
- Pre-eclampsia.
- Assistive reproductive techniques.

Q16. Define chordee.
- Chordee is a strand of connective tissue which is stretched like a cord between the meatus and glans penis, giving rise to bowstringing.
- There are three theories for the cause of penile curvature:
  - Urethral plate is abnormally developed.
  - Abnormal fibrotic mesenchymal tissue at the urethral meatus.
  - Disproportionate growth of corpora or differential growth between normal dorsal corpora cavernosa tissue and abnormal corporal tissue ventrally.

Q17. What are the grades of chordee?
Mild: Chordee not seen normally, in erect penis there is slight bending.
Moderate: Chordee apparent in flaccid penis but more obvious on erection.
Severe: Chordee obvious in flaccid condition.

Q18. What is chordee without hypospadias?
There is congenital short urethra and corpus spongiosum not fully developed.

Q19. How do you release chordee?
Steps of chordee release (**Fig. 17.9a–d**):
- A traction suture is applied in the glans penis and an infant feeding tube no. 8 is placed in urethra.

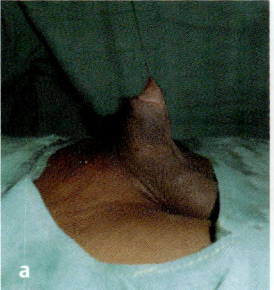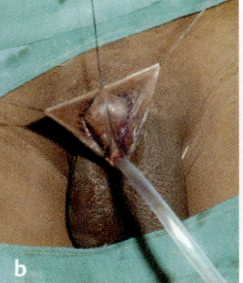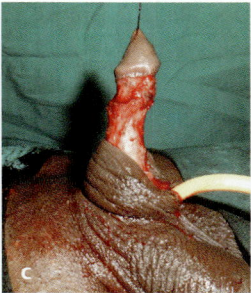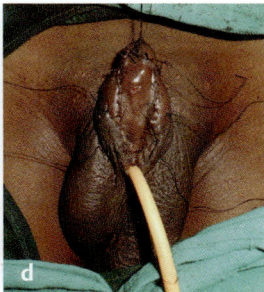

Fig. 17.9 (a–d) Chordee release and penile skin degloving.

- For hemostasis, 1 in 100,000 adrenaline solution may be infiltrated along the chordee (adrenaline safe dose is 1 mL/kg) or tourniquet may be applied at the base of the penis (tourniquet time: 20–60 min).
- Two parallel incisions enclosing the chordee are given, extending from approximately 2 mm proximal to meatus and distally up to the corona.
- Distally, the incisions are continued circumcoronal just proximal (2–3 mm proximally for having enough skin during final suturing).
- Penis is degloved along these incisions. Dissection should be in the plane deep to Buck's fascia. At this stage, Gittes test is done to assess the degree of chordee.
- Excise the whole of urethral plate along with fibrous chordee. Proximally, the excision extends 1 mm proximal to urethral meatus. Gittes test is repeated to check the complete correction of chordee.
- Once tourniquet is released and hemostasis is achieved, in two-staged procedures, at the time of chordee release during the first stage, penile skin flaps are stitched to form the urethral plate.

Q20. What is Gittes and Mclaughlin test?

- This test is used during surgery to check the complete correction of chordee after release.
- Tie the root of penis with soft clamp or tourniquet.

- With 26-gauge needle and a scalp vein set, 10 mL of normal saline is injected in corpora cavernosa.
- Then look for erection of penis and its straightened appearance.
- The two corpora are connected by vascular anastomosis so injection into one is enough.

Q21. In how many layers is urethroplasty done?

Urethroplasty is done in three layers:

- First layer urethra formation.
- Second layer—Stitch dartos in midline as second layer or use as a transposition flap.
- Third layer—Preputial skin.

Q22. How do we assess on table, how much wide should be the incision?

We assess the width of incision by pinching the skin over infant feeding tube.

Q23. What are the disadvantages of narrow tube and wide tube?

- Disadvantages of narrow tube:
  - May not be able to form the tube.
  - Patient may develop urethral stricture and meatal stenosis in postop period.
- Disadvantages of wide tube:
  - Urethra will be patulous which leads to stasis of urine which further causes infection and stones.

Q24. How far is the undermining done over the medial side of incision?

No undermining is done under urethral plate.

Q25. What will you do for the ventral curvature with hypospadias?

The following is the stepwise algorithm for straightening the ventral curvature (**Algorithm 17.1**).

Q26. What are the surgical options according to the site of hypospadias?

- The surgical options in hypospadias depend not only on the location of meatus but also on the presence/absence of chordee (**Algorithm 17.2**).
  - Distal →
    - MAGPAI (meatal advancement and glanuloplasty incorporated).
    - GAP (Glans approximation procedure).

- Mathieu flip-flap.
- TIP (tubularized incised plate urethroplasty) (Snodgrass).
- Proximal →
  - Onlay island flap.
  - Two-stage reconstruction.
  - TPIF (transverse preputial island flap) devised by Duckett in 1981.

Q27. What is MAGPI procedure?

MAGPI → Meatal Advancement and Glanuloplasty by preputial incorporation (**Fig. 17.10**).
- Indications:
  - Glanular, coronal, and subcoronal variety.

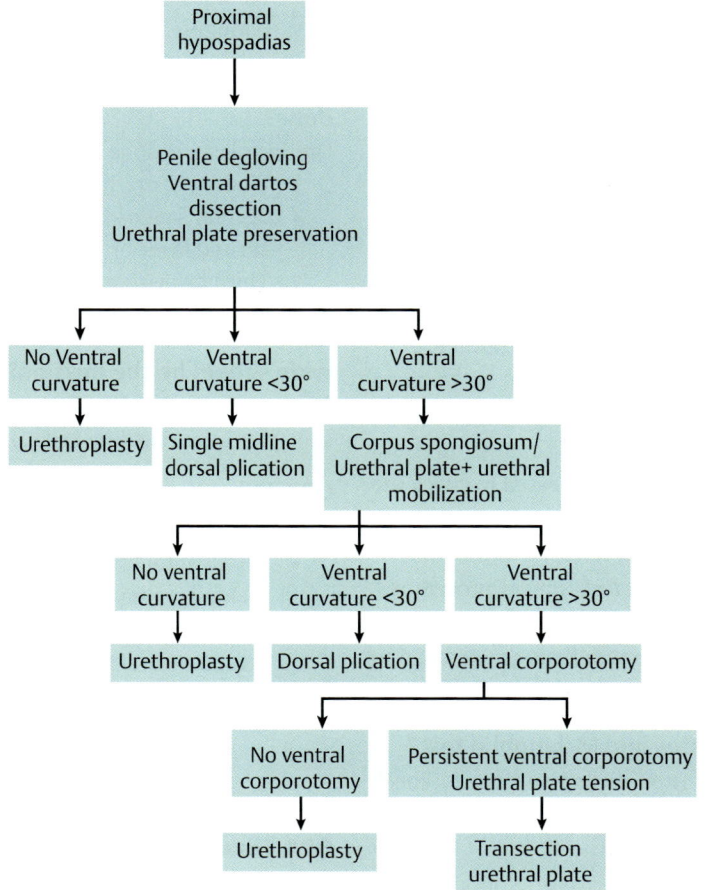

Algorithm 17.1 Algorithm for straightening ventral curvature (VC) with hypospadias

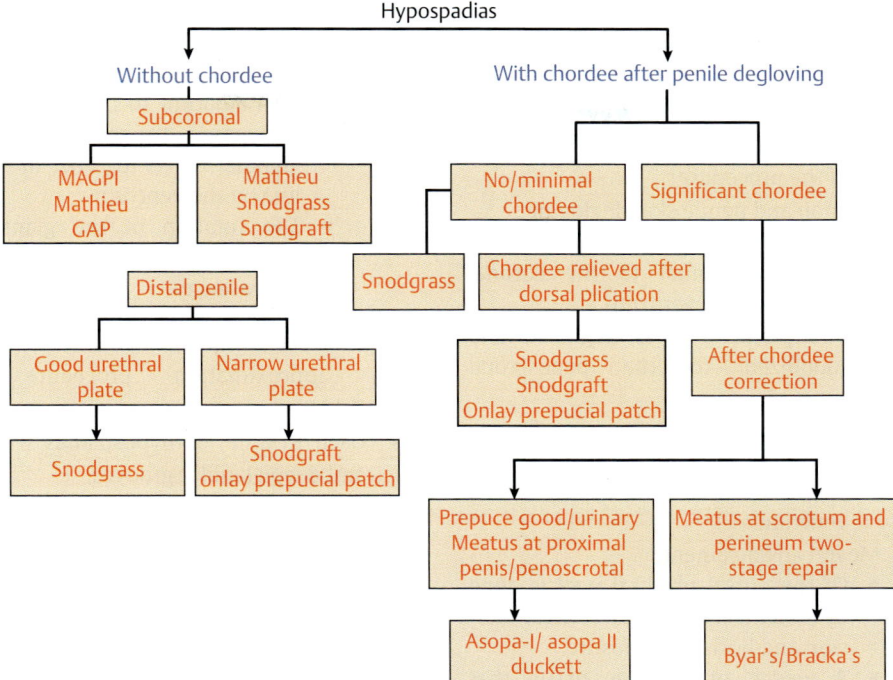

Algorithm 17.2 Surgical options according to the site of hypospadias

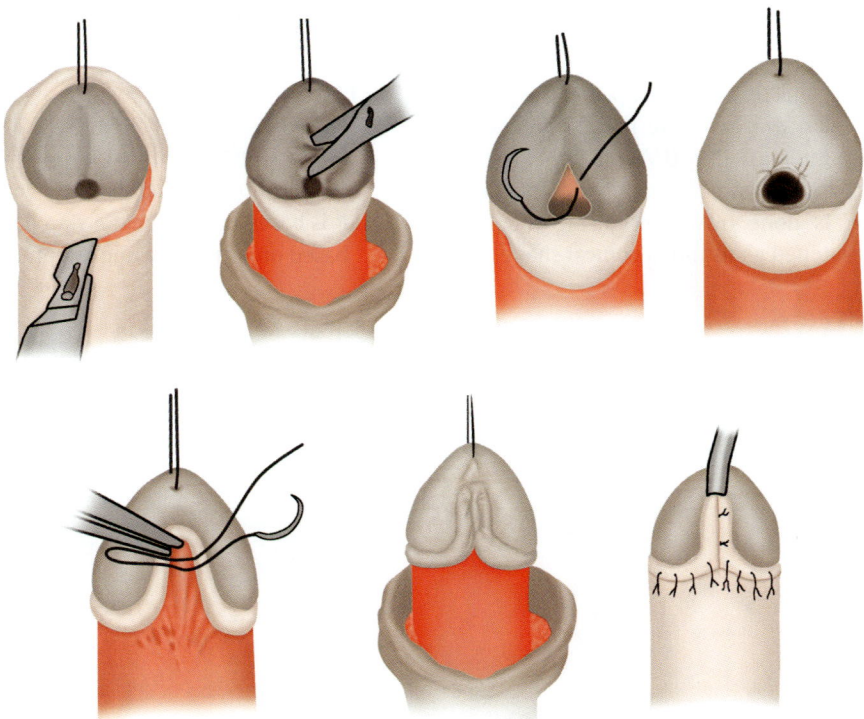

Fig. 17.10 Meatal advancement and glanuloplasty MAGPI procedure.

- Criteria for MAGPI:
  - Normal ventral wall of urethra should be there.
  - Urethra must be mobile, so that it can be advanced into the glans.
- Steps of the procedure:
  - Incision and penile skin degloving:
    - A circumferential incision is made 5 mm proximal to the coronal margin on the ventrum.
    - The penile skin is degloved and mobilized to the penoscrotal junction.
    - Penis is straightened by freeing any tethering fibers of the skin and subdartos fascia, particularly on the ventrum.
  - Meatal advancement:
    - Of the dorsal urethral wall is done by a Heineke-Mikulicz vertical incision and horizontal closure.
    - A wedge of glanular tissue that includes the glanular meatal wall is removed.
    - The horizontal closure flattens out the glanular bridge.
    - Dorsal urethra advanced onto the glans tissue to the apex of the glanular groove where it is sutured with interrupted 7–0 Vicryl.
  - Glanuloplasty:
    - Is done by reconfiguring the flattened glans into a conical shape.

- By rotating lateral wings to the midline proximal to the meatus, a proper conical glans shape is made.
- Skin adjacent to the glanular edges is excised to reapproximate the glanular wings together in the midline on the ventrum.
- The rotation of the glans wings gives a nearly normal glanular appearance.

Q28. What is GAP procedure?

Glans approximation procedure (GAP) (**Fig. 17.11**):
- Used in anterior hypospadias with wide and deep glanular grooves.
- Steps:
  - Exposure of glans mesenchyme by de-epithelialization of tissue, which is critical for a two-layer glans closure, allowing for good support of the urethroplasty.
  - Tubularization of the neourethra over a stent followed by glans closure.

Q29. What is Mathieu flip-flap procedure?

Mathieu Flip flap (perimeatal-based flap) (**Fig. 17.12**):
- It is done when the meatus is too proximal on the shaft to perform a MAGPAI or when there is no deep glanular groove for GAP.
- It is based on perimeatal skin flap which is based on intrinsic blood supply.

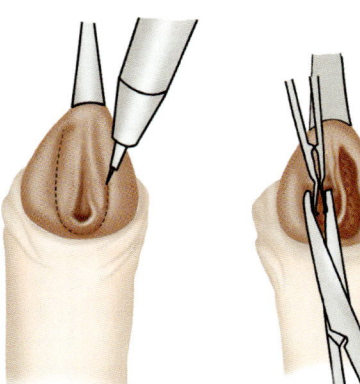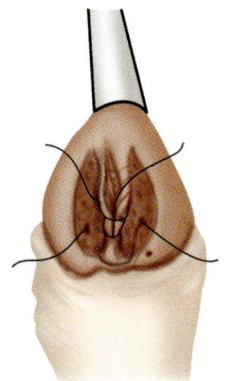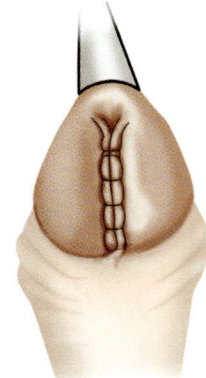

Fig. 17.11 Glans approximation procedure (GAP) procedure.

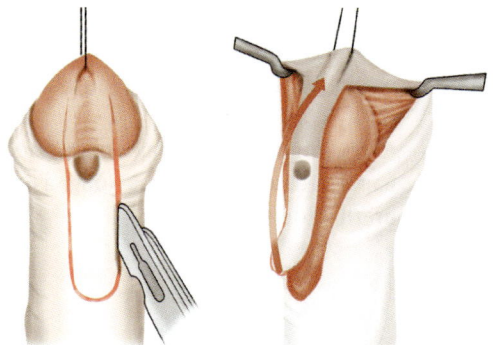

Fig. 17.12 Mathieu flip-flap technique.

- For viability, the length-width ratio should not exceed 2:1.

Q30. What is Snodgrass procedure?

Snodgrass tubularized incised plate (TIP) urethroplasty (**Fig. 17.13**):

- Two important criteria for Snodgrass surgery:
  - Urethral plate should be at least 1 cm wide.
  - No distal deep chordee should be there.
- Steps of TIP procedure:
  - Skin incision and penile skin degloving:
    - A circumferential skin incision is made 1- to 2-mm proximal to the meatus and the shaft skin is degloved.
    - A U-shaped incision is made extending along the edges of urethra plate from glans tips to 2 to 3 mm proximal to meatus.
  - Mobilization of the glans wings:
    - While avoiding damage to the margins of the urethral plate.
  - Incision in urethral plate:
    - A relaxing incision is made in the midline from distal extent of the plate to the meatus.
    - The incision should not reach the tip of glans.
    - The depth of the relaxing incision depends on the plate width and depth.
  - Tubularization of urethra:
    - Done with 7–0 polyglactin suture with a two-layer running subepithelial closure.

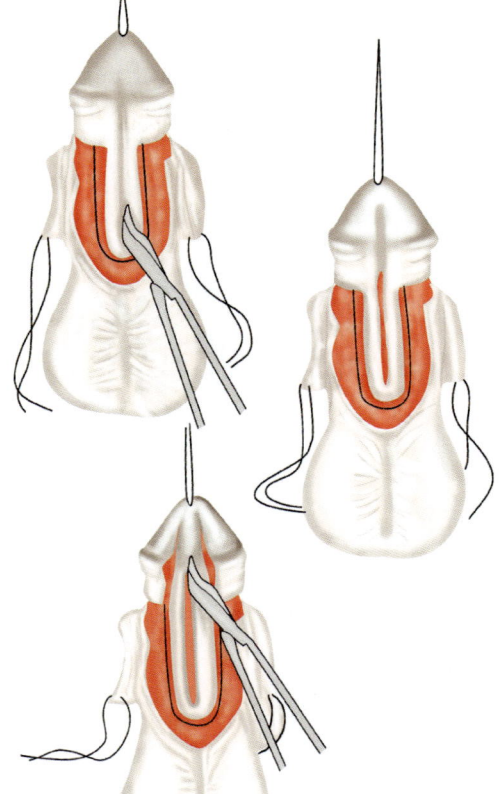

Fig. 17.13 Snodgrass technique.

  - Adjacent dartos tissues are used to cover the neourethra:
    - A dartos pedicle is developed from the dorsal shaft skin and button holed.
    - It is then transposed to the ventrum to additionally cover the repair.
  - Approximation of the margins:
    - The coronal margins of the glans are approximated with subepithelial 6–0 polyglactin.
    - The skin edges of the glans are sutured, and the meatus with 7–0 polypropylene.
- Advantages of TIP: Improved appearance of meatus creating a vertical slit neomeatus.

Q31. What is the contraindication of TIP?

A flat and a narrow urethral plate less than 1 cm is a contraindication of TIP.

Q32. What is onlay island flap?

The onlay island flap (**Fig. 17.14**):

- In 1987, Elder reported the first one-stage hypospadias repair using an island onlay.
- It allows for repair of subcoronal and mid-shaft hypospadias.

- Steps of the procedure:
  - A near-circumferential incision is made on the penile shaft preserving the urethral plate.
  - A rectangular preputial onlay flap is harvested, measuring as long as the urethral defect.

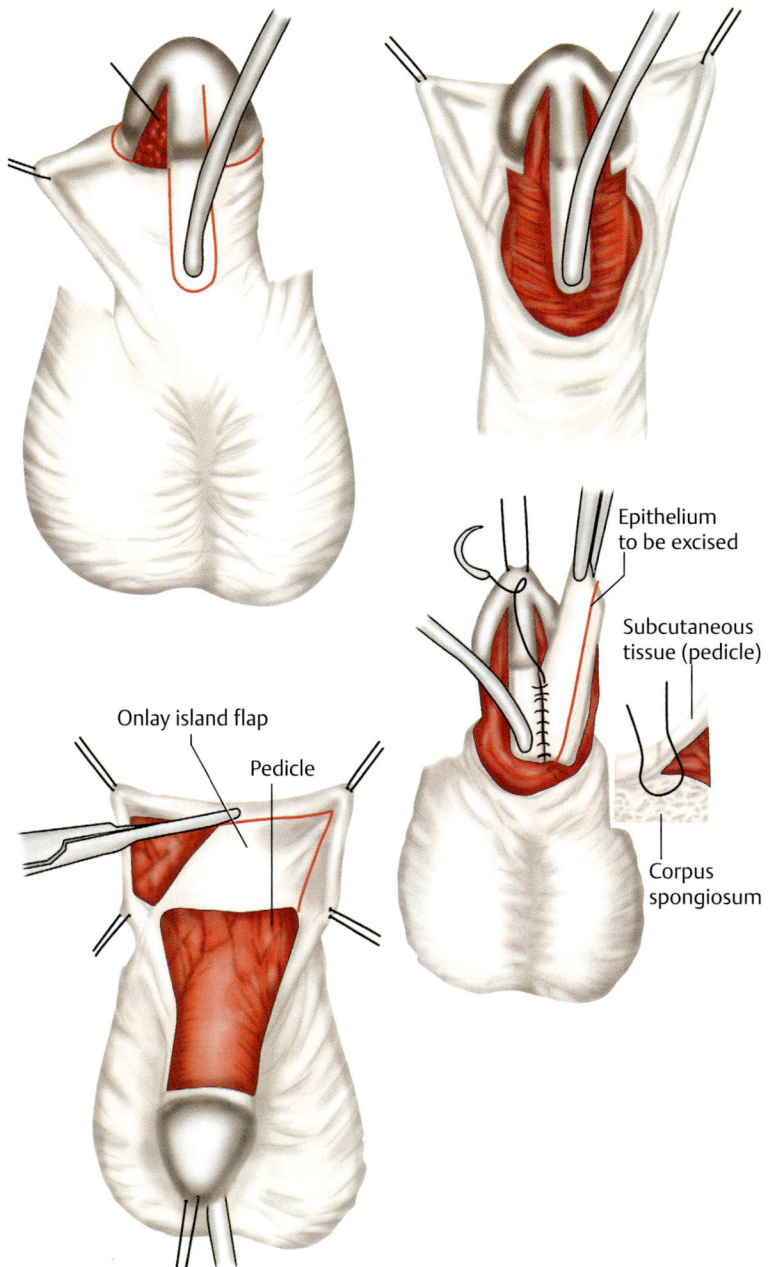

Fig. 17.14 Onlay island flap procedure.

- Dissection of the preputial skin is done preserving its pedicle to the base of penis.
- Anastomosis of the onlay flap is done on the urethral plate.
- In case of insufficient urethral plate, tubularization of the flap is performed.
- A second layer of coverage of the neourethra is then performed with dartos or tunica vaginalis.

Q33. What are the two-stage surgical procedures in hypospadias?

Two-stage repair includes two surgical procedures for correction of hypospadias:
- First stage → Chordee correction is done.
- Second stage → Urethroplasty is done by Bracka or Byars procedure.

- Bracka procedure:
  - In the first stage, a circumferential incision is made 1 to 2 mm proximal to the coronal sulcus, then chordee is excised.
  - Artificial erection test is done for confirmation of penile straightening and removal of all chordee tissue.
  - Buccal mucosa or inner preputial skin is used as a free graft (**Fig. 17.15**).
  - The second stage is performed after 6 to 12 months in which previously transferred skin or mucosa is used to reconstruct the glans and urethra.
- Byars procedure:
  - Byars stresses the point that the maximum surface of the available preputial tissue should be utilized by

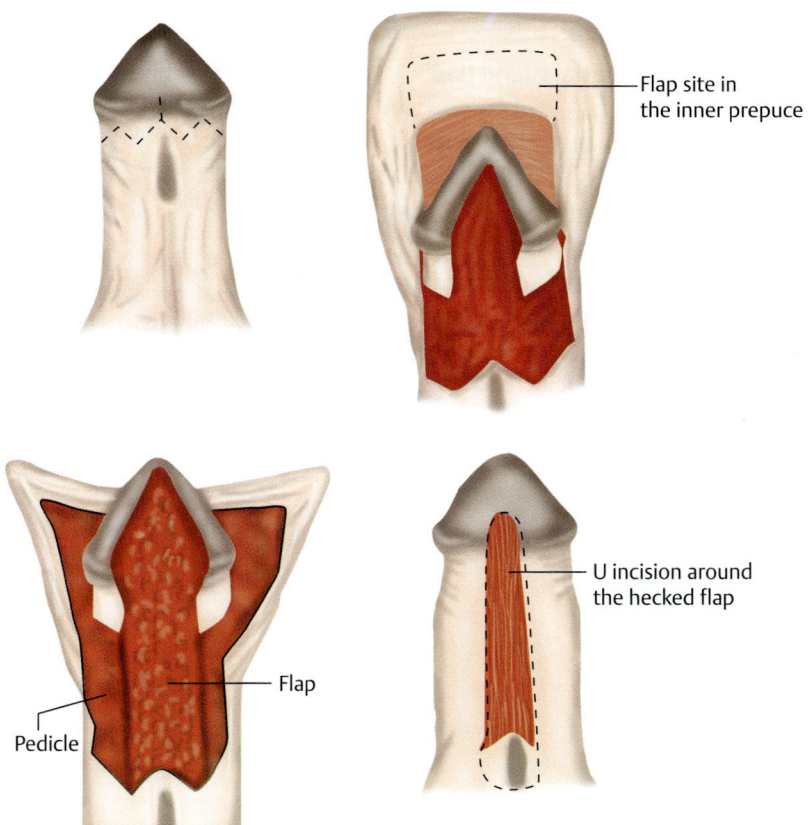

Fig. 17.15 Bracka procedure.

transforming all of the preputial skin to the ventral side of the organ.

– The first stage consists of the correction of the chordee. This initial surgery is usually carried out at 3 years of age.

- Urethral plate formation by preputial skin flap (**Fig. 17.16**):

  – An incision is then made through the full-thickness of the unfolded prepuce from the midline to the coronal sulcus.

  – These flaps of prepuce are transferred ventrally to resurface the area between the retracted urethral meatus and the glans.

  – Since the preputial tissue will be used to construct a new urethra, it must be brought to all areas where the new urethra will be formed.

- In the second stage urethral tube is reconstructed around a 14-Fr catheter.

Q34. What is transverse preputial island flap (TPIF)?

The meatus is assessed, and a cut back is made to widen the meatus.

- A subcoronal incision is made around the glans.

- The penile and preputial skin is dissected free off the shaft from distal to proximal close to the Buck's fascia preserving the arteries that constitute the pedicle to the preputial flap.

- A 1.5-cm-wide rectangular flap from preputial skin is prepared. The length must suffice the gap between the meatus and the tip of the glans.

- The flap is tubularized around a 10-Fr catheter and sutured into the meatus (**Fig. 17.17**).

Q35. What is Asopa technique?

- Asopa technique (dorsal inlay urethroplasty):

  – Asopa described the inlay of a graft (preferably buccal mucosa) into Snodgrass's longitudinal urethral plate incision using a ventral sagittal urethrotomy approach.

  – It is indicated in urethral stricture reconstruction, where the plate is scarred and the blood supply compromised, so epithelialization from the edge is typically poor.

- Asopa II technique (vascularized double-skin island technique):

  – Asopa technique is inner transverse preputial skin tube urethroplasty (**Fig. 17.18**).

  – Indications:

    ▪ Midpenile, proximal penile, penoscrotal hypospadias with considerable chordee and good and adequate prepuce.

    ▪ Congenitally short urethra with good prepuce.

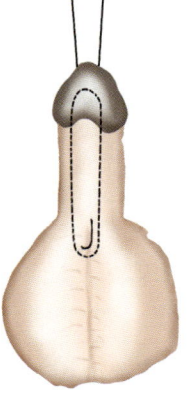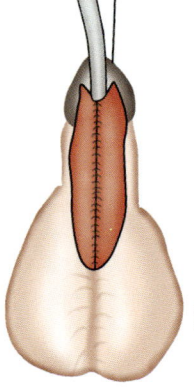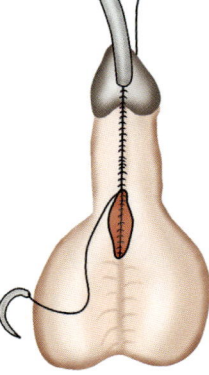

Fig. 17.16 Steps of Byars second-stage surgery.

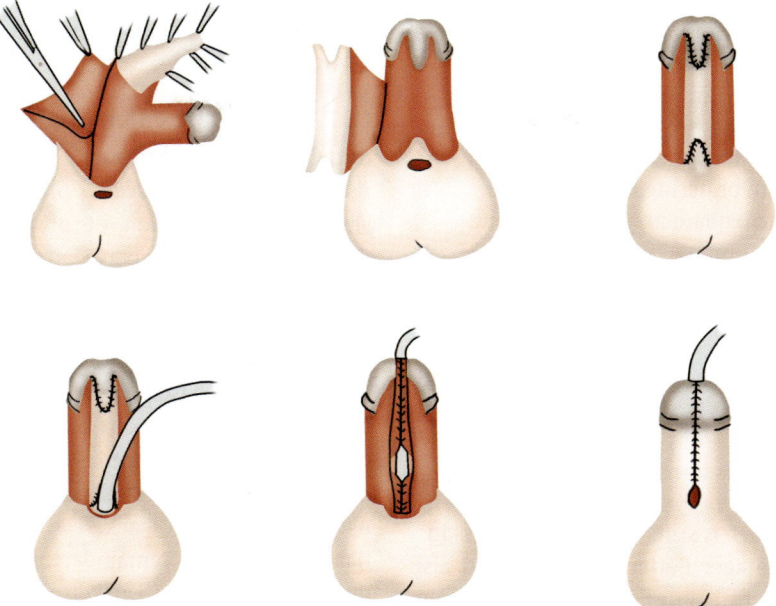

Fig. 17.17 Transverse preputial island flap (TPIF).

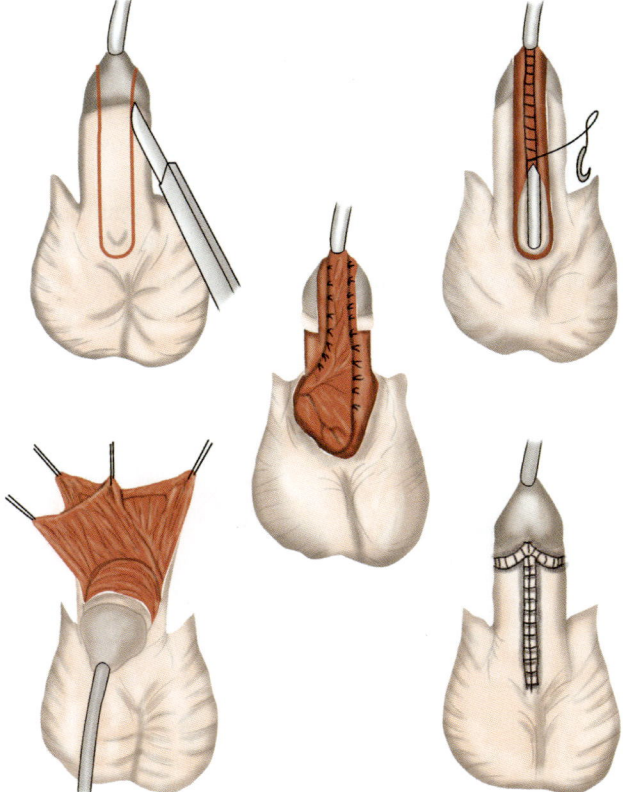

Fig. 17.18 Asopa technique.

- Patients with earlier surgery and complications with minimal or unscarred prepuce.
  - Contraindications:
    - Patients with severe chordee and proximal meatus at the level of scrotum or perineum.
    - Inadequate prepuce.
    - Circumcised patients.
  - Technique:
    - Inner and outer preputial layers are separated from the penile skin as a double island flap and then both layers are separated from each other.
    - Tube is formed from inner prepuce.
    - Outer prepuce forms a cover over it which is stitched to the penile skin.
  - Advantage: Better aesthetics and also the suture lines do not overlap each other.

Q36. What is Duckett's procedure?

Duckett's procedure is also known as transverse tubularized island flap (**Fig. 17.19**).

- Indications are same as that for Asopa.
- The inner preputial flap is dissected from the outer preputial skin up to the base of penis protecting the vascularity.
- Outer preputial skin is incised midline to give a midline closure.
- Better cosmetic results are obtained than Asopa.

- Both Asopa and Duckett have problems of diverticulum formation and meatal stenosis.

Q37. What is the difference between Asopa and Duckett's techniques?

Asopa used the transverse preputial skin as a single-stage correction of proximal hypospadias based on the superficial dorsal vessels of the penis. He described a double-faced preputial island flap where he used the adjacent skin flap covering the mucosal flap of the neourethra. Both flaps are based on the superficial dorsal vessels. In 1981, Duckett used the same principle and described the tubularized preputial island flap. The Duckett island flap differed from Asopa's flap in that Duckett isolated the preputial tube from the remainder of the dorsal skin on a vascular pedicle. Duckett used a glans channel when he described the technique. This is no longer recommended as meatal stenosis is liable to occur.

Q38. What are the principles for hypospadias repair?

General principles for hypospadias repair are:

- Fine microvascular instruments are necessary.
- Optical magnification of 2 to 2.5×.
- Sutures like 6–0 or 7–0 Vicryl (polyglactin 910), Monocryl (polyglecaprone 25), PDS (polydioxanone) are used for urethroplasty.

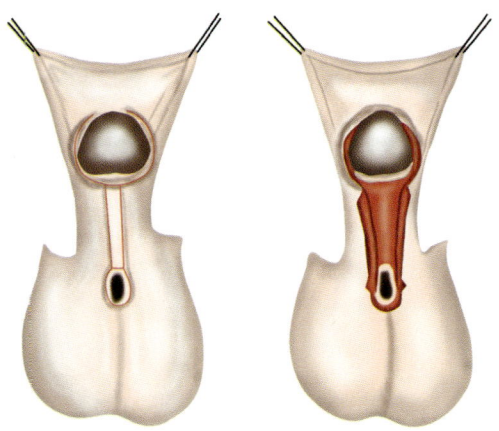
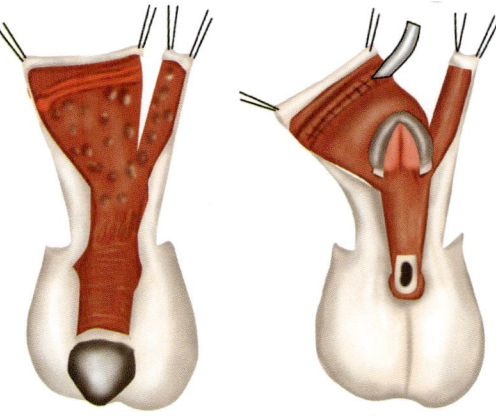

Fig. 17.19 Duckett's technique.

- Tourniquet or epinephrine (1:100000) in 1% lidocaine is used for minimizing the bleeding.
- Urethroplasty should be performed around a 10-Fr catheter to avoid subsequent stenosis. A compressing dressing is applied postoperatively.
- Silastic foam or Tegaderm dressing for 2 to 5 days.
- 6-Fr Silastic catheter for 7 to 10 days.
- Minimal and atraumatic tissue-handling.
- Careful hemostasis.
- Good surgical assistance.

Q39. Is there any role of preoperative hormonal stimulation?

- Hormone stimulation has the following effects:
    - Increases penile size.
    - Reduces ventral curvature.
    - Improves vascularity.
- One regimen is intramuscular testosterone enanthate 2 mg/kg given 5 and 2 weeks preoperatively.
- Others are:
    - Human chorionic gonadotropin (HCG):
        - In proximal hypospadias 6 to 8 weeks preoperatively.
        - Stimulates the glans size preoperatively to allow better tubularization of the urethral plate and decrease the incidence of glans dehiscence.
        - In children <1 year, 250 IU twice weekly is the recommended dose.
        - In children 1 to 5 years, 500 IU twice weekly is the dose.
    - Testosterone ointment:
        - Can be applied to glans penis for 2 weeks before surgery.

Q40. What do you mean by hypospadias cripple?

It is the deformity used to describe the patient who has undergone multiple, unsuccessful hypospadias repair attempt, with significant resultant penile deformity.

Q41. What are the complications of urethroplasty?

- Fistula: Most common complication (**Fig. 17.20**). Two-layer subepithelial closure of the neourethra and subsequent coverage with dartos reduce the chances of fistula formation.
- Meatal stenosis: The most common cause is tubularization of the urethra too far distally. To avoid this, urethra should not be tubularized beyond midglans point.
- Bleeding and hematoma: It is due to inadequate hemostasis.
- Neourethra stricture: The most common site is at the proximal anastomosis of the neourethra to native urethra.
- Dehiscence causes could be:
    - Technical factors like suture material, and technique used in glansplasty.
    - Glans size.
    - Traumatic catheter placement.
    - Wound infection.
- Diverticulum: It occurs due to distal obstruction, turbulent urinary flow.
- Infection.
- Balanitis xerotica obliterans.
- Recurrent penile curvature.

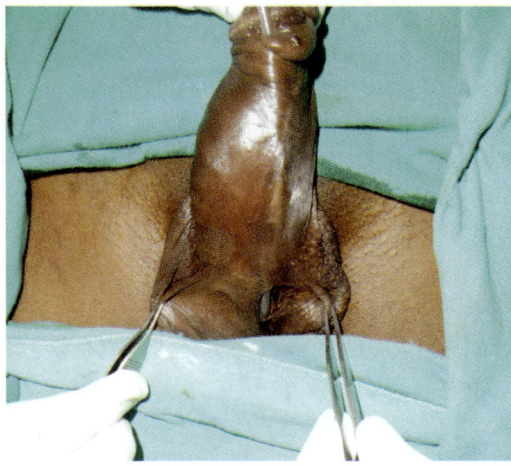

Fig. 17.20 Urethra-cutaneous fistula in a penoscrotal hypospadias.

Q42. What are the other methods of hypospadias repair?

- Duplay → The two techniques of Duplay (**Fig. 17.21**) are:
  - The first technique is a modification of Thiersch.
    - The chordee having been relieved at a previous stage, a flap of skin is outlined, formed into a tube, and covered by the penile skin.
  - The second technique is similar, but:
    - The flap of the skin is not made large enough to be brought around the catheter.
    - Epithelial growth of the buried skin allows a complete tube to form.
- Ombredanne's technique (**Fig. 17.22a, b**):
  - He recommended a button-hole type of preputial hood flap to transfer to the ventral penile surface (first stage).
  - He recommended a distally based flap at the urethral meatus, brought forward with a purse-string suture to the tip of the penis (second stage).

- Denis-Browne operation (**Fig. 17.23**):
  - First stage is done at about 18 months of age. Three important elements of the first stage of repair are:
    - Meatotomy.
    - Resection of the chordee tissue.
    - Transfer of dorsal penile skin to the ventral surface.
  - Second stage of surgery is completed at about 4 to 5 years of age.
    - The chordee having been released, an incision is made outlining a strip of skin from around the urethral meatus to the glans penis.
    - After giving lateral incisions, margins of the skin are elevated.
    - These are closed over the skin strip.
    - Wire sutures are used to take tension off the suture line.
    - These sutures are secured with glass beads.
- Cecil-Culp technique (**Fig. 17.24**):
  - The penile skin flap is formed into a tube with a running suture and the

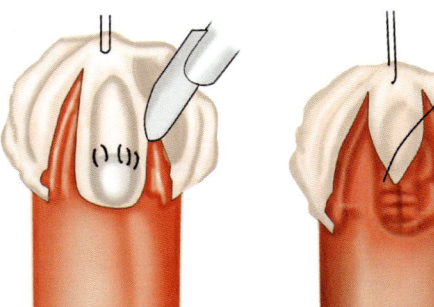
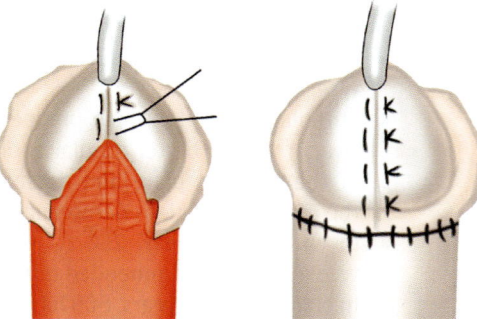

Fig. 17.21 Duplay's technique.

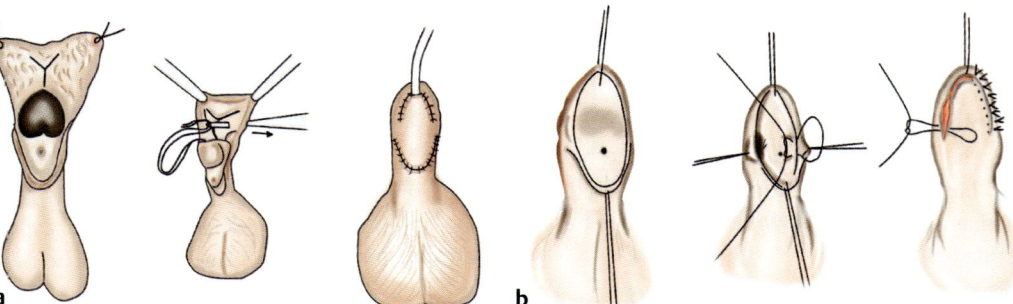

a   b

Fig. 17.22 **(a, b)** Ombredanne's technique.

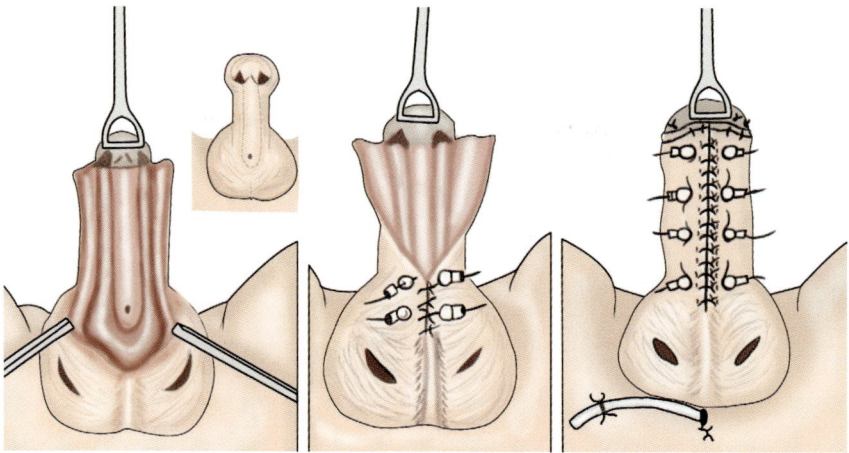

Fig. 17.23 Denis-Browne procedure.

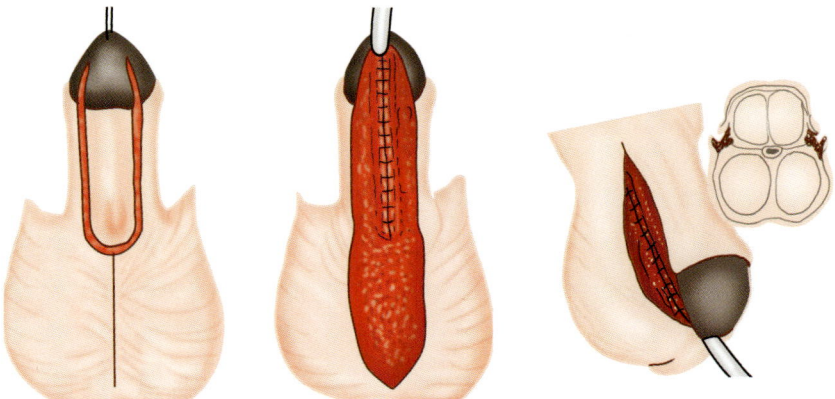

Fig. 17.24 Cecil-Culp procedure.

edges of the skin of the penis and scrotum are undermined.

– The penis is sutured to the scrotum in two layers, attaching the subcutaneous tissue of the scrotum to the tunica albuginea of the corpora cavernosa and the skin of the scrotum to the skin of the penis.

– Two to three months later the skin of the scrotum is incised and the penis freed up, and the defect is closed with silk sutures.

Suggested Readings

1. Baskin L. Development of the penile urethra. in: Baskin L.S. Hypospadias and genital development. Kluwer Academic/Plenum, Philadelphia 2004: 87-100.
2. Partin AW, Wein AJ, Kavoussi LR, Peters CA. Campbell-Walsh urology E-book. Elsevier Health Sciences; 2015:Chapter 130; 3503–3536

Learning Objectives

At the end of the chapter, the students will be able to:
1. Recognize the presentation of various types of syndactyly.
2. Demonstrate the preoperative markings for release.
3. Understand the principles of management.
4. Perform the surgical procedures for syndactyly correction.

Introduction

Syndactyly (fused digits) is the most common congenital anomaly of upper limb. It is a disorder of separation and occurs due to failure of "programmed cell death" between the digital rays. It may be seen as an isolated anomaly or in association with various syndromes. The most commonly affected is third web space in the hand and second web space in the foot. The least affected is first web space as thumb separates earlier than fingers.

History Taking

Details of the patient: Name, age, sex, gender, hand dominance, whether informant is mother/father.

Chief Complaints

- Fusion of fingers/toes in hand/foot.
- Short fingers.
- Bending of fingers in a grown-up child.

History of Present Illness

- Informant is usually mother.
- Child was having these problems since birth.
- In older children, enquire whether the child is able to do the routine activities.
- Ask about presence of any other congenital anomaly: Facial abnormality, cleft lip and palate, genital abnormality.

Antenatal History

- Ask about the duration of pregnancy: Full term or preterm.
- Ask about the maternal age at pregnancy.
- Whether delivered by normal vaginal delivery or cesarean section.
- History of maternal diabetes and hypertension.
- History of intake of any fertility drugs and in vitro fertilization.
- History of intake of antiepileptic drugs.
- Smoking history of mother.
- Alcohol intake by the mother.
- Ask about the birth weight of the baby.

Family History

- History of similar problems in other siblings.
- History of syndactyly on maternal and paternal side.

Immunization History

Whether all vaccines have been received for the age as per national immunization program.

General Examination

- In case of child, anthropometry is very important to assess the normal development of the child. Measure the height and weight of the child.
- Look for other congenital anomalies in the body like:
  - Examine chest and face as syndactyly may be associated with Poland's syndrome and Apert's syndrome.
    - Feature of Poland's syndrome:
      - Absence of the sternocostal portion of the pectoralis major muscles.
      - Hypoplasia of the hand, forearm, and upper arm.
    - Features of Apert's syndrome should be looked for as it is commonly associated with syndactyly:
      - Examine face: Orbits may be shallow.
      - Exorbitism.
      - Forehead may be deeply furrowed.
      - Parrot-beaked nose may be there.
      - High-arched palate.
      - Crowding of maxillary teeth and tongue.

Local Examination of Hand

Inspection

1. Involvement of hand: Right, left, or bilateral.
2. Which web space is involved: first, second, third, fourth, or multiple.
3. Whether it is complete or incomplete.
   - Incomplete: The fusion is not up to the tip of the fingers (**Fig. 18.1**).
   - Complete: The fusion extends up to the tip of the fingers (**Fig. 18.2**).
     - Separation of nails is possible but less pulp on the joined side after separation. There will be sharing of the nail between the two fingers.
4. Whether simple or complex:
   - Simple: The fusion of fingers is only skin deep.
   - Complex: Along with the skin, bony fusion is also there (**Fig. 18.3**).
     - Usually, the bone fusion is distally leading to a tapered appearance of the two joined fingers.
     - There will be sharing of the nail between the two fingers evident by abnormal nail ridge or confluence.
     - It causes angulation and buckling due to disproportionate growth of the digits.
   - Complicated: Presence of abnormal bony structures like hypoplastic bone or joints, missing bones, abnormal shape of

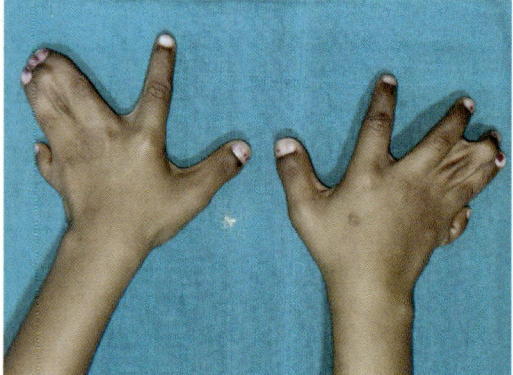

Fig. 18.1 Incomplete simple syndactyly (third web space, right hand).

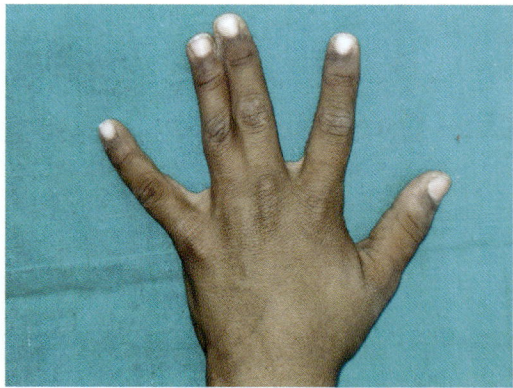

Fig. 18.2 Complete simple syndactyly.

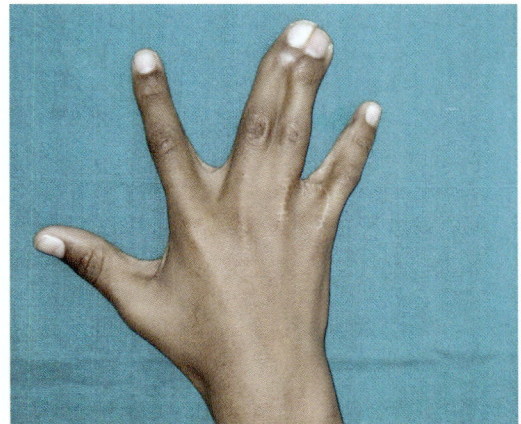

Fig. 18.3 Complex syndactyly.

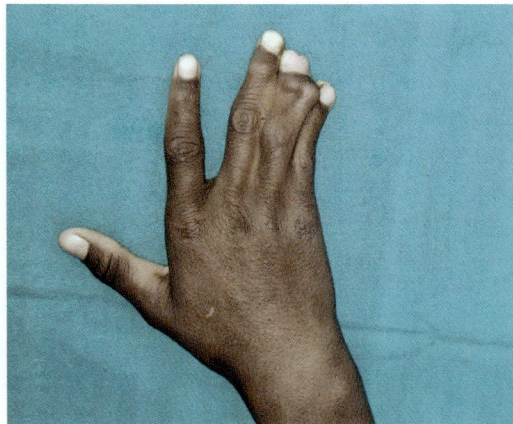

Fig. 18.4 Complicated syndactyly.

the bones (more confirmatory on X-ray) (**Fig. 18.4**).

5. Whether the skin bridges are lax or tight: Helps in assessing the amount of skin available for covering the joints.

6. Condition of nails: Whether shared between the fused fingers (**Fig. 18.5**). Look for the other deformities in the nails.

Palpation

1. All findings on inspection must be corroborated.

2. To confirm if there is bony fusion between the fingers.

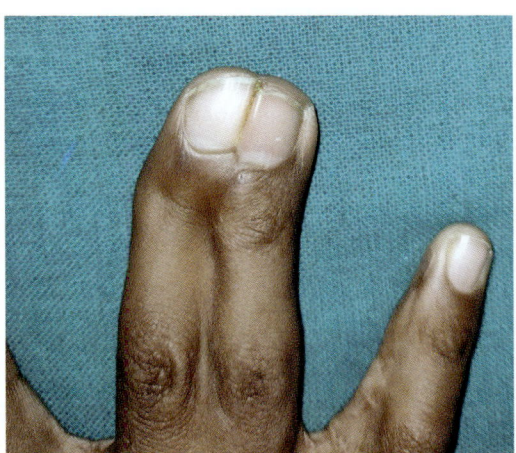

Fig. 18.5 Condition of nail in syndactyly.

Systemic Examination

- Abdomen.
- Respiratory system. ⎤ Refer to chapter 3
- CVS.   ⎟ "Carcinoma Oral
- CNS.   ⎦ Cavity"

X-ray: If X-ray is available, it must be seen before making a provisional diagnosis.

Provisional Diagnosis

This is a case of a 2-year-old child with simple, complete syndactyly of second and third web space of right hand and simple incomplete syndactyly of third and fourth web space of left hand with no other congenital anomaly.

Important points to mention in diagnosis:

- Hand: Right or left or bilateral.
- Simple, complex, or complicated.
- Complete or incomplete.
- Which web spaces are involved: First, second, third, fourth, or multiple.

Investigations Suggested

- Hemoglobin, TLC, DLC, PT/INR.
- Renal function tests.
- Viral markers (HBsAg, HCV, HIV1 and 2).
- X-rays of the affected hand: Anteroposterior (AP) and oblique views.
- USG abdomen, chest X-ray (CXR)/Echo as per advice by the pediatrician.

Questions

Q1. What are the X-ray findings in syndactyly?

Following findings may be present in the X-ray hand:

- Bony fusion, if present can be seen.
- Joints in patients with syndactyly may be incompletely developed, angulated, ankylosed, or even fused in a wide range of variations.
- Phalanges may be crooked, broad, short, long, or fused. These patterns are more common in the hereditary forms of syndactyly.
- The proximal phalanx of thumb may be triangular (delta) or trapezoidal in shape instead of a rectangular bone.
  - X-ray is mandatory for the confirmation of a complex and complicated syndactyly (**Fig. 18.6a, b**).

Q2. What are the deformities seen in the nail?

The deformities seen in the nails are:

- Nails are usually dysplastic.
- There may be a ridging, flaking, or poor growth of the nails.
- The deformity may be more diffuse with nearly complete loss of nails.

Q3. What is the ideal time of surgery?

Timing of surgery usually varies with the complexity of the deformity and the web space involved.

- Complicated and complex webbing of the adjacent fingers with different growth potential should be released by 1 year of age.
- Complete webbing of the first (thumbindex) and fourth (ring small) web spaces should be released between 6 and 12 months of age.
- Simple syndactyly can be corrected between 1 and 2 years of age.

Whatever is the type of syndactyly, the upper age limit of correction is 24 months, as the prehensile function is usually established by that time.

Q4. Can release of syndactyly be done bilaterally?

In case of nonambulatory children who are younger than 12 to 14 months, bilateral procedures should be performed.

- In older patients, bilateral procedures should be avoided as they become totally dependent on their family members for their daily activities, which should be avoided.

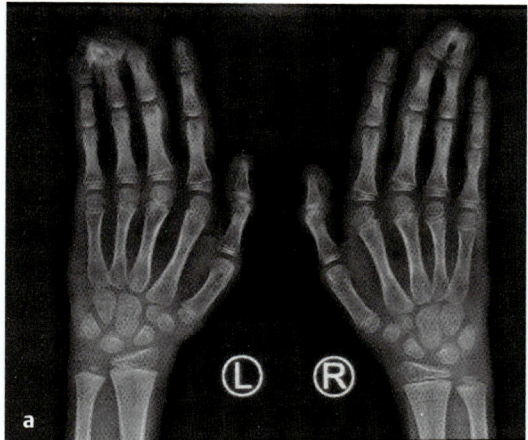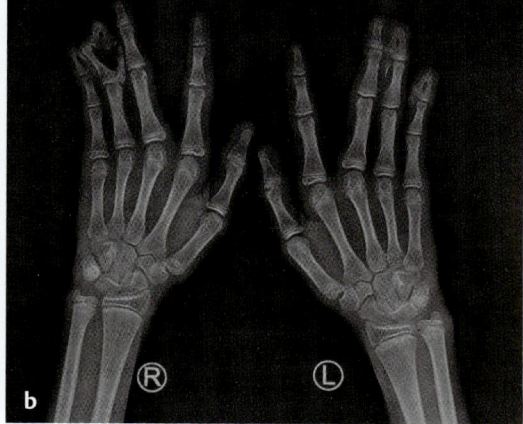

Fig. 18.6 X-ray in various types of syndactyly. **(a)** Complex syndactyly, **(b)** complicated syndactyly.

Q5. What are the principles of syndactyly release?

Following are the principles:

- Zig-zag incisions should be used on the palmar surfaces to avoid contracture.
- Commissure should be placed at a dorsal to palmar 45-degree angle at level of the proximal phalanx.
- Full-thickness tissue should be used for commissure reconstructions.
- Raw area should be covered with full-thickness skin grafts which should be equally distributed.
- One side of the digit should be operated at one time to avoid damage to the vessels.
- Nails and nail folds should be constructed near to normal.
- Skeletal deformities should be corrected earlier when there is no danger of injuring growth centers.
- Postoperative stents to be used at night to maintain web configuration.
- Adequate immobilization should be there postoperatively in the form of cast.

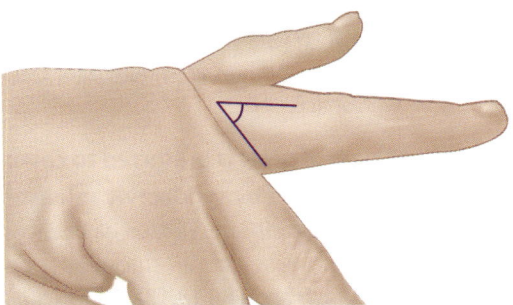

Fig. 18.7 A normal web space of hand.

Q6. What is the normal position of the web space?

The normal web space should have a dorsal-palmar slope of 45 degrees and extends from the metacarpal heads to the mid of proximal phalanx (**Fig. 18.7**).

- The second and fourth web spaces are comparatively wider than the third.
- The first web space is diamond-shaped.

Q7. Show the markings of syndactyly release.

Upton's marking of syndactyly release (**Fig. 18.8a, b**):

- Mark the dorsal and palmar levels of web space as compared to the other web spaces.
- A large, dorsal, truncated rectangular flap is marked, used for the creation of the web space.
- Dorsal flap should extend to the proximal interphalangeal (PIP) joint extension crease.
- The palmar flap is triangular.
- Distal zig-zag incisions are marked for triangular flaps. Mirror images are created on the two sides of each finger.
- Angles of the triangular flaps should be sharp and acute.
- In complete syndactyly with nail folds:
  - Buck-Gramcko pedicled pulp flaps are used for the reconstruction of the nail fold using the pulp of the adjacent finger (**Fig. 18.9a, b**).

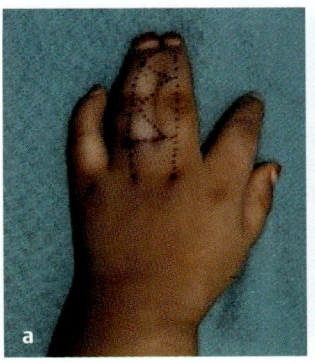
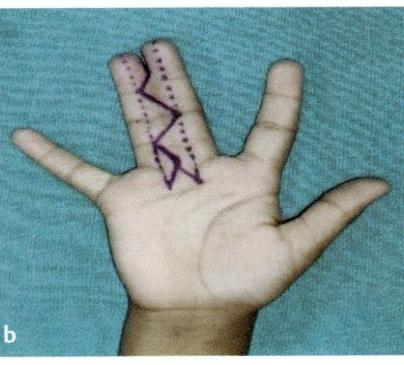

Fig. 18.8 (a) Marking on the dorsal aspect. **(b)** Marking on palmar aspect.

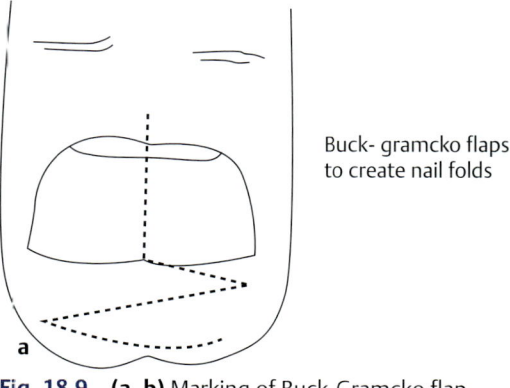

Buck- gramcko flaps to create nail folds

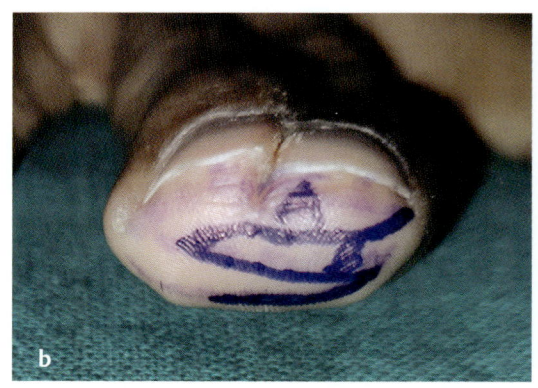

Fig. 18.9 **(a, b)** Marking of Buck-Gramcko flap.

Q8. What are the flaps used for syndactyly release?

- For small defects, Z-plasty transposition flaps are used.
  - For first web space, four-flap Z-plasty (**Fig. 18.10a, b**) is preferred because it provides excellent length and contour within the depth of the web space.
- V-Y flaps.
- Dorsal transposition flaps.
- Dorsal rotation.
- Rotation advancement flaps.

Q9. What are the various flaps used for web space creation?

- Dorsal flap: Most commonly used flaps for creating web in syndactyly.
- Palmar flap: Second most commonly used flap.
- A combination of both dorsal and palmar flap.
- Cloverleaf or manta ray-type flap:
  - In this technique, flaps are taken from the more proximal part of the dorsum.
  - The wings in cloverleaf flap help in covering some part of the lateral side of the proximal phalanx.
- Dorsal metacarpal flap may also be used.
  - Advantage of this flap is that no skin graft is required.
  - Primary closure of the raw areas over the fingers can be done.

Q10. Why do we release on one side of a digit at one time in case of syndactyly in adjacent digits?

There are two reasons for that:

- The common digital artery gives branches to the adjacent digits usually through the commissure. While releasing the syndactyly and deepening the commissure, if we need to sacrifice the digital artery of a finger, so at least one digital artery per digit should be preserved.
- Scarcity of dorsal flaps as usually the amount of dorsal flaps are enough for only one web space.

Q11. What type of graft is preferred to cover the raw areas caused by syndactyly release?

Full-thickness skin graft is preferred as chances of contracture are less in full-thickness skin grafts (**Fig. 18.11a, b** and **Fig. 18.12a, b**).

Q12. What are the key points to be taken care of during the postoperative dressing?

Grafts and suture lines should be covered with innermost layer of nonadherent dressing followed by compressible synthetic foam or moistened cotton placed as a stent within the interdigital web space.

- Fingers should be kept abducted throughout the dressing to avoid any kinking of the commissure flaps.
- Then a bulky fluffy dressing should be applied with a circumferential bandage.

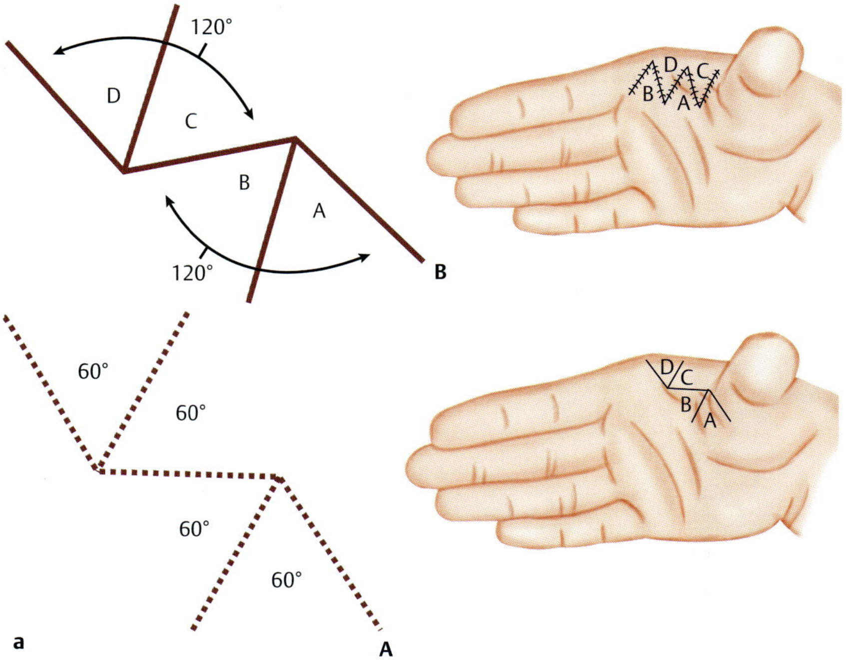

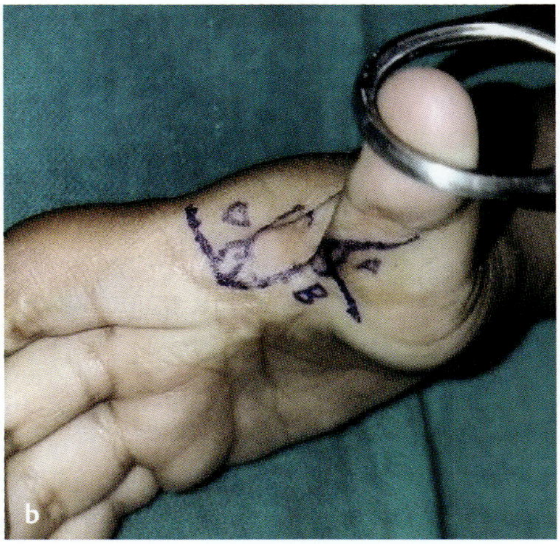

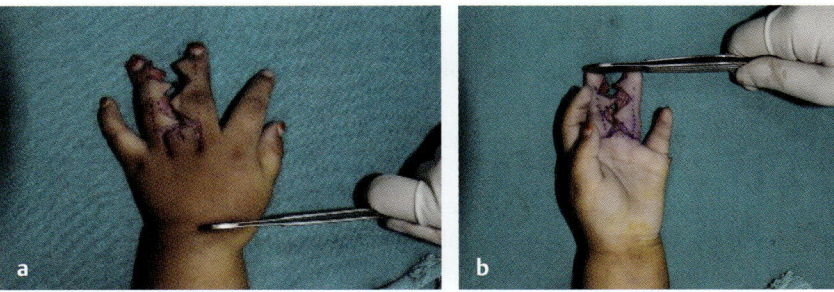

Fig. 18.10 (**a, b**) Four-flap Z-plasty for the first web space.

Fig. 18.11 (**a, b**) Intraoperative separation of digits.

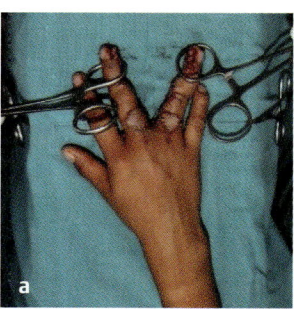
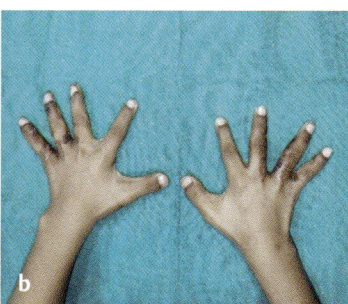

Fig. 18.12 (a, b) Application of full-thickness graft after syndactyly release and postoperative appearance.

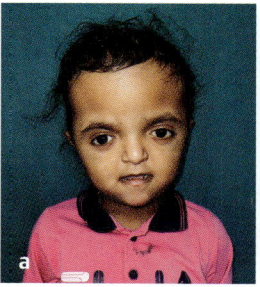
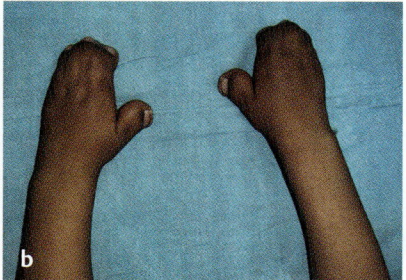
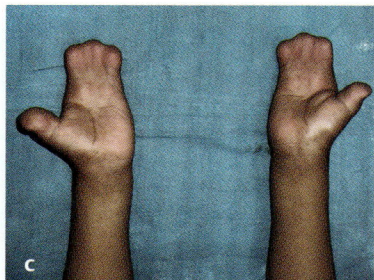

Fig. 18.13 (a–c) Appearance of hands in Apert's syndrome.

- In no condition, there should be any tight dressing around the digits as it may lead to venous compromise which may in turn lead to distal loss of digits.
- Finally, immobilization of the limb should be done with above-elbow splint with elbow in 90-degrees flexion.

Q13. What is the incidence of syndactyly?
- One in every 2000 live births.
- More common in boys.
- Third web space is most commonly involved—50%, followed by:

Fourth web space	–	30%
Second web space	–	15%
First web space	–	5%

Q14. What is the embryological basis of syndactyly?
- At fourth intrauterine week, upper limb bud develops.
- At 5 to 6 weeks of intrauterine life, the interactions between the apical ectodermal ridge and the underlying mesenchymal tissue within the hand plate result in a distal to proximal cleft formation between the rays of hand.
- The soft tissue between the longitudinal cartilaginous rays of the hand disappears by the process of "apoptosis" or "programmed cell death" and separation of digits and thumb occurs.

Q15. What are the syndromes associated with syndactyly?
At least 28 syndromes are associated with syndactyly. Most common are:
- Poland's syndrome (absence of the sternocostal portion of the pectoralis major muscles, hypoplasia of the hand, forearm, and upper arm, simple complex or incomplete syndactyly and short fingers).
- Apert's syndrome (acrocephalosyndactyly)—Characteristics of hand deformity in Apert's syndrome are (**Fig. 18.13a–c**):
  - Brachy-clinodactyly of the thumb.
  - Complex syndactyly of index/long/ring finger.

- Symbrachyphalangism.
- Simple syndactyly of fourth web.
- Three types:
  - Type I spade hand.
  - Type II constricted cupped "mitten" hand.
  - Type III coalesced "rosebud" hand.
- Surgical sequence in correction— Release of thumb and index or deepening of the first web and separation of digit 4 and 5, followed by separation of other digits and correction of clinodactyly of the thumb.

- Constriction ring syndrome.
- Multiple facial syndrome.

Suggested Readings

1. Upton J. Management of disorders of separation syndactyly. In: Mathes SJ, Hentz VR, eds. Plastic surgery: the hand and upper limb, part 2. Vol. 8. 2nd ed. Saunders Elsevier; 2006:139–184
2. Steven ERH, van Nieuwenhoven CA. In: Neligan PC, ed. Plastic surgery: hand and upper extremity. Vol. 6. 4th ed. Canada: Elsevier; 2018: 624–630

19 Camptodactyly

Veena K. Singh

Learning Objectives

At the end of this chapter, the students will be able to:
1. Describe the clinical presentation of camptodactyly.
2. Understand the pathophysiology of camptodactyly.
3. Understand the different options and decision-making in camptodactyly.
4. Demonstrate the surgical correction of camptodactyly.

Introduction

Camptodactyly refers to permanent flexion contracture at the proximal interphalangeal joint. Most cases are limited to fifth-finger involvement. The pathological basis is anatomical imbalance between the extrinsics and anomalous insertion of the intrinsic muscles. Although common, the treatment of camptodactyly is controversial. So, a detailed clinical examination to assess the severity of the deformity will help in the selection of a patient who will actually benefit from surgery.

History

Particulars of the patient: Name, age, gender, address.

Chief Complaints

- Presence of angulated/bent finger(s) since birth/in adolescence age.
- Sometimes, pain may be an associated complaint if recent trauma history is there.

History of Present Illness

- In case of child, the parents generally give a history of flexion (bent finger) deformity at birth or during infancy.
- Sometimes, it is first noticeable during childhood that is gradually progressive.
- There may be a history of worsening of deformity during the adolescent growth spurt.
- Any history of physiotherapy or splintage during infancy or childhood.
- Ask about trauma or other deformities elsewhere in the body (see the differential diagnosis).

Past History

Any relevant medical illness or surgery performed in the child for some other ailment.

Antenatal History

A complete antenatal history needs to be taken from the mother if the presentation is during infancy or childhood.

Family History

History of similar problems in other siblings or in family.

Immunization History

Whether immunization is updated as per the national immunization program for the age of the child.

History of Allergy

To any food or medication.

General Physical Examination

Look for other deformities (see the differential diagnoses).

Systemic Examination

- Abdomen.
- Respiratory system.
- Cardiovascular system (CVS).
- Central nervous system (CNS).

Refer chapter 3 "Carcinoma Oral Cavity"

Local Examination of the Hand

Exposure

After proper exposure of B/L hands up to forearm in adequate light with proper explained informed consent.

Inspection

Attitude of the Hand and Fingers

1. Inspection in outstretched hands with elbow rested on the top of a table.
2. Note the flexion deformity at the proximal interphalangeal (PIP) joint of affected fingers of both hands (**Fig. 19.1**).
3. Any fixed deformity which may be carefully looked for by asking the patient to actively flex and extend the PIP joint.

Scar

From trauma or from previous surgical intervention. It needs to be mentioned in detail.

Palpation/Movements

1. Look for whether the child is able to make a full fist.
2. PIP joint—Check for active range of motion and passive range of motion.
   - Try to differentiate a flexible deformity from a fixed flexion contracture.
3. Check for change in the passive extension of PIP joint on flexion of wrist and metacarpophalangeal (MCP) joint.
4. Do the central slip tenodesis test:
   - The central slip tenodesis test is done to determine the integrity of the central slip in a flexible deformity.
     - With the elbow rested on a table top, hold the MCP joint in flexion and look for the change in extension at PIP joint of the affected finger.
     - If there is complete PIP joint extension it indicates the ability of the extrinsic extensors to achieve active PIP joint extension.
     - Any extension lag during this maneuver infers central slip attenuation that may require augmentation at the time of surgery.

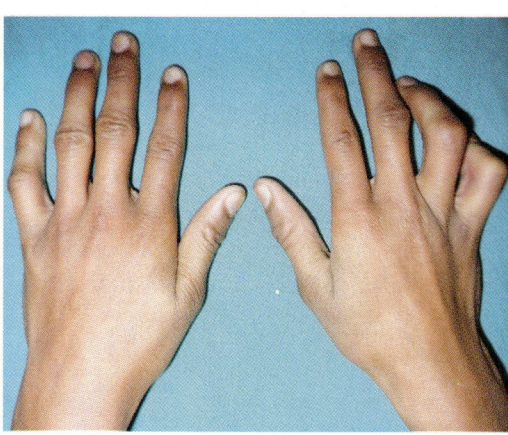

Fig. 19.1 Examination of fingers in camptodactyly.

5. Function of flexor digitorum superficialis (FDS) and flexor digitorum profundus (FDP) of the involved fingers must be assessed individually.
   - At times, FDS of ring and little finger may be interconnected and hence PIP joint of little finger may not be able to flex independently.
   - In these cases, ring finger may be kept free to recheck the flexion at PIP joint of little finger.
6. Document for intact sensation and vascularity of affected finger.

Measurements

- Measure the angle at PIP joint of the affected finger(s) with a finger goniometer.
- PIP joint—Flexion.
  - Extension lag

X-ray: If available, please check before making the final diagnosis.

Provisional Diagnosis

This is a case of a 11-year-old female with camptodactyly of the left little finger, type II category without fixed joint deformity.

Questions

Q1. How will you proceed?
- Since it is a severe type of camptodactyly >60 degrees of flexion at PIP joint with preserved mobility, I would like to go for corrective surgery.
- The baseline investigations will be done for preanesthetic fitness.
- An X-ray of the affected finger in a lateral view will be done to see the bony changes in the middle phalanx.
- Preoperative counseling of the patient and family members will be done regarding the expected outcome, risk of compromising the flexion at the expense of gain in extension, and long-term compliance of splintage and physiotherapy.

Q2. How do you classify camptodactyly?
Camptodactyly occurs in less than 1% of the population. It is divided into three categories:
- Type I deformity:
  - Most common.
  - Becomes apparent during infancy.
  - Isolated deformity.
  - Involves mostly fifth finger (**Fig. 19.2**).
- Type II deformity:
  - Same features as type I.
  - But not apparent until preadolescence.
  - Develops between 7 and 11 years of age.
  - Affects girls more than boys.
  - Does not improve spontaneously.
  - May progress to severe flexion deformity.
- Type III deformity:
  - Severe form of deformity.
  - Usually involves multiple digits of both extremities (**Fig. 19.3**).
  - Associated with variety of syndromes.
  - Involvement of hand is asymmetrical.
  - This is a camptodactyly which can occur in conjunction with craniofacial disorders, short nature, and chromosomal abnormalities.

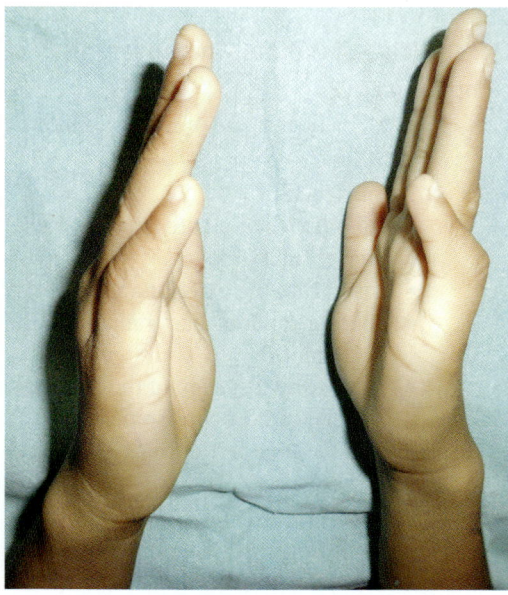

Fig. 19.2 Type I deformity.

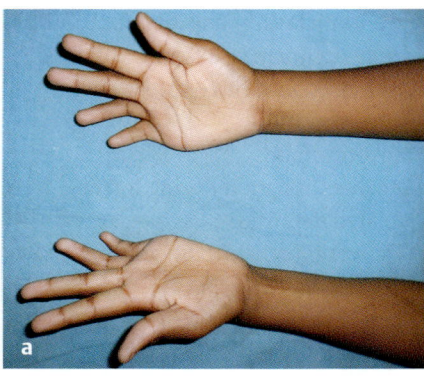 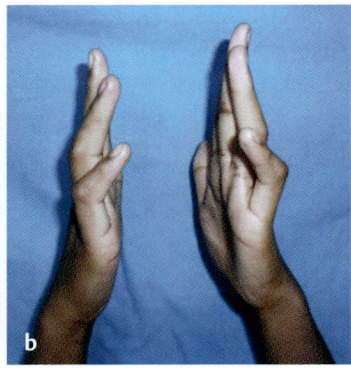

Fig. 19.3 (a, b) Type III deformity.

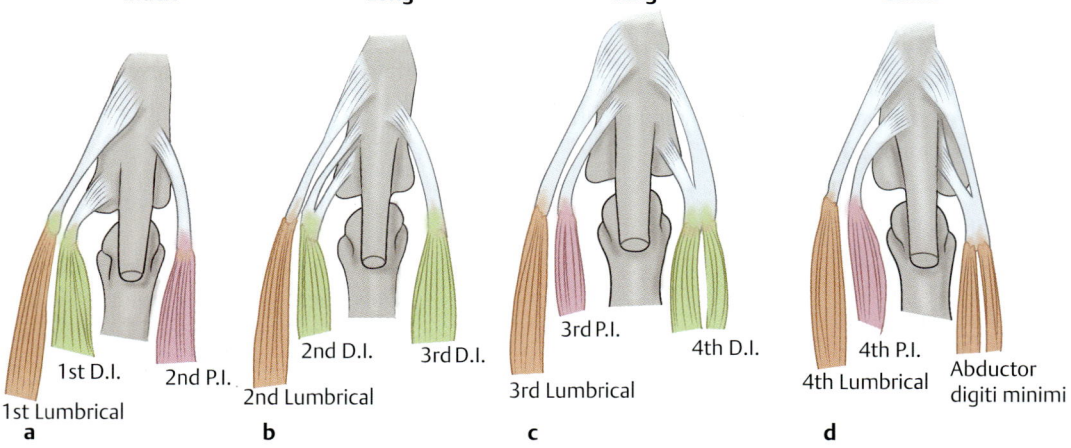

Fig. 19.4 (a-d) Normal intrinsic muscle anatomy. Abbreviations: DI, dorsal interossei; PI, palmar interossei.

Q3. What is the pathogenesis of camptodactyly?

- Normal intrinsic muscle anatomy (**Fig. 19.4**):
  - **Lumbricals:**
    - All muscles originate from the radial side of the FDP.
    - Insert into the exterior aponeurosis.
    - All four tendons pass radially to the MCP joint.
    - Origin and insertion of the first lumbrical is almost consistent.
    - It is variable in the third and fourth lumbricals.
  - **Interossei:**
    - Each finger has two interossei with exception of the fifth finger which has abductor digiti minimi.

- Three palmar interossei adduct the middle, ring, and little fingers toward the index finger.
- Four dorsal interossei abduct the digits.
- Distal insertions of interossei are classified into:
  - Superficial/distal—into extensor aponeurosis.
  - Deep/proximal—into the bone.
- The first dorsal interosseous muscle inserts into the bone (proximal or deep).
- The third dorsal interosseous inserts into the extensor.
- Second and fourth dorsal interossei have mixed insertions.
- Palmar interossei have predominantly superficial insertions

into the extensor aponeurosis on the ulnar side of the index finger and radial sides of ring and small fingers.

- **Abnormal intrinsic muscle anatomy (Fig. 19.5a, b):**
  - The etiopathogenesis of camptodactyly is the dynamic imbalance due to abnormal intrinsic muscle anatomy.
  - Most common factors responsible for it are that instead of inserting into the lateral band, abnormal lumbrical insertion is there either:
    - Into the superficialis tendon distal to the MCP joint.
    - Or, into the fibrous flexor sheath.
    - Or, capsule of the MCP joint.
  - Other abnormal anatomical findings are:
    - Tight superficialis muscle-tendon unit.
    - Absent or hypoplastic FDS with abnormal insertions.
    - Contracture of collateral ligaments and palmar plate.
    - Tight palmar skin.
    - Slowly retracting flexor tendon.
    - Deficient extensor tendons over the PIP joint.
    - Also, fibrous strands beneath the skin.

Q4. What is the clinical presentation of camptodactyly?

- The term camptodactyly was introduced by Tamplin.
  - It is derived from a Greek term meaning "bent finger."
  - The term describes the flexion deformity of the PIP joint in an anteroposterior direction.
  - It is differentiated from clinodactyly in which there is deviation in radioulnar plane.
  - In decreasing order of frequency, camptodactyly occurs in the ring, middle, and index finger.

Q5. What are the radiological features in camptodactyly?

- A true lateral view is required (**Fig. 19.6**):
  - Dorsal and palmar flattening of the normal circular surface of the condyle of the proximal phalanx.
  - Narrowing of the joint space.
  - Indentation in the neck of the proximal phalanx.
  - Base of the middle phalanx may be broad and may show greater subchondral bone density.

Q6. What are the key points in the management of camptodactyly?

- **Conservative management:**
  - Can be done in young children.
  - Passive stretching exercises and splinting are taught to the parents.
  - Parents are counseled to accept the deformity for as long as possible.
  - It is also important to keep in mind that the deformity may worsen during adolescent growth spurt.
- **Indication for surgical management:**
  - Older children and adults with PIP joint contractures 50 to 70 degrees.
  - Children having progressive deformity in spite of conservative management and the deformity has stabilized.
- **Planning for surgery:**
  - The surgery for significant contractures involves four logical steps:
    - Planning of skin incision.
    - Examination of abnormal lumbrical, interosseous, and superficial flexor tendon anatomy.
    - Release of secondary contractures.
    - Rebalancing it with tendon transfer, if indicated.
    - Surgical techniques:
      - **Incision:**
        - i. A longitudinal palmar approach in the distal palm with extension to the digit.

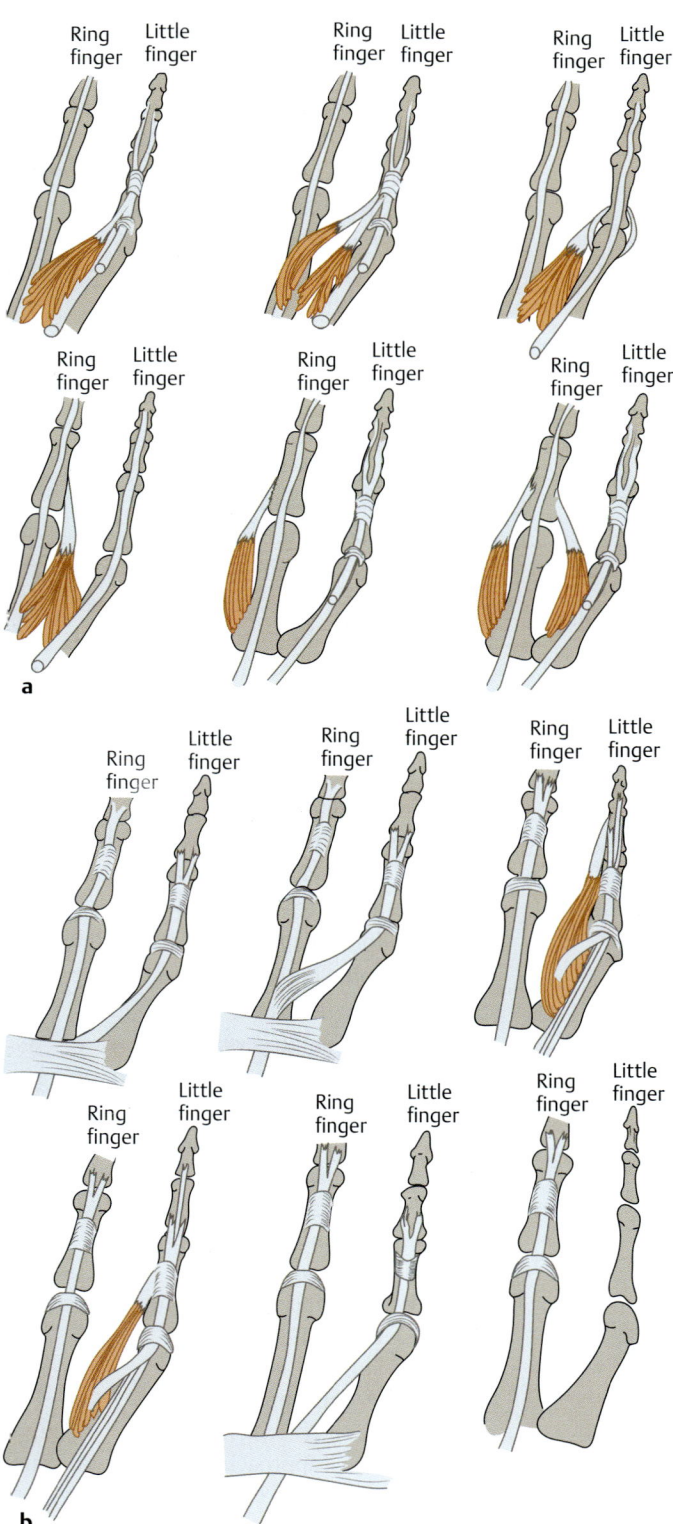

Common variations in lumbrical anatomy.

a. bipennate origin and insertion into flexor tendon and sheath.

b. extra muscle from ring finger FDP and insertion into flexor sheath.

c. bipennate origin and insertion into MCP joint collateral ligament.

d. bipennate muscle and insertion into ring finger.

e. absent 4th lumbrical and intact extrinsic flexor tendons.

f. unipennate muscle insertion into ulnar side of ring finger proximal phalanx.

Variations in flexor digitorum superficialis anatomy

a. origin from transverse carpal ligament.

b. origin from adjacent FDP of ring finger.

c. origin from lumbrical to little finger.

d. origin of both lumbrical and FDS from radial side of 5th metacarpal.

e. origin in the distal forearm proximal to transverse carpal ligament.

f. complete absence of FDS.

Fig. 19.5 (a, b) Anomalous insertion of intrinsic muscles.

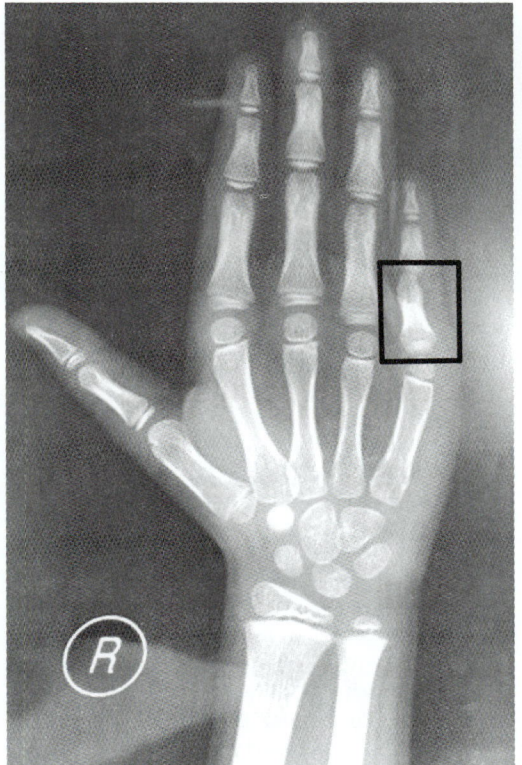

Fig. 19.6 X-ray findings in camptodactyly.

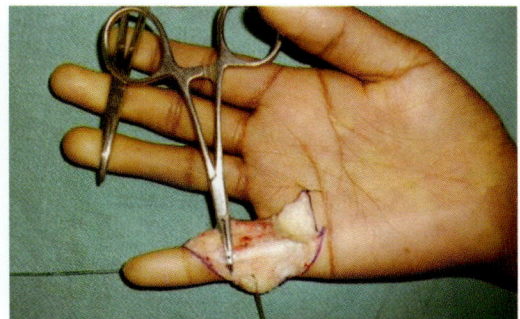

Fig. 19.7 Tight and hypoplastic flexor digitorum superficialis (FDS).

– **In older patients with significant bone changes and PIP contractures of 90 degrees.**
  ▪ Corrective osteotomy at the neck of proximal phalanx may achieve.
– **PIP joint extension without loss of flexion:**
  ▪ If fixed contracture, arthrodesis and shortening in functional position may be considered.

Q7. What is the postoperative care?
• K-wires are used to hold the PIP joint in extension for 2 weeks.
• After 2 weeks, physiotherapy and an extension splint is given once k-wires are removed.
• Night splints are worn for 3 to 6 months.

Q8. How will you classify the outcome after treatment for camptodactyly?
• **Excellent**—Correction to full extension.
  – With <15-degree loss of PIP joint flexion.
• **Good**—Correction to within 20 degrees of full PIP joint extension or >40 degrees of increase in: PIP joint extension.
  – With >30-degree loss of PIP joint flexion.
• **Fair**—Correction to within 40 degrees of full PIP joint extension or >20 degrees of increase in: PIP joint extension.
  – With <45-degree loss of PIP joint flexion.

ii. Incisions must be planned in such a way that it allows z-plasty closure at several levels.
– **Release of structures responsible for contracture:**
  ▪ Tight and hypoplastic superficialis tendon—to be released (**Fig. 19.7**).
  ▪ Anomalous lumbrical insertion—to be released.
  ▪ Any soft tissue fiber responsible for contracture—to be released.
– **Rebalancing with tendon transfer:**
  ▪ A tight flexor can be converted into a PIP joint extensor by transferring the two slips of FDS to the lateral band and central slip via the lumbrical canal.
  ▪ In long-standing cases, palmar plate release and collateral ligament shortening may be required.

- **Poor**—<20-degree improvement in PIP joint flexion or <40 degrees of total PIP joint motion.

Q9. What is the most worrisome complication after camptodactyly surgery?

- Loss of PIP joint flexion at the cost of extension at PIP joint is most worrisome complication after surgical correction of camptodactyly.
- It should be clearly explained to the parents and patients and therefore operative treatment is only reserved for a severe deformity that has failed conservative management.

Q10. What are the differential diagnoses of camptodactyly?

- Pterygium syndrome—multiple pterygia including knee and elbow.
- Arthrogryposis congenita:
  - Multiple joint.
  - Underdeveloped muscles.
  - Ulnar deviation of digits.

- Symphalangism:
  - No active/passive joint motion.
  - Absent skin creases.
- Boutonniere:
  - H/o trauma and pain.
  - Joint swelling.
  - Distal interphalangeal (DIP) joint hyperextension.
- Trigger fingers—MCP joint is involved.
  - Palpable click on finger extension.

Suggested Readings

1. Steven ER, van Nieuwenhoven CA. In: Neligan PC, editors. Plastic surgery: hand and upper extremity. Vol. 6. 4th ed. Canada: Elsevier; 2018: 624–655.
2. Upton J. In: Mathes SJ, ed. Plastic surgery: the hand and upper limb. Part 2. Vol. 8. 2nd ed. Canada: Elsevier; 2006: 265–322.
3. Singh V, Haq A, Priyadarshini P, Kumar P. Camptodactyly: An unsolved area of plastic surgery. Arch Plast Surg 2018;45(4):363–366
4. Siegert JJ, Cooney WP, Dobyns JH. Management of simple camptodactyly. J Hand Surg [Br] 1990;15(2):181–189

Introduction

Basal cell carcinoma is a one of the common cutaneous malignancies seen in plastic surgery consultation room. It is a very slowly progressive and locally invasive lesion with rare neurovascular involvement. A detailed examination will differentiate it from the other skin malignancies and help in making correct diagnosis and management plan.

Chief Complaints

- Ulcer over the face (upper lip, cheek, medial eyelid, etc.).
- On and off bleeding.
- Pigmentation on the face.

History of Present Illness

- Onset: Sudden/insidious appearance.
- Ask about the color to start with and the present color.
- Progression in the size and any other associated features like change in color, discharge, etc.
- Pain: The lesion may be initially painless but as the size increases and ulcer develops, there may be associated intermittent/persistent mild/dull aching pain over the ulcer. Pain may also increase during eating and speaking if ulcer is around the areas of upper and lower lip. Requirement of medication must also be asked as it indicates the severity of pain.
- Bleeding may be associated with the ulcer, spontaneous or on trivial trauma like scratching.
- History of (History of) any ointment application and dressing.
- History of any drooling of saliva or difficulty in chewing/swallowing food or any change in quality of speech (in cases of BCC lip).
- In BCC upper lip, patient finds difficulty in speaking loudly as the air passes over the ulcer making it painful and in cases of large ulcer, there may be escape of air.
- History of neck swelling, if any.
- Inquire about sleep/appetite/any weight loss.
- Negative History of cough/hemoptysis/joint pain/headache/nausea.

Past History

- If any similar swelling/ulcer which subsided by itself.

- History of diabetes mellitus, tuberculosis, hypertension, or any surgical or medical intervention for the ulcer.

Family History

Similar history in the family or history of skin malignancy in other members.

Personal History

- Special focus on the nature of occupation if it involves long hours of sun exposure especially in a fair-skinned patient.
- Whether history of smoking present or not.

Treatment History

- Any intake of immunosuppressive drugs.
- History of allergy to food or medications.

General Examination

The subheadings must remain same in all the long and short cases.
- Level of consciousness, alertness, whether cooperative.
- Decubitus.
- Build.
- Nutrition.
- Facies.
- Pallor.
- Cyanosis.
- Jaundice.
- Clubbing.
- Pedal edema.
- Pulse.
- Blood pressure (BP).
- Respiration.
- Temperature.
- Neck veins.
- Neck nodes.
- Any other deformity/scars.
- Any skin abnormality—naevus, angioma, hyperpigmentation.
- Any other.

Systemic Examination

- Examination of abdomen.
- Respiration system.
- Cardiovascular system (CVS).
- Central nervous system (CNS).

Refer chapter 3 "Carcinoma Oral Cavity"

Local Examination of an Ulcer

For details, see Carcinoma Oral Cavity. (chapter 3)

Inspection (in cases of ulcer)

1. Site.
2. Size.
3. Shape.
4. Margins.
5. Edge.
6. Floor.
7. Discharge, smell.
8. Surrounding skin.
9. In case of lips, intraoral examination:
   - Teeth hygiene.
   - Mouth opening.
   - Oral mucosa.
10. Facial nerve exam.
11. Neck swelling.

Inspection (in cases of swelling)

1. Site.
2. Size.
3. Shape.
4. Number.
5. Extent.
6. Surface.
7. Margin.
8. Skin over the swelling.
   - Scar, pigmentation, prominent veins, any ulcer, satellite nodule.
9. Surrounding area, if any deformity.

Palpation

1. Temperature.
2. Tenderness.

3. Inspectory findings to be corroborated.
4. Margins.
5. Base of ulcer.
6. Induration.
7. Whether ulcer is mobile/fixed to the underlying structures. To check mobility, feel the base of the ulcer by holding it in between the thumb, index, and middle fingers and move both in vertical and horizontal planes.
8. Whether bleeds easily on touch.

Lymph Node (LN) Palpation

1. Cervical L.N. can be palpated both from the front and back.
2. It is easier to palpate from back as it is uncomfortable for the examiner to sit in front of the patient for long.
   - The examiner stands behind the patient with patient sitting on a stool.
3. The neck is slightly flexed to the side of the examination to relax the sternocleidomastoid muscle (SCM); stabilizing the patient's head with the left hand, the examiner starts palpating the lymph node with his/her right hand.

Levels of Lymph Nodes in the Neck

- Level Ia (submental L.N.):
  - Lie in submental triangle.
  - Palpated in the submental triangle with the pulp of the fingers.
- Level Ib (submandibular L.N.):
  - Located in submandibular triangle and palpated there.
- Level II (upper jugular L.N.). Lie along the internal jugular vein (IJV) in the upper third from the level of carotid bifurcation to the skull base.
- Level III (middle jugular L.N.). In the middle third from the carotid bifurcation above to the cricothyroid below.
- Level IV (lower jugular L.N.). In the lower third of IJV between cricothyroid above and clavicle below.

Level II, III, IV: With the pulp of fingers, palpated along the IV.

Level V: Posterior triangle L.N. or supraclavicular L.N.
- Located in the posterior triangle.
- Anteriorly, posterior border of SCM; posteriorly, anterior border of trapezius.
- Boundaries of posterior below lateral half of the clavicle.
- Level V L.N. are palpated in the posterior triangle in the supraclavicular fossa with the pulp of the fingers.
- Both sides can be palpated simultaneously.
- To make it prominent, patient may be asked to shrug the shoulders.

Level VI (anterior compartment group):
- Includes Pre-and paratracheal L.N., perilaryngeal and pericricoid L.N.
- Located from suprasternal notch up to the hyoid bone and extends laterally up to the anterior border of SCM.
- Both sides can be palpated simultaneously. If a palpable L.N. is found (usually when L.N. size >1 cm) look for:
  - Size.
  - Tenderness.
  - Surface.
  - Fixity to the overlying skin or underlying structure.
  - Margin.
  - Consistency.
  - Number.

Measurement

- With a scale/measuring tape, the size of ulcer or swelling is measured in both vertical and horizontal dimensions.
- Distance of ulcer margins from the anatomical landmarks should also be measured.
- Mouth opening will be measured as interincisal distance with the help of a scale.

Provisional Diagnosis

This is a case of a 1-year-old ulceroproliferative lesion involving left medial canthus, nose, upper eyelid, and cheek, which is most likely to be BCC without any palpable lymph nodes in a 65-year-old male patient (**Fig. 20.1**).

Questions

Q1. How will you proceed further?

To confirm the diagnosis, a biopsy from the ulcer is needed. In case of:

- Small ulcer: Excisional biopsy (excision of the entire ulcer with health margins).
- Large ulcer: Incisional biopsy (four-quadrant wedge biopsy).
- Routine investigation for anesthesia fitness will include:
  - Complete blood count, prothrombin time (PT)/international normalized ratio (INR).
  - Electrocardiogram (ECG), in 12 leads.
  - Chest X-ray (CXR)—posteroanterior (PA) view.

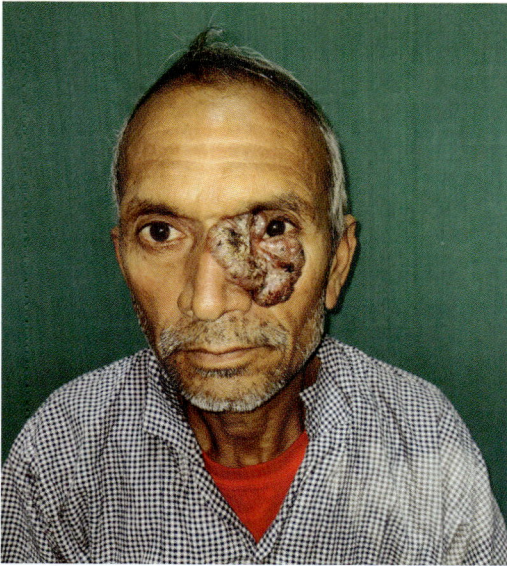

Fig. 20.1 Basal cell carcinoma involving left medial canthus, nose, upper eyelid, and cheek.

- Liver function tests (LFTs)/kidney function tests (KFTs) (as patients are elderly).
- Orthopantomogram (in cases, where ulcer is near the bone or ulcer base is fixed to the bone).

Q2. What are the points in favor of BCC?

- Slowly progressive.
- In the tear drop area.
- Over the sun-exposed areas like face and neck.
- Rolled-out edges with typical appearance of a rodent ulcer.

Q3. What are the various forms in which a BCC can present?

Or

What is the most common complaint of the patient?

A shiny skin colored swelling over which tiny blood vessels may be seen:

- Brown, black lesion.
- A flat or scaly raised patch with ulceration.

Most commonly, the patient complaints that it is sore which is not healing.

Q4. What are the etiological factors responsible for BCC?

BCC is the most common malignant tumor of the skin.

- The main cause is exposure to sunlight, especially the ultraviolet rays:
  - UV-A—320-nm wavelength.
  - UV-B—290-nm wavelength.

Indian skin is Fitzpatrick skin type IV (dark brown) which rarely burns but tans easily, so BCC is uncommon as compared to western skin (Fitzpatrick skin type I-II, very fair, fair) that has a tendency to burn rather than to tan.

- Other risk factors include exposure to arsenic, poor immune system, chronic wounds, and scars.
- BCC may occur in the background of diseases like xeroderma pigmentosa and basal cell naevus syndrome.

Q5. What is the origin of BCC?

Both BCC and squamous cell carcinoma (SCC) have their genesis from pluripotent cells in the epithelium and hair follicles.

- The growth and spread of BCC depends on the connective tissue stroma.
- It is more common in men but recently females are also being affected due to more involvement in outdoor activities.

Q6. What are the premalignant lesions for BCC and SCC?

- Actinic keratosis (SCC).
- Leukoplakia (SCC).
- Xeroderma pigmentosum (BCC, SCC, melanoma).
- Keratoacanthoma (SCC).
- Bowen's disease (SCC) (erythroplasia of Queyrat).
- Naevus sebaceous of Jodassahn.

Q7. What are the clinical features of BCC?

- About 85% of all tumors are present in head and neck region. The most common site being the nose.
- In Asians, BCC is usually associated with burns, chronic wounds, or albinism.
- BCC occurs as an isolated lesion but metachronous lesions are also common and 40% of patients develop another skin malignancy within a period of 10 years.
- Growth is very slow with actual growth at the periphery associated with cellular apoptosis and central ulceration and necrosis. Therefore, it becomes of utmost importance that a wide margin of 0.5 to 1 cm is excised as the cells in the marginal areas are most aggressively behaving cells.
- Long-standing BCC may invade along the tissue planes periosteum and nerves and embryonic fusion planes like nasolabial or naso-orbital regions are more susceptible to tumor invasion.
- BCC has rare incidence of metastasis (<0.1%) as the survival and multiplication of the cells require connective tissue stroma. The metastatic spread is via blood to lung and bones.

Q8. What are the types and their clinical presentations?

Based on the histology, BCC is divided into five subtypes:

- Nodular.
- Superficial.
- Micronodular.
- Infiltrative.
- Morpheaform.

Nodular BCC:

- Most common type (50% of all BCCs).
- Presents as a small nodule with tiny blood vessels on its surface.
- With time, it enlarges in size and ulcerates, representing its description as rodent ulcer because the irregular margins give the appearance of the tissue being bitten by a rodent.
- This lesion has raised, rolled-out edges with central ulceration and necrotic tissue.

Superficial BCC:

- ~10% of all BCC.
- Have flat, scaly, and reddish appearance.
- More commonly occurs on trunk.
- The lesion may initially expand but later ulcerate also.
- This is the type of BCC with chances of spontaneous regression in the form of flat scars.

Pigmented BCC:

- ~5% of all BCCs.
- They contain melanin giving them a brown appearance and may be confused with melanoma as melanocytes are present in epidermis and in hair matrix in 75% of skin tumors.
- Their behavioral pattern is same as nodular BCC except for color.

Morpheaform or sclerosing BCC:

- Clinical presentation may vary from flat whitish to yellow plaques-like lesion with ill-defined borders.

- Surface is shiny and scar-like, and because of its confusing appearance, it is often misdiagnosed, undertreated, and recurrent.

Q9. What are the high-risk factors in basal cell carcinoma?

There are various factors which are the predictors of high risk in BCC:

- Location: Tumors on the central region of the face, around the eyes/ears, hand, and feet.
- Size:
  - >5 mm on above-mentioned anatomical sites.
  - >10 mm on scalp, forehead, cheek, and neck.
  - >20 mm on limbs and central trunk.
- Histopathology:
  - BCC subtypes: Morpheaform, infiltrative, micronodular.
- Clinical presentation:
  - Ill-defined borders.
  - Recurrence.
  - Immunosuppression.

Q10. What are the treatment options?

The options are many: **Table 20.1**

- Curettage and electrodessication.
- Surgical excision.
- Moh's surgery (chemosurgery).
- 5-Fluorouracil.
- Radiation therapy.
- Cryosurgery.

- Chemotherapy.
- Photodynamic therapy.

Surgical excision:

- It is indicated in both high-risk and low-risk cases.
- Wide local excision (WLE) should be done with negative margins of 5 mm in lesions of <1 cm size and 1 cm in lesions of >1 cm size.
- Reconstruction of the defect can be done according to the reconstructive principles in involved areas. As most of the patients are elderly, the laxity of skin over the face allows closure of defect with Limberg's flap (**Fig. 20.2a, b**), other local flaps (**Fig. 20.3a–c**, **Fig. 20.4a–d**).

Principles of reconstruction with a Limberg flap:

- The lesion must be excised in a rhomboid shape (a rhombus is a quadrilateral with all sides parallel and equal to each other; its two opposite angles are obtuse at 120 degrees and the other two opposite angles are acute at 60 degrees). In a circular lesion, to create such a shape of the defect, some normal tissue might need to be sacrificed. So, always first excise the lesion with standard wide margins and then reshape the defect in a rhomboid fashion.
- The short diagonal bisecting the obtuse angles is extended to a length equal to one of the sides.

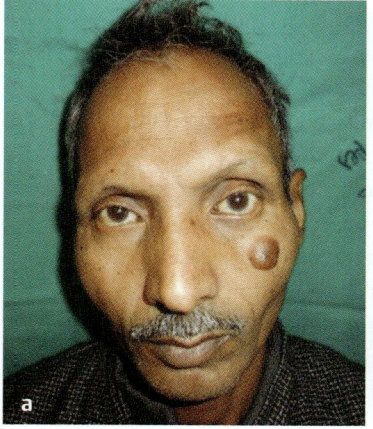
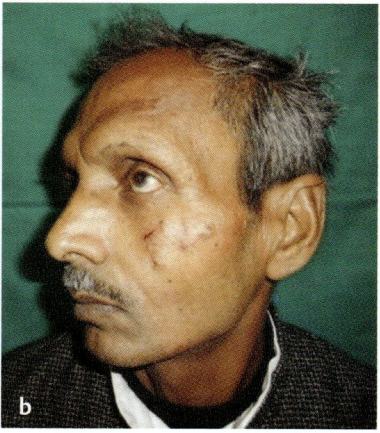

Fig. 20.2 (a, b) Basal cell carcinoma on left cheek in a 67-year-old male and postoperative appearance after excision and reconstruction with Limberg flap.

Table 20.1 Treatment of basal cell carcinoma

Treatment	Indications	Advantages	Disadvantages	Cure Rate
Surgical excision	Most tumors	Wounds closed primarily: better cosmetic result; single stage	Higher recurrence rates in some types compared with Moh's surgery; removes some normal tissue; limited histologic control	Up to 98% for nodular, primary 80% for recurrence
Moh's surgery	Large, invasive (Morpheaform), or recurrent; high-risk areas; when patient is not a candidate for surgery	Histologic control of tumor excision	May leave large defects requiring surgical repair; time-consuming; requires special techniques and training	Up to 99% for primary
Curettage and electrodessication	Small (2–4 mm), primary, localized tumors; superficial multicentric	Commonly available, widely used	Poor histologic control; hypertrophic scarring, hypopigmentation; delayed wound healing	100% (<2 mm) 50% (>3 cm)
5-FU	Superficial, multicentric (very limited)	Noninvasive	Long treatment; pigmentation changes; not for invasive or recurrent tumors	Low
Radiation therapy	Nonsurgical candidates; inoperable tumors; palliation	"Spares" normal tissue	Requires special expertise; ulceration; poor cosmesis	95% (<5 mm), 85% (15 mm) 75–90% recurrent
Cryosurgery	Localized, primary tumors; patient at poor surgical risk	"Spares" normal tissue	"Blind" treatment; not effective for sclerosing tumors or recurrences	Up to 95% (<2 cm) in primary lesions
Chemotherapy	Uncontrolled local and metastatic disease	May prolong survival; palliation	Toxicity	N/A
Photodynamic therapy	Superficial lesions	Noninvasive	Limited penetration of light source; lack of histologic control; patient photosensitized	10–40% in nodular, higher in superficial

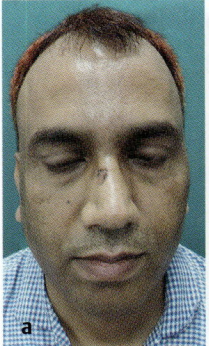
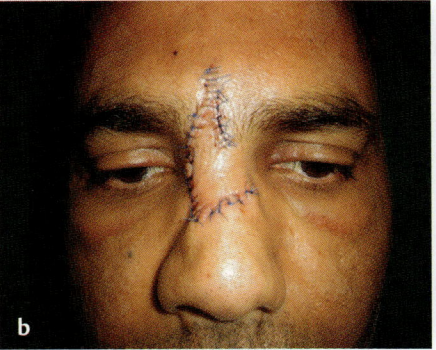
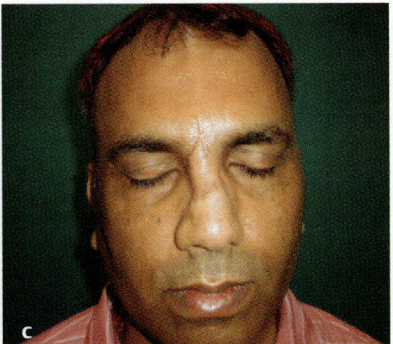

Fig. 20.3 **(a–c)** Lesion at dorsum of nose and postoperative appearance after excision and local flap.

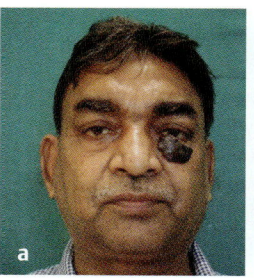 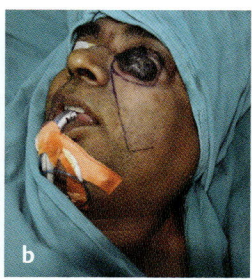 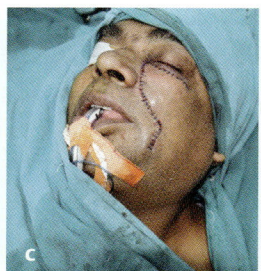 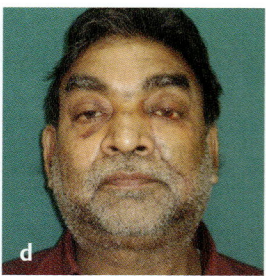

Fig. 20.4 (a–d) Excision of basal cell carcinoma at cheek-eyelid junction and reconstruction with local cheek flap.

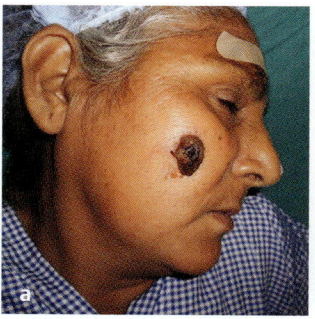 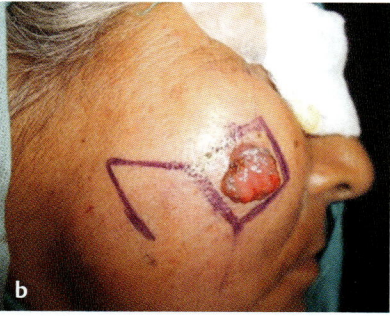 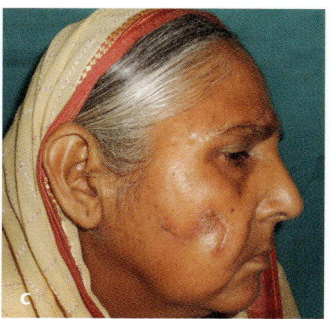

Fig. 20.5 (a–c) Basal cell carcinoma (BCC) over right cheek, marking of Limberg flap, closure of donor defect and final scar.

- Another line is drawn from the end of the extended diagonal which is parallel and equal in length to one of the sides.
- The choice of the flap depends on:
  - There can be four possible Limberg flaps in one rhomboid defect but it is always marked on the side where tissue laxity is present for primary closure of the secondary defect.
  - There should not be any distortion of the important structures once flap is transposed into the defect.
  - The position of final scar must lie in one of the relaxed skin tension lines (RSTLs) (**Fig. 20.5a–c**).

Moh's micrographic surgery:

- It is indicated in high-risk BCC located at anatomically complex areas, especially over face where excision with clinically negative margin may result in deformity or difficult reconstruction.

- The lesion is excised all around its margins and sent for histological examination of not only the margins but the base also. Serial excisions are continued till margins and base are free of tumor.
- Its disadvantages are long duration surgery and high expenses involved with repeated histopathological examinations.

Q11. What is basal cell naevus syndrome? (Nevoid BCC syndrome/Gorlin syndrome)

- It is an autosomal-dominant inherited disorder.
- It is characterized by multiple BCCs, pitting surfaces of palm and sole, jaw cysts and other musculoskeletal and neurologic abnormalities.
- Presence of BCC over the palm is a strong evidence in favor of basal cell naevus syndrome.

- Treatment options include surgical excision and careful monitoring.

Q12. What are the aesthetic units of cheek?

- Zone I—Suborbital.
- Zone II—Preauricular.
- Zone III—Buccal mandibular area.

Suborbital: Extends along lateral border of the nose to the nasolabial fold.

- Across the cheek below gingival sulcus.
- Up to anterior sideburn to lateral crow's foot line.
- Along the lower eyelid cheek junction.
- Wound in this area may be closed by rhomboid, circular, bilobed flaps.

Preauricular:

- Extends from helical junction with cheek across to sideburn to overlap with Zone I at molar prominence.

- Includes tissues over parotid-masseteric fascia and extends inferiorly to mandibular angle and lower mandibular border.

Buccomandibular: Extends from vertical division at middle cheek down to mandibular margin and from oral commissure back up to a horizontal division line half-way up the chest.

Suggested Readings

1. Barton R M. Malignant tumors of the skin. In: Mathes SJ, Hentz VR, editors. Plastic surgery. Vol. 5. 2nd ed. Saunders Elsevier; 2006:273-304.
2. Ogawa R. Benign and malignant non melanocytic tumors of the skin and soft tissue. In:Chang J, Neligan PC,editors. Plastic Surgery: Principles. Vol. 1. 4th ed. Canada: Elsevier; 2018. P.554
3. Ceradini D J, Blechman K M. In ; Thorne CH, editors. Grabb and Smith's Plastic Surgery: Dermatology for Plastic Surgeons II - Cutaneous Malignancies. 7th ed. Wolters Kluwer; 2014. P 115-126.

Microtia

Veena K. Singh

Introduction

The incidence of microtia is 1 in 6000 livebirths. Absence of normal ear in a newborn child is devastating to the entire family and at a grown-up stage, the child is also aware of the problem and wants it resolved as much as the family does. A good counseling of the parents about the timing and stages of reconstruction, donor options, complications, and overall outcome is of utmost importance. Plastic surgery trainee must have a thorough understanding of the location of new ear and technical details involved in each stage to ensure successful outcomes.

History

Particulars of the patient (same as for general case like name, age, sex, gender, occupation, residence, etc.).

Chief Complaints

- Deformity of ear—since birth or posttraumatic, one/both sided.
- Absent ear.
- Difficulty in hearing/loss of hearing.
- Deformity of the face.

History of Present Illness

- Present since birth or after any trauma of infection.
- History of other congenital deformities in the body.
- History of any difficulty in biting, eating, chewing.
- Negative history—pain or discharge from the ear, difficulty in hearing, history suggestive of facial nerve weakness.
- Antenatal history:
  - In detail, in cases of children.
  - Ask about the duration of pregnancy: full term or preterm.
  - Ask about the maternal age at pregnancy.
  - Whether delivered by normal vaginal delivery or cesarean section.
  - History of maternal diabetes and hypertension.
  - History of intake of any fertility drugs and in vitro fertilization.
  - History of intake of antiepileptic drugs.
  - Smoking history of mother.
  - Alcohol intake by the mother.
  - Ask about the birth weight of the baby.

Past History

- History of any medical illness.
- Any history of surgery anywhere else in the body.

Personal History

In cases of adult patients presenting with ear deformities, enquire about the education, occupation, marital status, socioeconomic status, any addiction.

Family History

History of any similar illness in the family.

Immunization History

Whether as per national immunization program for the age of the child.

Treatment History

Any medication for ear discharge or surgical intervention for the current problem. **History of allergy to food or medication.**

Examination

General Physical Examination

- In case of child, anthropometry is very important to assess the normal development of the child. Measure the height and weight of the child.
- Congenital anomalies like type of facies.
- Look for other congenital anomalies in the body.

Systemic Examination

- Abdomen.
- Central nervous system (CNS).
- Cardiovascular system (CVS).
- Respiratory system.

Local Examination of Face

Inspection

Ear

1. Either completely absent ear or smaller than normal sized ear: Always compare with the other side ear in case of unilateral deformity or ears in a same age child in case of bilateral deformity.
2. Ear may be vestigial like a vertically oriented nubbin.
3. Condition of ear lobule and location—whether superiorly placed to the level of other side.
4. Condition of external auditory meatus.
5. Level of hairline.

Face

1. Look carefully for signs of facial nerve palsy.
2. Compare the face on the affected side with the other side for signs of hemifacial microstomia (**Fig. 21.1**).
3. Check for occlusion and type.
4. Level of angle of mouth.

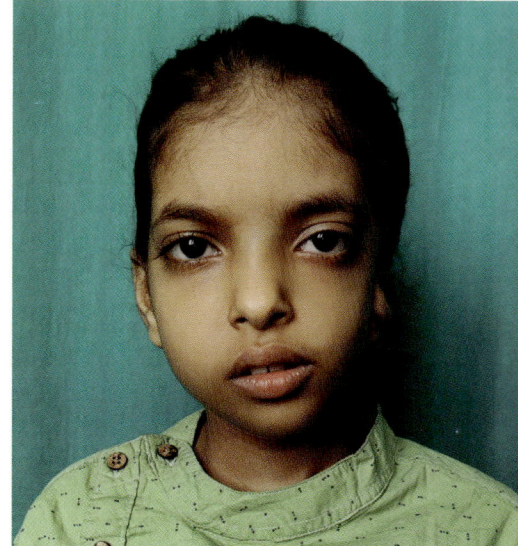

Fig. 21.1 Hemifacial microsomia in a microtia patient.

Palpation

1. Corroboration of all inspectory findings.
2. Look for Cantt: Place a wooden spatula or ice-cream stick in between the molars on both side and see the angle of elevation of both jaws on the affected side as compared to the normal side (**Fig. 21.2**).
3. Hearing tests: Using a tuning fork, both Rinne and Weber tests need to be performed.

Measurement

1. Measure the distance between:
   - Lateral canthus and helical root on normal side.
   - Lateral canthus and proximal point of the vestige or lobule on affected side.
2. Draw a line on the affected side parallel to the nasal profile. The ear's axis is roughly parallel to nasal profile.
3. In the frontal profile, mark the position of lobule on normal side. The reversed auricular pattern is traced 6 mm below the lobule on affected side.
   - Take a rough X-ray film and draw the pattern of the normal ear and then place it on the affected side in a reversed pattern.

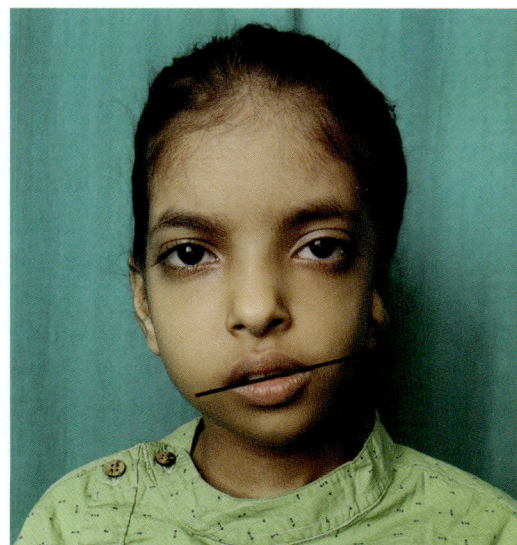

Fig. 21.2 Measurement of Cantt.

Provisional Diagnosis

A case of left-sided microtia (Tanzer's type IIa) in a 7-year-old girl with features of facial nerve palsy, hemifacial microsomia and hearing loss.

Questions

Q1. What is your plan?
- My plan is to counsel the parents regarding the stages of ear reconstruction and prepare the patient for the first stage surgery.
- For the anesthetic fitness, I would like to go for the baseline investigations:
  - Complete blood count (CBC).
  - Prothrombin time/International normalized ratio (PT/INR).
  - Viral markers (human immunodeficiency virus [HIV] 1 and 2, hepatitis B surface antigen [HBsAg], hepatitis C virus [HCV]).
- In adults patients—chest X-ray (posteroanterior [PA] view) to check for the ossification of the costal cartilage.

Q2. What preoperative counseling will you do for parents?
The preoperative counseling for parents will be done under the following points:
- Stages of surgery and interval between stages must be explained.
- Use of endogenous rib cartilage for ear framework reconstruction and scar at the chest. Also, information regarding alloplastic materials along with the merits and demerits need to be discussed.
  - Alloplastic ear will obviate the significant morbidity associated with autologous cartilage.
  - Chances of exposure and susceptibility to trauma is more in alloplastic materials.
- Age of reconstruction must be explained, in case a child presents early at age.

- Ideally, ear reconstruction must begin before the child starts going to school and the body image concept also starts forming around 4 to 5 years of age.
- But to balance between the age of the child and amount of cartilage required, the recommended age of surgery is around 8 years.
- Sometimes, if the patient is small for age or opposite ear is large, the surgery may be postponed for few more years.

Q3. How are you going to do the markings for surgery?

- For the preoperative markings, the following aspects must be taken into consideration (**Fig. 21.3**):
  - Compare the height of the vestigial ear with that of normal ear on frontal view. Mark the position of lobule also.
  - From side view, mark the axis of the ear which is roughly parallel to the nasal profile.
  - The distance between the lateral canthus and the helical root of the normal ear is measured.
- In pure microtia, the position of new ear can be marked easily as vestige-to-canthus distance mirrors the helical root-to-canthus distance of the normal side.
- Once the positions are marked, the tracings of the normal ear are marked on the normal ear and this pattern is reversed to design the framework pattern for the new ear.
- In cases of bilateral microtia, the tracings are marked on another patient of same age and height.
- These patterns are sterilized and used as guidelines for the framework fabrication during surgery.

Q4. Can you tell us the steps of ear cartilage framework placement surgery?

- Cartilage harvest:
  - The cartilage for creation of the ear framework is harvested from the contralateral chest ribs so that natural configuration of the ribs is used.
  - In males, incision is given in the seventh intercostal space for good access to sixth, seventh, and eighth rib, but in females, the incision is slightly higher up in the sixth intercostal space so that the scar lies over the future inframammary fold (**Fig. 21.4**).

Distance between these 2 lines is equal to one ear ↘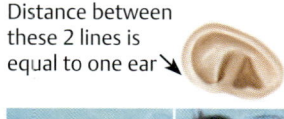

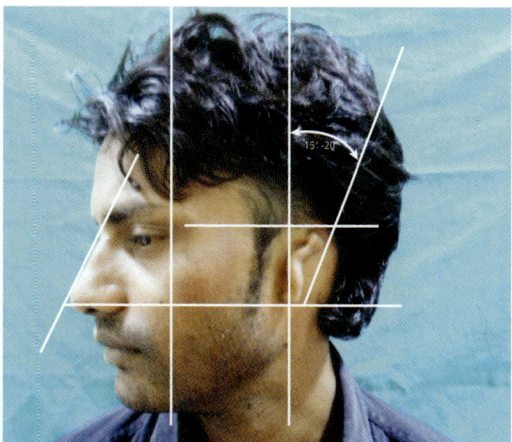

Fig. 21.3 Markings of new ear.

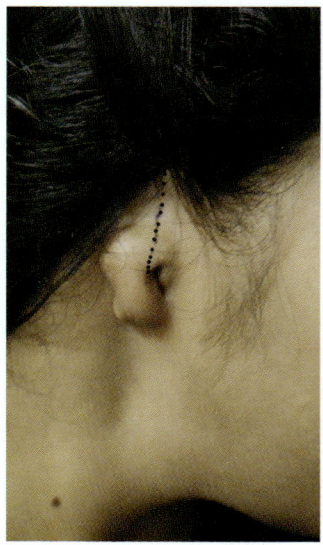

Fig. 21.4 Marking of incision.

- Synchondrosis of the sixth and seventh ribs is used for the creation of antihelix (**Fig. 21.5**).
- First free floating rib (usually the eighth rib but may be the ninth rib in cases it is the first free floating rib) is used for helical rim (**Fig. 21.6**).
- A thin rim of the sixth rib cartilage on its upper border is left behind to prevent subsequent chest deformity when the child grows up.

- Fabrication of ear framework:
  - Using the sterilized X-ray pattern of normal ear, ear framework is carved manually with blade and carving chisels as power-assisted tools will damage the chondrocytes.
  - While thinning the cartilage for helical rim, the direction of thinning is on its convex surface and care is taken to preserve the perichondrium on the lateral outer aspect of the framework to facilitate its adherence to the surrounding tissues.

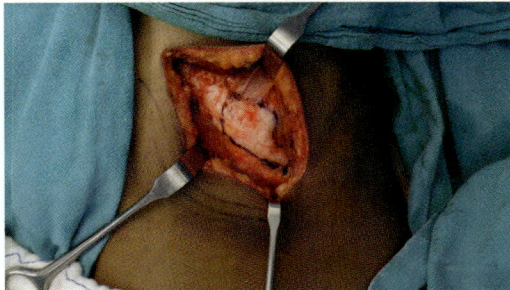

Fig. 21.5 Synchondrosis of sixth and seventh costal cartilages.

- 4–0 Nylon or Prolene sutures are used to fix the cartilage framework and knots are placed inside or on the undersurface of the framework (**Fig. 21.7**).

- Creation of subcutaneous pocket for placement of the framework:
  - A small incision is placed posterior to the auricular vestige and a thin subcutaneous pocket is created.
  - The plane of dissection is subfollicular so as to preserve the subdermal plexus.
  - Native cartilage may be excised and discarded.
  - The pocket should be 1 to 2 cm larger than the framework marking so that the slack skin is available to wrap well around the framework without any tension.

- Dressing: A small size number 12 F negative suction drain or a mini-RomoVac is used to create negative suction inside the subcutaneous pocket. This keeps the skin contoured to the underlying cartilage framework.
  - Dressing:
    - Small pieces of wet and loose cotton is used to conform to the convolutions.
    - This layer is placed over a nonadherent paraffin gauze.
    - Pressure dressing is avoided on all costs to prevent pressure necrosis of the skin.
    - A bulky, noncompressive dressing is applied.

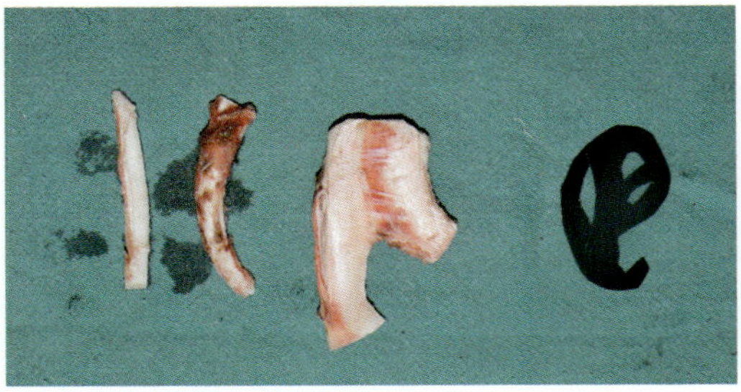

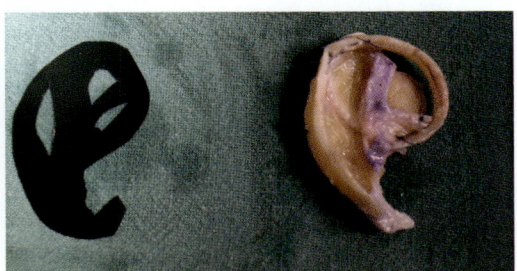

Fig. 21.6 Floating rib.

Fig. 21.7 Carving of cartilage framework according to the template.

Q5. What is the postoperative protocol?

The postoperative protocol is as follows:

- On postoperative day (POD) 1, the drain bag is charged every 4 to 6 hours to maintain the negative pressure on a continuous basis (**Fig. 21.8**).
- First dressing is done on POD2 and then on regular intervals.
- Drain can be removed after 2 weeks.

Q6. What are the immediate postoperative complications?

- Signs of infection may be observed by looking for local erythema, edema, pain, and fever. Irrigation with antibiotic can help.
- Skin flap necrosis may result from:
  - Small and tight pocket.
  - Bolster sutures, if used.
  - Damage to subdermal vascularity.
- If necrosis occurs, prompt action needs to be taken:
  - Smaller necrosis generally heals with good local care and dressing with antibiotic ointment to prevent cartilage desiccation.
  - Major skin flap necrosis would require a coverage with local transposition flap or small fascial flap with skin graft.
- Patient is instructed not to sleep on the side of reconstructed ear.

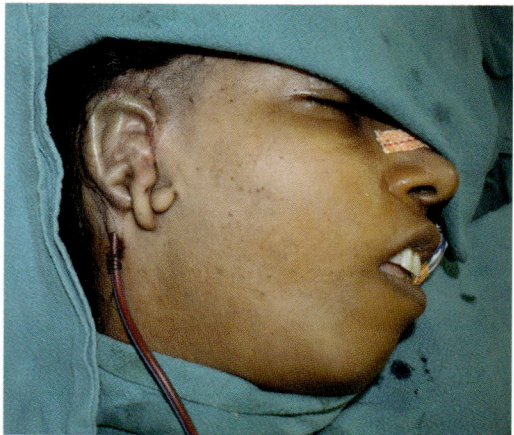

Fig. 21.8 Redraping of subcutaneous pocket after negative suction is charged.

- Patient may protect the newly reconstructed ear from trauma.
- Sports activities can be resumed only after 3 to 4 weeks of chest scar healing.

Q7. How will you decide in a case of microtia associated with hemifacial microsomia?

- In severe hemifacial microsomia, since the vestigial ear is much closer to the eye, the position of the new ear is marked at an appropriate position so that it is neither very close to eye nor very far back on the head.
- In cases where bony work for hemifacial microsomia is done first, the scars must not lie in the region of future ear reconstruction.

Q8. What are the other congenital abnormalities associated with microtia?

The other congenital abnormalities associated with microtia are:

- Classic microtia is associated with canal atresia and ossicular abnormalities.
- Middle ear deformities like fused, hypoplastic ossicular, failure of mastoid cell pneumatization.
- Hemifacial microsomia.
- Facial nerve palsy.
- Microstomia.
- Cleft lip, cleft palate.
- Urogenital defects.
- Cardiovascular malformations.

Q9. How do you classify microtia/ear abnormalities?

Tanzer classified the congenital ear defects which correlates with both the embryologic development and approach for surgical correction:

- Anotia.
- Complete hypoplasia (microtia).
  - With atresia of external auditory canal.
  - Without atresia of external auditory canal.
- Hypoplasia of middle third of auricle.
- Hypoplasia of superior third of auricle.
  - Constricted ear (cup and lop ear).
  - Cryptotia.

- Hypoplasia of entire superior third.
- Prominent ear.

Q10. What are the other steps of Brent's ear reconstruction?

The other stages of ear reconstruction are:
- Rotation of lobule.
- Elevation of the ear framework.
- Tragal construction and deepening of conchal.
- Rotation of lobule:
  - The lobule is elevated based on a narrow inferiorly based triangular flap which is transposed by Z-plasty (**Fig. 21.9a, b**).
  - Nagata and Firmin transposed the ear-lobe by:
    - Using skin from the lobule's posterior surface to line the framework tragal strut during the first stage surgery.
    - It produces excellent appearance of the tragus but there are high risk of skin necrosis.
- Elevation of the ear framework:
  - Creation of the auricular-cephalic sulcus includes separation of the ear from the head and coverage of its undersurface with medium thickness split-skin graft.

- Incision is made behind the rim taking care to preserve a layer of connective tissue layer on the cartilage framework (**Fig. 21.10**).
- The retroauricular skin is well advanced into the newly created sulcus and SSG is applied over the posterior surface of the framework.
- Bolster dressing of the graft is done.
- If cartilage was banked during the first stage surgery, then it is placed as a wedge behind the elevated ear which is covered with soft tissue for better graft taken. This gives a better projection to the new ear.
- The banked cartilage wedge can also be covered with a turnover "book flap" of occipitalis fascia.
- Tragal contraction and conchal deepening:
  - A chondrocutaneous composite graft harvested from the concha of opposite ear is used to form the tragus and deepening of concha both.
  - In bilateral microtia cases, tragus construction is done by incorporating the tragus strut in the original cartilage framework during the first stage surgery.

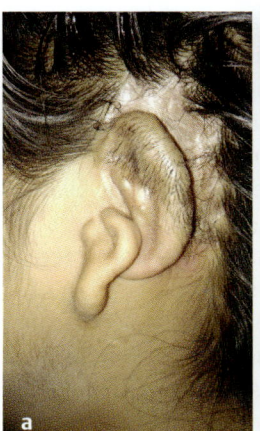
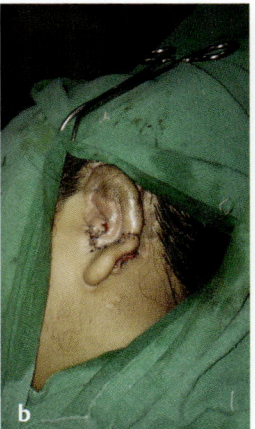
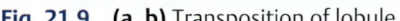

Fig. 21.9 (a, b) Transposition of lobule.

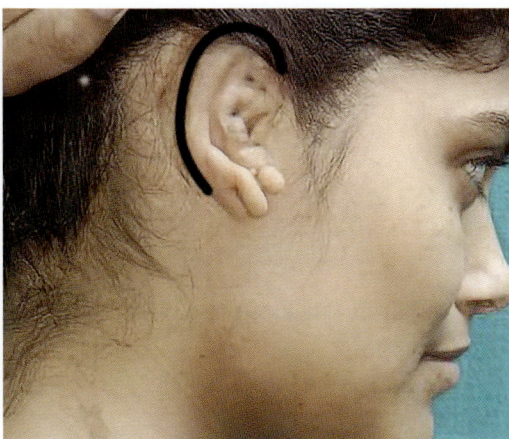

Fig. 21.10 Markings for ear elevation.

- Another option in bilateral microtia is modified Kirkham method in which an anteriorly based conchal flap is doubled on itself.

Q11. What are the sites where cartilage can be banked during the first stage?

- Underneath the chest incision during the first stage surgery.
- Underneath the scalp posterior to the main pocket.
  Advantages of scalp site:
  - Can be conveniently retrieved while performing the ear elevation.
  - Provides comparatively better nourishment to the banked cartilage.

Q12. What is Nagata classification of auricular deformity?

Lobule type	Ear remnant +
	Malpositioned lobule
	Concha—absent
	Acoustic meatus—absent
	Tragus—absent
Concha type	Ear remnant +
	Malpositioned lobule
	Concha—present
	Tragus—present
	Antitragus—present
Small concha type	Ear remnant +
	Malpositioned lobule
	Concha—absent (instead, a small indentation is present)
Anotia	Only a minute or no ear remnant
Atypical microtia	Deformities which do not fit into any of the above categories

Q13. What is Nagata's technique of ear reconstruction?

- Nagata's technique includes ear reconstruction in two stages.
  - Stage I: Cartilage framework placement, tragus construction, and lobule transposition (combining first, second, and third stages of Brent's ear construction).
  - Stage II: Ear elevation using a cartilage block which is covered by a fascial flap and skin graft.
- Advantages: Obviates several stages of surgery as in Brent's technique.
- Disadvantages:
  - Increased chances of tissue necrosis due to extensive soft tissue manipulation.
  - The quality and appearance of earlobe is not that good as compared to Brent's technique as Nagata used the earlobe's back side skin for lining of tragus.
  - More rib cartilages are required and excised from the chest with chest wall deformity.
  - Nagata's second stages use the superficial temporal vessel containing fascial flap for coverage of cartilage in the auricular-cephalic sulcus. The second stage also involves the harvest of cartilage wedge from chest again causing chest discomfort second time.
  - In Nagata's technique, a third stage is actually required at times to match the frontal symmetry of both ears.

Q14. How will you manage a case of bilateral microtia?

- Bilateral microtia is commonly seen in patients with Treacher Collins-Franceschetti syndrome, bilateral craniofacial microstomia, and other uncommon craniofacial malformations.
- Principles of ear reconstruction in bilateral microtia:
  - Auricular reconstruction must precede the middle ear surgery.
  - Cartilage framework procedures are performed on each side several month apart to avoid splintage effect on chest and respiratory distress.
  - Both sided earlobes can be transposed during single procedure.

- The stage of ear separation and middle ear surgery can be combined together.

Q15. How will you manage constricted ear, cryptotia, and prominent ear?

- Constricted ear:
  - Group of ear anomalies in which the encircling helix seems tight as if constricted by a "purse string."
  - Also known as "cup or lop" ears or helical and scaphal hooding.
  - Treatment:
    - Minimal height discrepancy:
      ○ Overhanging tissues can merely be excised.
      ○ Cartilage lid can be used as a "banner flap" to increase the height.
    - Moderate height discrepancy: Augmentation of cartilage height by modifying the ipsilateral ear cartilage or using contralateral conchal cartilage grafts.
    - Severe height discrepancy (>1.5 cm): Add both cartilage and skin as in a microtia reconstruction.
- Cryptotia:
  - Upper pole of the ear cartilage is buried underneath the scalp.
  - Characterized by the absence of auriculocophalic sulcus in the superior pole.
  - Manage nonsurgically by applying an external conforming splint before 6 months of age.
  - Surgical repairs may include addition to skin in retroauricular sulcus by skin grafts, Z-plasty, V-Y advancement, or rotational flaps.
- Prominent ear:
  - Pathology:
    - Prominent ear arises when antihelix fails to fold during the development phase of the ear.
    - There may be only flattening of superior crus, but in severe cases, the rolling of the helical rim is absent which protrudes a flat, shell-like ear with no convolutions.

- It is usually bilateral and frequently noted in siblings and parents.
  - Management:
    - Repair should be symmetrical in bilateral cases and convolutions should appear smooth.
      End points of repair:
      ○ Most lateral point of the repair should be between 1.7 and 2.0 cm from the head.
      ○ From the frontal view of both ears, the helix should be visible behind the antihelix.
    - In upper third protrusion due to weak antihelix, exaggeration of antihelix may be done.
    - If middle third is affected, concha can be recessed by either cartilage excision or suture fixation.
    - If lobule protrudes, resection or retroposition of cartilage tail of helix can be done.
  - Techniques:
    - Dieffenbach procedure (conchal alteration): Excision of skin from the auricular-cephalic sulcus and suturing the conchal cartilage to the mastoid periosteum.
    - Luckett procedure (restoring the antihelical fold): Restoration of antihelix fold by excising a crescent of medial skin and cartilage.
    - Mustarde procedure (altering the cartilage medial surface):
      ○ Placement of permanent mattress sutures through the cartilage without any actual cartilage incisions.
      ○ Useful in pliable ear cartilages but recurrence rate is high.
    - Kaye procedure (altering the cartilage lateral surface): Combination of both lateral cartilage scoring and fixation with permanent sutures.

Q16. What are the parts of a normal ear?

Parts of a normal ear are shown in **Fig. 21.11a, b**.

- Vascular supply: Superficial temporal and posterior auricular vessels.

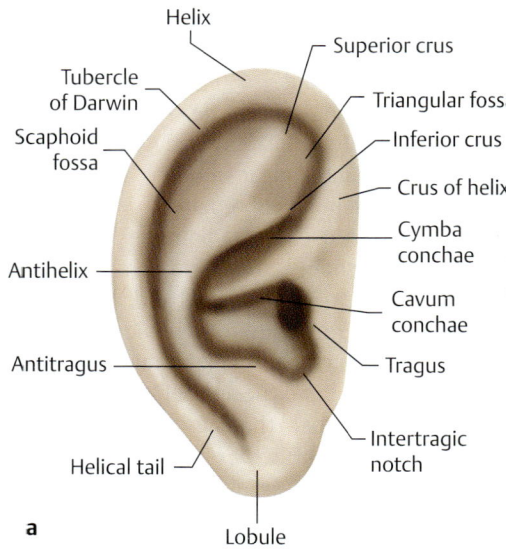

Fig. 21.11 **(a, b)** Anatomy of ear.

- Sensory supply (**Fig. 21.12**):
  - From greater auricular nerve which supplies the inferior portions of the ear.
  - Lesser occipital and auriculotemporal nerves which supply the superior portions of the ear.
  - Conchal regions supplied by vagal nerve.

Q17. What is the embryological development of an ear?

- Middle ear and external ear are developed from the first (mandibular) and second (hyoid) branchial arches.
- The auricle is formed from six "hillocks" of tissue that lie along these arches and can be seen in a 5-week embryo.
- The inner ear develops at 3 weeks of gestational period from the tissues of ectodermal origin. It is because of this difference in the development that inner ear is spared in microtic cases.
- Theory of in utero tissue ischemia from either an obliterated stapedial artery or hemorrhage into local tissues leads to development of ear abnormalities.

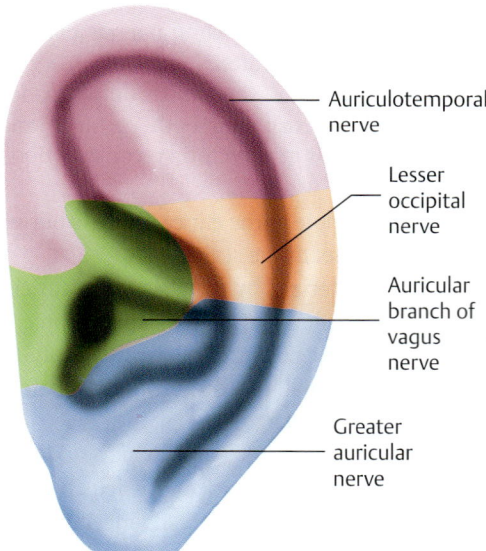

Fig. 21.12 Sensory supply of the ear.

Q18. What are the middle ear problems associated with microtia?

- Aural atresia is the most common middle ear deformity associated with microtia.
- Some degree of hearing loss is also associated.

Q19. What type of hearing loss is seen in patients with microtia?

- Conductive hearing loss is seen in microtia due to atresia of middle ear and normal development of inner ear.
- It can be confirmed by hearing tests—Rinne and Weber using 512-Hz tuning fork.
- Rinne test:
  - Strike a tuning fork and place it on the mastoid bone behind normal ear.
  - When the patient can no longer hear the sound, move the tuning fork next to ear canal.
  - Note the time for which the patient hears sound at each site.
  - Repeat the same on the side of microtia.
- Weber test:
  - Strike a tuning fork and place it on the middle of the patient's head.
  - Note where the sound is best heard: the left ear, the right ear, or both equally.
- Interpretation:
  - On Rinne test, normal hearing will show an air conduction time that is twice as long as the bone conduction time. In microtia (conductive hearing loss), the bone conduction is heard longer than the air conduction sound. If you have sensorineural hearing loss, air conduction is heard longer than bone conduction, but may not be twice as long.
  - On Weber test, normally, there will be equal sound in both ears but in microtia where conductive loss is there, it will cause the sound to be heard best in the abnormal ear. Sensorineural loss will cause the sound to be heard best in the normal ear.

Q20. What is the incidence of microtia?

- Incidence of microtia is 1 in 6000 births. It is higher in Japanese children (1 in 4000).
- Twice more common in males.
- Twice more common on right side.
- Incidence of bilateral microtia is 10 to 20 in microtic cases.

Q21. What are the features of hemifacial microsomia?

The most common classification used to enumerate the features of hemifacial microsomia is OMENS classification:

- Orbit:
  - 0_0—Normal orbit size and position.
  - 0_1—Abnormal size.
  - 0_2—Abnormal position.
  - 0_3—Abnormal size and position.
- Mandible:
  - M_0—Normal mandible.
  - M_1—Mandible and glenoid fossa are small.
  - M_2—Mandibular ramus short and abnormally shaped.
  - M_{2A}—Glenoid in acceptable position.
  - M_{2B}—Temporomandibular joint medially displaced.
  - M_3—Complete absence of ramus, glenoid fossa, and temporomandibular joint.
- Ear:
  - E_0—Normal.
  - E_1—Mild hypoplasia and cupping.
  - E_2—Absence of external auditory canal.
  - E_3—Malpositioned lobule with absent auricle.
- Nerve:
  - N_0—No facial nerve involvement.
  - N_1—Upper facial nerve involvement.
  - N_2—Lower facial nerve involvement.
  - N_3—All branches affected.
- Soft tissue:
  - S_0—No soft tissue deformity.
  - S_1—Minimal (mild) tissue deformity.
  - S_2—Moderate tissue deformity (between the two extremes).
  - S_3—Major (severe) subcutaneous and muscular deficiency.

Q22. What is Firmin algorithm for ear reconstruction?

- Francoise Firmin described an algorithm to optimally utilize the available auricular skin (Ref: article on Firmin).

– The main goal of the classification provided by Firmin is to plan a skin approach for ear cartilage framework to be placed in such a way so as to be covered with tension-free and well-vascularized flaps (**Fig. 21.13**).

■ Type I is a Z-plasty with transposition which is incorporated by one of the flaps of the lobule.

■ Type II is a transfixion incision of the microtic ear (transfixes the skin and fibrocartilage horizontally, splitting remnants into two halves).

■ Type III exposes the cartilage remnants through a cutaneous incision.

○ Type IIIa: Accessing the native cartilage (deformed) through a direct incision and replacing with a framework (one-stage).

○ Type IIIb: Enough skin not available to accommodate the framework into the remnants. So, entire framework is buried and elevated in second stage.

– Firmin has also classified the microtia according to the **types of anomalies**.

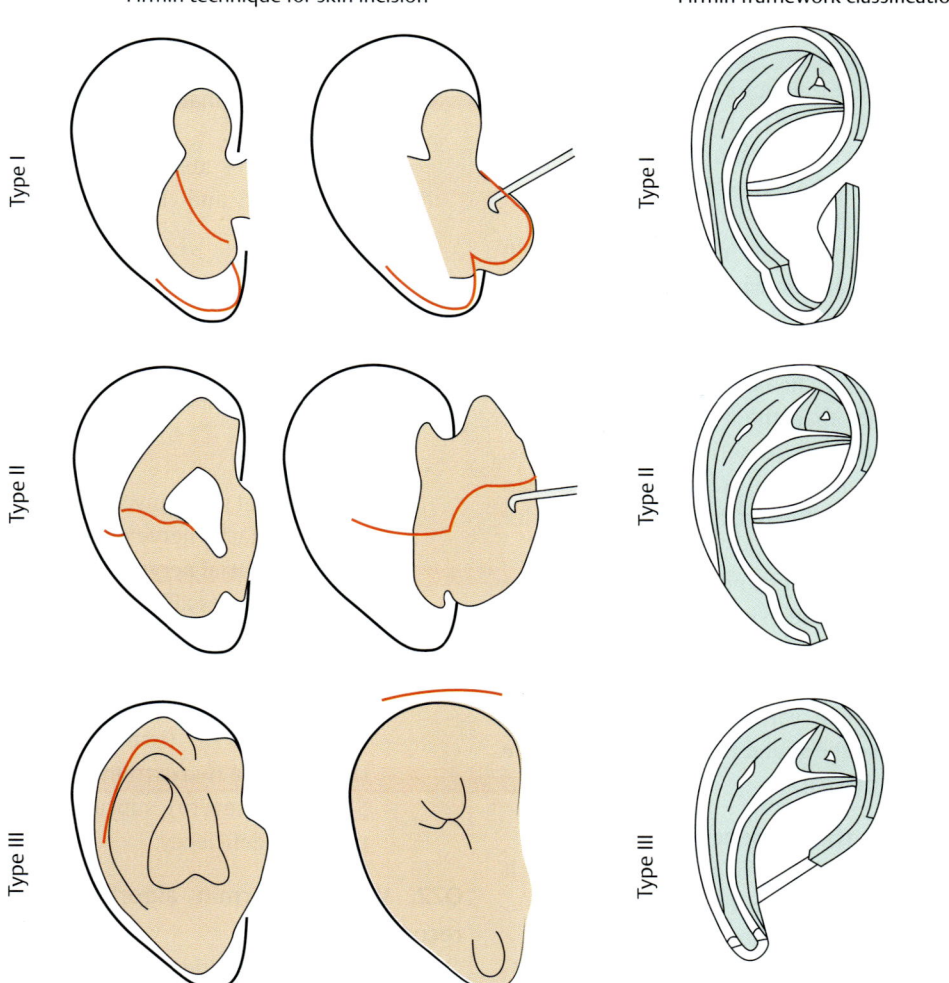

Firmin technique for skin incision

Firmin framework classification

Type I

Type II

Type III

Fig. 21.13 Firmin classification to plan the skin approach for ear cartilage framework placement.

According to the anomalies, framework has also been classified into Type I, II, and III.

- Microtia without tragus.
- Microtia with tragus but without antitragus.
- Microtia with good tragus-antitragus.

- Firmin classification of the **different types of projection pieces** added to the undersurface of the base of cartilage framework during the first stage:
  - P1—Positioned under root of helix and tragus.
  - P2—Positioned under antihelix.
  - P3—Positioned so as to compensate for a hypoplastic mastoid.

Q23. What is Firmin modification of Nagata's technique?

- In Nagata's technique during the second stage the cartilage framework is raised along with a layer of soft tissue, but in Firmin's modification of Nagata's technique, the posterior surface of the base is exposed and then the additional pieces of cartilage are added.

- Advantages of this modification:
  - Framework can be mobilized to do some adjustment of axis, if required.
  - Direct coverage of framework posterior surface without intervening soft tissue results in a thinner ear when looked from behind.
  - Removal of wire sutures and thinning of framework can be done if required.

Suggested Readings

1. Thorne CH, ed. Grabb and Smiths's plastic surgery: congenital anomalies and paediatric plastic surgery. 7th ed. Wolters Kluwer; 2014: 283–294
2. Yamada A, Harada T. In: Neligan PC, ed. Plastic surgery: craniofacial, head and neck surgery, and pediatric plastic surgery. Vol. 3. 4th ed. Canada: Elsevier; 2018:181–213
3. Brent BD. In: Mathes SJ, ed. Plastic surgery: the head and neck. Part 2. Vol. 3. 2nd ed. Canada: Elsevier; 2006:633–698
4. Firmin F, Marchac A. A novel algorithm for autologous ear reconstruction. Semin Plast Surg. 2011 Nov;25(4):257-64. doi: 10.1055/s-0031-1288917. PMID: 23115531; PMCID: PMC3312152.

22 Ptosis

Saurabh K. Gupta and Veena K. Singh

Learning Objectives

At the end of the chapter, the students will be able to:
1. Recall the anatomy of eyelids and etiology of ptosis.
2. Understand the assessment of a patient with congenital ptosis.
3. Make decision on the surgical options for correction of ptosis.
4. Explain the common surgical procedures for ptosis.

Introduction

Upper eyelid ptosis is a condition that affects individuals of all ages, ranging from a newborn to an elderly patient. Its etiology can be various—congenital, posttraumatic, involutional, or neoplastic—but the most common underlying cause is inability of levator muscle to lift the tarsal plate. Assessment of function and integrity of levator is important in choosing the correct surgical option. Equally important is the assessment of the lid level, levator function, muller muscle function, and tear production.

Chief Complaints

- Drooping of upper eyelid.
- Tired appearance of the face.
- Blurred vision, double vision.
- Increased tearing.

History of Present Illness

- Onset of drooping of eyelid—whether at the time of birth or later in the course of life.
- Whether in single eye or both eyes.
- Any aggravating or relieving factors.
- Any diurnal variation, for example, worsening in the evening or not.
- Any difficulty in vision either blurred vision or difficulty in seeing farther object clearly.
- Increased tearing in the affected eye or use of handkerchief to wipe off tears at shorter intervals.
- Any complaints of double vision or seeing two images of the same object.
- Any history of body fatigue.
- Any progression or worsening of symptoms in due course of time.
- Any redness of eye or itchy sensation.
- History suggestive of decreased social interaction because of the disability.
- Enquire about the emotional and mental status of the patient.
- Whether history of tilting neck upward to maintain the forward vision.
- History suggestive of any infection or facial cellulitis.
- Any change in sleeping habits or appetite.

Past History

- Any history of diabetes mellitus, hypertension, tuberculosis, or any other medical illness.
- Any surgical history.
- Any history suggestive of head or facial trauma.

Personal History

- Marital status of the patient.
- Number of kids.
- History of smoking, drinking, or any substance abuse.
- Patient's status in the society, social obligations, employment status.

Family History

- Any relevant details need mentioning.
- Number of family members dependent on the patient.
- Any member suffering from the same problem.
- History of congenital or hereditary ptosis in the family.
- Any history of ocular myopathies.

Treatment History

Whether any treatment taken previously for the same problem, either medical or surgical.

Allergic History

- Any allergy to drug intake.
- Any allergy to food.

General Physical Examination

- Remains same as for other cases except head and neck examination which has to be done in detail.
- Neck nodes to be palpated in every case.

System Examination

- CNS.
- CVS.
- Abdomen.
- Respiratory system.

Local Examination of the Face

Inspection

Eyebrow

- Position of eyebrow.

Eyelid

- Position of eyelid.
- Discrepancy in lid position of both eyes.
- Position of eyelid crease.
- Size of palpebral aperture on both sides.
- Movements of both eyelids during excursion.
- Any lid lag noted in both eyes (with head held steady, the patient is asked to look up and down, presence of lagophthalmos is noted).
- Fatiguability of eyelid (in upward gaze for 60 s).
- Visible lesions.
- Any thickening.
- Any loss of eye lashes.
- Any abnormal movement association should be noted like jaw-winking phenomenon (aberrant connections between CN III and V3).

Pupil

- Pupils are compared to each other for symmetry.
- Pupillary reflex is evaluated.
  - Anisocoria or abnormal pupillary reflex may occur in Horner's syndrome or CN III palsy.

Palpation

1. Visual acuity is examined first.
2. Measurement of lid fold from ciliary margin (normally 7–9 mm).
   - If crease is blunted/or distance from the margin is greater, then the normal separation of levator aponeurosis from the

overlying orbicularis should be taken into consideration.

- If deep fold is there (sulcus deformity—separation of levator from tarsal plate), suspect levator dehiscence.

3. Position of upper lid should be documented.
   - Pupillary light reflex and upper lid margin. (This distance should normally be 3–4.5 mm.)
   - Lid margin should rest halfway between the pupillary aperture and the superior margin of the corneoscleral junction.
4. Measurement of levator function.
   - Examiner sits directly in front of the patient.
   - Examiner places his or her left thumb over the eyebrow to stabilize and holds a millimeter scale in right hand over the lateral midline of the palpebral fissure.
   - The difference between the eyelid apertures from upgaze to downgaze is a measure of levator excursion and function.
5. Tear function.
   - The most commonly used procedure is Schirmer test.
6. Examine:
   - Extraocular muscles and facial muscles.
   - Cranial nerves.

Provisional Diagnosis

This is a case of a 12-year-old male child with congenital ptosis without any associated abnormality.

Questions

Q1. How will you proceed?
I will first assess the levator excursion and accordingly choose the appropriate surgery for the patient.

- Before surgery, I will also go for evaluation by an ophthalmologist and a visual acuity test.
- For surgery, I will get the routine investigations done for the patient and the preanesthetic fitness.

- Routine surgery for ptosis in adults is done under local anesthesia.

Q2. How to measure levator function?
Levator function is assessed using Berke's method.

- Measurement of upper eyelid excursions from downgaze to upgaze with frontalis muscle function negated by stabilizing the head.
- The amount of lid elevation is recorded in millimeters (mm) of levator excursion.
- Classifications:

Normal	>15 mm lid elevation
Good	12–14 mm lid elevation
Fair	5–11 mm lid elevation
Poor	0–4 mm lid elevation

Q3. How to measure excursion of eyelid?
Excursion of upper eyelid is measured as the range of eyelid movement from full elevation to closure.

- It is usually greater than 12 mm.

Q4. What are the different measurements in examining a case of ptosis?
- The different measurements are (**Fig. 22.1**):
  - Marginal Reflex Distance 1 (MRD1):
    - The distance between the central corneal light reflex and upper eyelid margins with eyes in primary position.
    - Normal MRD1 is 4 to 5 mm.

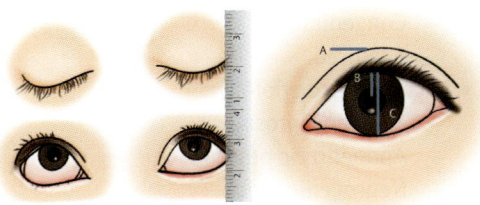

Fig. 22.1 Showing measurement of upper eyelid excursion. Top Left: Margin of upper eyelid at 20 mm. Bottom Left: Fully elevated at 33 mm (normal eyelid excursion at 13 mm). Right side: A - Normal eyelid crease. B - Upper Marginal Reflex Distance. C - Palpebral fissure.

- Margin Reflex Distance 2 (MRD2):
- Distance between central light reflex and lower eyelid margin with eyes in primary position.
  - Palpebral fissure height (PFH):
    - Distance between the upper and lower eyelid margins at the axis of the pupil.
    - The sum of the MRD1 and the MRD2 should equal the vertical PFH.

Q5. What are the tests for ptosis?

- Fatigue test:
  - MRD1 should be measured first.
  - Patient is asked to look up for 2 minutes.
  - Then MRD1 is measured again.
  - Worsening of ptosis is seen in:
    - Myopathies.
    - Myasthenia.
    - Senile aponeurotic ptosis.
- Tensilon test:
  - In cases of suspected myasthenia, 2 mg of edrophonium is injected IV slowly in 15 to 30 seconds.
  - The needle is left in situ, and later 8 mg is injected slowly if no adverse reaction is noted.
  - In case of myasthenia, ptosis improves after the injection.
- Phenylephrine test:
  - Sympathomimetic agents, such as phenylephrine is instilled under the eyelid to test the function of Muller muscle.

Q6. How is ptosis classified?

- Can be classified into:
  - Congenital.
  - Acquired.
- According to etiology:
  - Myogenic ptosis.
  - Aponeurotic ptosis.
  - Neurogenic ptosis.
  - Neuromuscular ptosis.
  - Traumatic ptosis.
  - Mechanical ptosis.
  - Pseudoptosis.

Q7. What are the characteristic features of ptosis according to etiology?

- Myogenic ptosis:
  - When the muscles elevating the lid are dysfunctional.
  - Most commonly seen as congenital ptosis where there is levator palpebrae superioris (LPS) dysgenesis.
  - Generally unilateral.
  - Lid lag on downgaze.
- Aponeurotic ptosis:
  - Due to stretching/attenuation/dehiscence/detachment of LPS aponeurosis from its tarsal attachments.
  - Usually, bilaterally symmetric.
- Neurogenic ptosis:
  - Third nerve palsy and Horner's syndrome.
  - Damage to the sympathetic supply to the eye from tumors, aneurysms, or inflammations.
- Traumatic ptosis:
  - damage to LPS muscle.
  - Aponeurosis.
  - Neural input.
- Mechanical ptosis:
  - Excessive skin overhanging the eyelid.
  - Mass weighing down the upper lid.
- Pseudoptosis:
  - Enophthalmos.
  - Dermatochalasis.
  - Anophthalmus.
  - Contralateral lid retraction.
  - Brow ptosis.
  - Facial nerve palsy.

Q8. What are the anatomical layers of eyelid?

There is much similarity between upper and lower eyelid anatomy (**Fig. 22.2**).

- Each consists of:
  - Anterior lamella—skin and orbicularis muscle.
  - Posterior lamella—tarsus and conjunctiva.

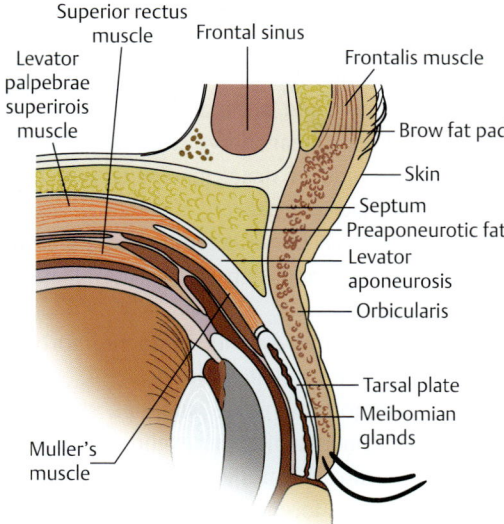

Superior rectus muscle
Levator palpebrae superirois muscle
Frontal sinus
Frontalis muscle
Brow fat pad
Skin
Septum
Preaponeurotic fat
Levator aponeurosis
Orbicularis
Tarsal plate
Meibomian glands
Muller's muscle

Fig. 22.2 Anatomy of upper eyelid.

- Eyelid mainly consists of five layers:
  - Skin and subcutaneous tissue.
  - Orbicularis oculi.
  - Tarsal plates.
  - Levator apparatus.
  - Conjunctiva.
- Skin and subcutaneous tissue:
  - The layer of skin is thinnest in the human body.
  - In the subcutaneous layer, there is loose connective tissue but no subcutaneous fat—the eyelids are readily distended by edema or blood.
  - The eyelashes are attached here with their accompanying modified sweat glands—the ciliary glands of Moll.
  - There are also sebaceous glands located in this layer, known as the glands of Zeis.
- Orbicularis oculi:
  - The orbicularis oculi muscle has three distinct parts: orbital, preseptal, and pretarsal segments.
  - Attachments:
    - Originates from the medial orbital margin, the medial palpebral ligament, and the lacrimal bone.

- It then inserts into the skin around the margin of the orbit, and the superior and inferior tarsal plates.
  - Actions:
    - Orbital (voluntary part): Winking and forced tight closure of the eyelids.
    - Preseptal (both voluntary and involuntary): Gently closes the eyelids (blinking).
    - Pretarsal (involuntary): Blinking and closure during sleep.
    - Both preseptal and pretarsal parts are involved in the drainage of tears.
  - Innervation: Facial nerve (CN VII, temporal and zygomatic branches).
- Tarsal plates:
  - The tarsal plates are present deep to the palpebral region of the orbicularis oculi muscle.
  - There are two plates: The superior tarsus (upper eyelid) and inferior tarsus (lower eyelid).
  - They are dense connective tissue and form the structural basis of the eyelids.
  - The superior tarsus also acts as the attachment site of the LPS.
  - In the tarsal plates, the Meibomian glands (also known as tarsal glands) are present.
  - These are a specialized type of sebaceous gland that secretes an oily substance onto the eye to slow the evaporation of the eye's tear film. The oily substance also prevents the eyelids from sticking together when closed.
- Levator palpebrae superioris:
  - Present in the upper eyelid.
  - Origin: From annulus of Zinn on lesser wing of sphenoid.
  - Insertion: Extends for 40 mm anteriorly and then forms an aponeurosis which fuses with orbital septum and gives fibrous strands to the dermis to form the lid crease. It finally inserts into superior tarsus (**Fig. 22.3**).
  - Function: Helps in opening of the eyelid.

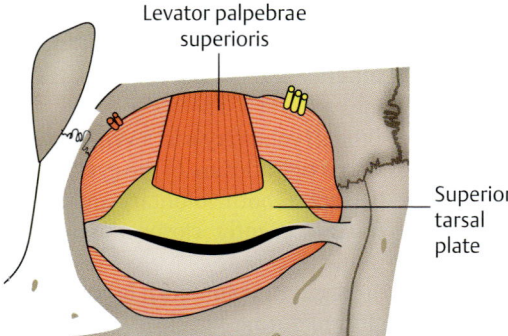

Fig. 22.3 Levator palpebrae superioris (LPS) and superior tarsal plate.

- – Innervation: By superior branch of the oculomotor nerve (CNIII).
- – Importance: Levator attenuation or dehiscence (aponeurosis transforms into fibrofilmy structure) leads levator to lose its grip on the tarsal plate, resulting in higher lid crease and dropping of lid margin.
- Muller muscle
  - – Also known as supratarsal muscle.
  - – Origin: deep surface of levator where muscle becomes aponeurotic.
  - – Insertion: into the superior tarsus.
  - – Importance: dehiscence of levator attachment to the tarsus leads to acquired ptosis only when Muller muscle attenuates.

Q9. What is the blood supply of eyelids?

Both internal and external arteries supply blood to the orbit and eyelids.

- Ophthalmic artery is the first intracranial branch of internal carotid and supplies the globe, extraocular muscles, lacrimal gland, ethmoid, upper eyelids, and forehead.
- Infraorbital artery is a continuation of maxillary artery (a terminal branch of external carotid artery) and exits 8 mm below the inferomedial orbital rim to supply the lower eyelid.

Q10. What is the nerve supply of eyelids?

The three branches of trigeminal nerve—ophthalmic (V1), maxillary (V2), and mandibular (V3)—provide sensory innervation to the periorbital region.

- Ophthalmic nerve divides into frontal, nasociliary, and lacrimal nerve.
  - – Infratrochlear nerve supplies the tip and side of nose, medial conjunctiva, and lacrimal sac.
  - – Lacrimal nerve supplies lateral conjunctiva and skin of the lateral upper eyelid.
  - – Frontal nerve divides into supraorbital and supratrochlear nerves.
  - – Supraorbital nerve supplies skin and conjunctiva of upper eyelid and scalp.
  - – Supratrochlear nerve supplies skin of glabella, forehead, medial upper eyelid, and medial conjunctiva.
- Maxillary division provides sensation to the skin of nose, lower eyelids, and upper lip.

Q11. What is jaw-winking phenomenon and its scientific basis?

- It is also known as Marcus Gunn phenomenon (MGP).
- A congenital uncommon condition characterized by synkinesis, when two or more muscles that are independently innervated have either simultaneous or coordinated movements.
- This was first described by Gunn in 1883.
- This unilateral synkinetic reflex retraction of the upper eyelid occurs during mouth opening or lateral excursions of the mandible to the contralateral side.
- It is also called pterygoid-levator synkinesis.
- Acquired forms of this condition is also known to have developed after eye surgery, syphilis, trauma, etc.

Scientific basis:

- The stimulation of the trigeminal nerve by contraction of the pterygoid muscles of jaw results in the excitation of the branch of the oculomotor nerve.
- It innervates the LPS ipsilaterally (on the same side of the face).

- So, the patient will have rhythmic upward jerking of their upper eyelid.

Q12. What are the different surgical procedures for ptosis?

In children, when there is risk of amblyopia, immediate surgery is required. A surgical algorithm is usually followed (**Table 22.1**):

- Transconjunctival Mullerectomy (Fasanella-Servat procedure):
  - Indications:
    - Mild congenital or acquired ptosis with good levator function.
    - Horner's syndrome.
    - Minor contour adjustment after any ptosis surgery.
  - Technique:
    - Upper border of the tarsus is excised with lower part of Muller muscle and the overlying conjunctiva.
- Muller muscle-conjunctival resection:
  - Indications:
    - Mild ptosis with good levator function.
    - Usually done in Horner's syndrome and mild congenital ptosis.
  - Techniques:
    - Excision of Muller muscle and overlying conjunctiva with reattachment of resected edges.
    - This procedure can achieve a maximal elevation of 2 to 3 mm.

- Levator repair or resection with advancement:
  - Indications:
    - Applicable to a wide range of severity as long as levator excursion is >5 mm.
    - It can be done in congenital as well as acquired ptosis.
  - Techniques:
    - Standard upper blepharoplasty incision is used.
    - Once levator aponeurosis is exposed, it is elevated off the Muller muscle and advanced over the tarsal border to simulate the levator advancement.
    - A general rule is that 1 mm of levator advancement corrects 1 mm of ptosis.
    - Alternatively, levator plication can also be performed in which instead of dividing the levator, vertical plication sutures are placed to tighten the aponeurosis.
- Frontalis sling:
  - Indications:
    - In patients with acquired ptosis having poor LPS function (<5 mm) or absent LPS with good frontalis action.
    - Congenital ptosis with poor levator function.
    - Neurogenic ptosis (**Fig. 22.4**).

Table 22.1 Ptosis algorithm: based on the extent of levator excursion and the degree of ptosis, the appropriate procedure can be systematically determined

Ptosis		Procedure		
		Mild (2–3 mm)	Moderate (3–5 mm)	Severe (>5 mm)
Excursion	Good (10–15 mm)	Levator advancement	Levator advancement	Levator advancement
		Levator plication	Levator plication	
		Tarsal conjunctival Mullerectomy		
	Fair (6–9 mm)	Levator advancement	Levator advancement	Levator advancement
	Poor (<5 mm)	Frontalis sling	Frontalis sling	Frontalis sling

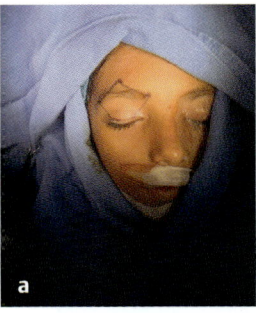
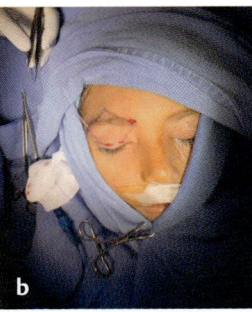
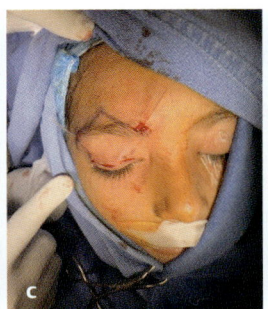
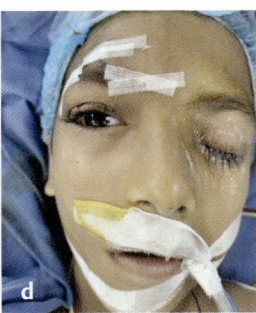
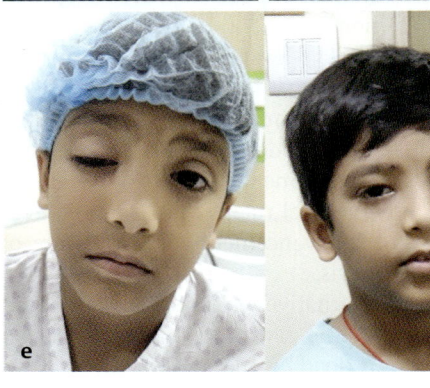

Fig. 22.4 **(a)** Planning of frontalis sling in a child with congenital ptosis (absent levator muscle). **(b)** Insertion of silicone rod. **(c)** Execution of procedure. **(d)** Immediate result on table after frontalis sling. **(e)** Before and after frontalis sling surgery.

- Techniques:
  - Tarsal plate is exposed via multiple stab wounds or eyelid crease incision.
  - The sling is passed in submuscular plane toward the brow.
  - Commonly used configurations:
    - A two-strand repair with four points of fixation to the tarsal plate and three points of fixation in the brow (double triangular and rhomboid design) (**Fig. 22.4a–e**).
    - A single-strand repair with two points of fixation to the tarsal plate and two points of fixation in the brow (single rhomboid design).
  - Sling materials can be:
    - Autogenous: Tensor fascia lata, temporalis fascia, palmaris longus.
    - Nonautogenous: Mersilene, Silicone.
- Complication:
  - Some lagophthalmos in the immediate postoperative period.

Q13. What are the complications of ptosis surgery?

- Complications of ptosis surgery:
  - Undercorrection.
  - Overcorrection.
  - Corneal exposure.
  - Infection.
  - Sling granuloma.
  - Notching of the eyelid.

Suggested Readings

1. Edmonson BC, Wulc AE. Ptosis evaluation and management. Otolaryngol Clin North Am 2005;38(5):921–946
2. Collin JR. Complications of ptosis surgery and their management: a review. J R Soc Med 1979;72(1):25–26
3. Zoumalan CI, Lisman RD. Evaluation and management of unilateral ptosis and avoiding contralateral ptosis. Aesthet Surg J 2010;30(3):320–328
4. Waller RR, McCord CD, Tanenbaum M. Evaluation and management of the ptosis patient. In: Oculoplastic surgery. New York: Raven Press; 1987:325–375

Gynecomastia

Rimpi Jain

Introduction

Gynecomastia or male enlargement of breast is caused by proliferation of ductal tissue, stroma with or without fat. The etiology in majority of cases is idiopathic and occurs as a response to hormonal changes during infancy, adolescence, and old age. A careful history and detailed physical examination including assessment of breast gland is the most important aspect of the management of gynecomastia.

History

Particulars of the patient (name, age, occupation, residence, etc.).

Chief Complaints

- Enlargement of one or both breasts.
- Pain in breasts.
- Heaviness in breasts and shoulder.
- Discharge from nipple.

History of Present Illness

- Patient was apparently well before 1/2 months/years back.
- Ask about the onset—whether sudden or gradual, on one side or both simultaneously.
- Ask about the progression of symptoms like swelling, pain, and heaviness.
- May present since birth in newborn babies due to exposure to maternal estrogen.

Negative History

- Any history of nipple discharge. Milky discharge from nipple may be seen in an individual having gynecomastia with a prolactin-secreting tumor.
- Ask about any history of drug intake, both prescribed and illegal.
- Neck swelling to rule out thyroid mass.
- Testicular swelling to rule out testicular mass.
- Any swelling in abdomen.

Past History

History of diabetes mellitus, tuberculosis, and hypertension.

Personal History

History of alcohol, smoking, and tobacco intake.

Any history of addition to illicit drugs like marijuana, heroin, etc. must be particularly enquired for.

Family History

Any family history of enlargement of breasts in father.

Treatment History

Whether he has received any treatment for this problem either in the form of surgery or medicines.

Allergy History

History of allergy to any drug or food materials.

Physical Examination

General Survey

Apart from examining the other points of general survey as mentioned in other chapters, look for the height and weight in particular.

Examine general buildup of the patient whether he is fatty as a whole or only has fatty breasts.

Local Examination of Bilateral Breasts

After proper consent, with adequate exposure and light.

Inspection

Breast

1. Must be done in anterior, lateral, and obliques views from both sides.

2. Look for the enlargement of breasts:
   - Whether unilateral (**Fig. 23.1**)/bilateral.
   - Symmetrical/asymmetrical.
3. Examine nipple: Size, position, shape, any retraction, discharge.
4. Examine areola: Size, shape, any discoloration.
5. Level of inframammary fold on both sides.

Axilla

1. Any visible swelling. If present, then examine in details.

Palpation

1. All the findings of inspection need to be confirmed on palpation.
2. Local temperature: Raised temperature indicates some inflammatory pathology.
3. Local tenderness over the breasts.
4. Any nipple discharges.
5. The consistency of the enlarged breasts. Look for any nodule and its size. If larger than 0.5 cm, then it is significant. Normally, the nipple-areola complex has an average diameter of 2.8 cm and it lies approximately 20 cm from the sternal notch.
6. Level of the inframammary fold—if any asymmetry is present.

Grading of Gynecomastia

Simon divided gynecomastia into four grades:
- Grade 1: Small enlargement of breast with no skin excess (**Fig. 23.2**).
- Grade 2a: Moderate enlargement of breast with no skin excess (**Fig. 23.3**).
- Grade 2b: Moderate enlargement of breast with extra skin (**Fig. 23.4**).

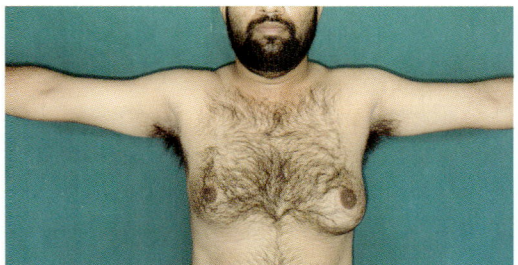

Fig. 23.1 Left-sided gynecomastia.

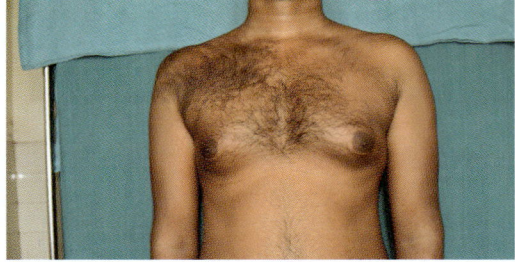

Fig. 23.2 Grade 1 gynecomastia.

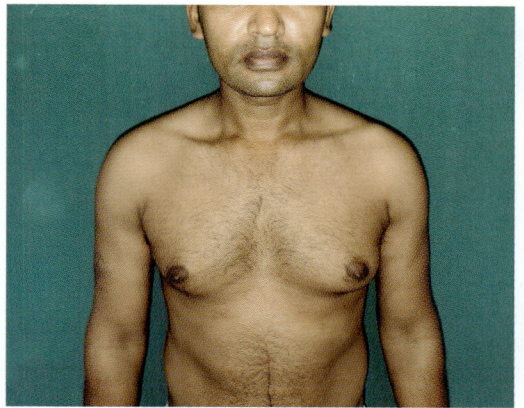

Fig. 23.3   Grade 2a gynecomastia.

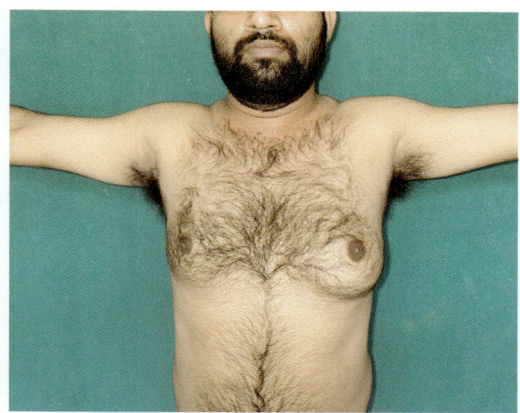

Fig. 23.4   Grade 2b gynecomastia.

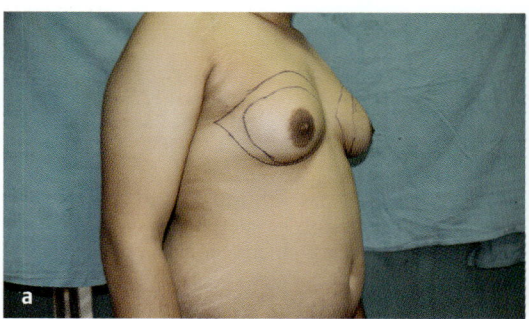

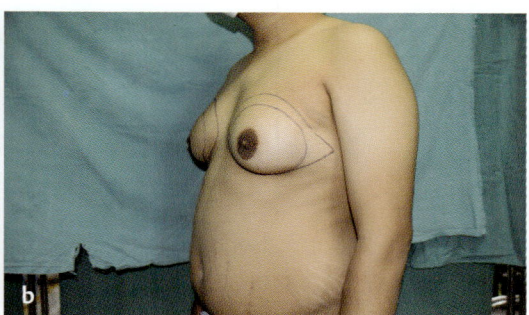

Fig. 23.5   **(a, b)** Grade 3 gynecomastia.

- Grade 3: Marked enlargement of breast with extra skin (looks similar to female breast) (**Fig. 23.5a, b**).

Another grading of gynecomastia, based on the ultrasound-assisted liposuction in the treatment of gynecomastia:

- Grade I: Minimal hypertrophy (<250 g of breast tissue) without ptosis.
- Grade II: Moderate hypertrophy (250–500 g of breast tissue) without ptosis.
- Grade III: Severe hypertrophy (>500 g of breast tissue) with grade 1 ptosis.
- Grade IV: Severe hypertrophy of breast with grade 2 or 3 ptosis.

Systemic Examination

Systemic examination is very important in gynecomastia to rule out other causes.

- Examine neck to rule out thyroid swelling.
- Examine genitourinary region to rule out any testicular mass.
- Examine abdomen to rule out any abdominal mass.
- Palpate for the liver to rule out hepatomegaly.

Provisional Diagnosis

This is a case of a 35-year-old man with bilateral gynecomastia grade 2b according to Simon's classification.

Questions

Q1. How will you proceed?

The basis of decision making in gynecomastia starts from detailed history, and examination is very important (**Flowchart 23.1**).

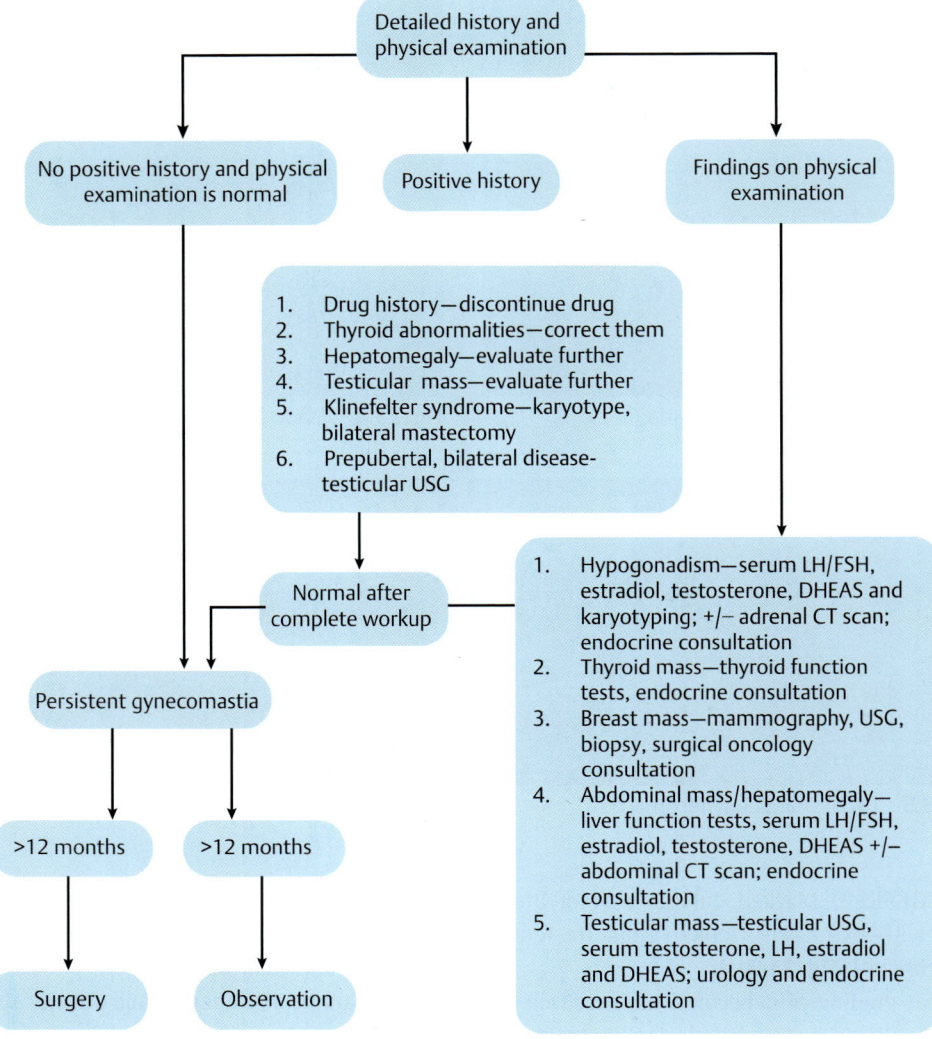

Flowchart 23.1 Flowchart showing decision making in gynecomastia

Q2. What investigations would you like to go for?

- Baseline investigations to assess fitness of the patient for surgery:
  - Blood for hemoglobin, total leukocyte count (TLC), differential leukocyte count (DLC), erythrocyte sedimentation rate (ESR).
  - Blood for sugar and renal function tests.
  - Chest X-ray.
  - Electrocardiography (ECG).
  - Viral markers.

Q3. How do you define gynecomastia ?

Gynecomastia is defined as abnormal enlargement of breast tissue in males. It is the most common breast pathology among males.

Q4. What is its incidence and how the trend has changed over time? Any particular reason for the increase in the number of cases in adolescents?

It has a prevalence of 30 to 70%, depending on the age group. In the past few years, the incidence of gynecomastia has increased in adolescents due to abuse of drugs, alcohol, and psychiatric medications. Another cause of increase is liver and other endocrine abnormalities. The presence of oxytocin in cow's milk, which is injected into dairy animals to increase the amount of milk, is also a reason.

Q5. What is the etiology of gynecomastia?

The most common cause is idiopathic. Other causes are (mnemonic—PENS-D):

- **Physiologic:**
  - Birth: Due to the increased level of maternal estrogens.
  - Puberty: Due to the imbalance of estradiol and testosterones.
  - Old age: Due to the decline in testosterone and increase in estrogen.
- **Endocrine:**
  - Pituitary: Pituitary failure.
  - Thyroid: Hypothyroid, hyperthyroid.
  - Adrenal: Cushing syndrome, congenital adrenal hyperplasia (CAH).
  - Testis: Hypogonadism, Klinefelter's syndrome.
- **Neoplasms:**
  - Pituitary.
  - Bronchogenic.
  - Adrenal.
  - Testis.
- **Systemic diseases:**
  - Malnutrition/starvation.
  - Cirrhosis.
  - Renal failure.
  - Adrenal.
- **Drug induced:**
  - Hormones: Estrogens, androgens.
  - Antiandrogens: Spironolactone, cimetidine, ketoconazole, ranitidine, flutamide.
  - Cardiovascular drugs: Amiodarone, digoxin, nifedipine, reserpine, verapamil.
  - Abused drugs: Alcohol, heroin, marijuana, methadone, amphetamines.
  - Stimulators of prolactin: Phenothiazines, reserpine, hydroxyzine.

- Antituberculosis drugs: Isoniazid, ethionamide, thioacetazone.
- Antireflux medications: Cimetidine, omeprazole, ranitidine.
- Chemotherapeutics: Methotrexate, imatinib, cyclophosphamide, alkylating agents, vinca alkaloids.
- Psychiatric medications: Benzodiazepines, phenothiazines, tricyclic antidepressants, olanzapine, haloperidol, and risperidone.

Q6. How starvation is associated with gynecomastia?

Starvation can cause gynecomastia due to decreased gonadotropin and testosterone levels, coupled with normal production of estrogens (and their precursors) from the adrenal glands. Again after refeeding, gonadotropins are increased which leads to testosterone secretion and estradiol production, which mimics normal puberty. Patients who develop gynecomastia after refeeding, therefore, are often described to be undergoing a **"second puberty."**

Q7. Is there any risk of breast cancer in patients with gynecomastia?

There is no increased risk of breast cancer in patients with gynecomastia except in cases of patients with Klinefelter's syndrome. They are 60 times more prone to develop breast cancer.

Q8. What are the types of gynecomastia?

Three types: Florid, fibrous, and intermediate.

- Florid: In this type there are more ductal tissues and there is increased vascularity.
- Fibrous: In this type there is more stromal fibrosis but few ducts.
- Intermediate: It is a mixture of the above two. The type of gynecomastia is usually related to the duration of the disorder. When the duration is 4 months or less then there is florid gynecomastia. After a duration of 1 year the fibrous type is usually present. The intermediate type is usually a progression from florid to fibrous and is usually seen between 4 and 12 months.

Q9. What are the treatment modalities of gynecomastia?

- Gynecomastia <1 year and normal history and physical examination—observation:
- If there is any history of drug, it should be discontinued.
- If any other abnormality is found on physical examination, work-up is indicated prior to consideration of surgery for gynecomastia.
- If the underlying condition is treated and the gynecomastia persists beyond 1 year, surgical correction is indicated.

Q.10 What are the surgical techniques for correcting gynecomastia?

The surgical technique used depends on the grading of gynecomastia and the distribution and proportion of the different breast components (fat, parenchyma, and looseness of the skin envelope).

- If only excess fatty tissue is present without substantial glandular hypertrophy then only liposuction may be sufficient (**Fig. 23.6**).
- Subcutaneous mastectomy is the most commonly used technique, which involves direct resection of the glandular tissue using a periareolar or transareolar approach, with or without liposuction. A combination of both has the advantage of resecting the glandular tissue through a small periareolar incision.

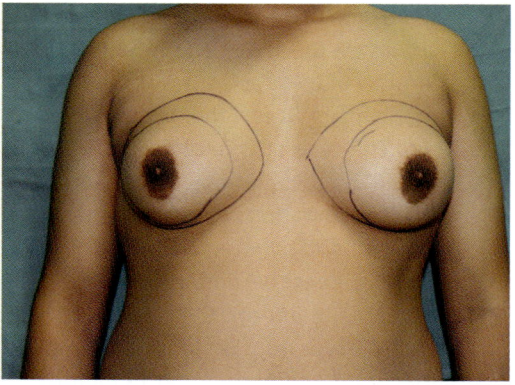

Fig. 23.6 Markings of liposuction in gynecomastia.

- Excision of skin is required for patients with marked gynecomastia and those who develop excessive sagging of the breast tissue.

Q11. How is grade 3 gynecomastia treated?

In grade 3 gynecomastia both liposuction and open surgery are required. Liposuction has multiple advantages before surgical excision. It causes pretunneling to facilitate the resection of tissue, reduces bleeding and bruising, and partially breaks down the breast tissue. After liposuction the tissue is resected via a number of techniques.

Q12. What are the markings in a case of gynecomastia and how will you assess the adequacy of procedure intraoperatively?

Various incisions are used, such as circumareolar and periareolar but the most commonly used technique is **Webster's technique**. In this technique a semicircular incision is made along the inferior margin of the nipple-areolar complex. During intraoperative period the weight of the resected gland and fat is measured and compared bilaterally. There should be no depression and asymmetry.

Q13. How will you correct excess skin in gynecomastia?

A number of techniques are available to reduce excess skin in gynecomastia. Most of these techniques are similar to those used in females.

Salient features of skin reduction surgery for gynecomastia are as follows:

Indications:
- Large gynecomastia (Simon's grade IIb or III).
- Ptotic breasts.
- Poor skin quality.
- Post massive weight loss.

Options for skin reduction:
- Concentric.
- Vertical scar (LeJour type).
- Elliptical.
- T-scar (Wise pattern).
- Lateral wedge.

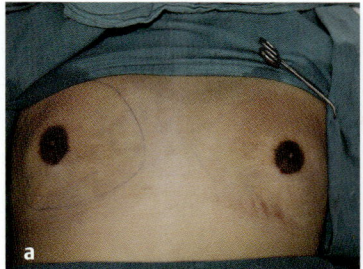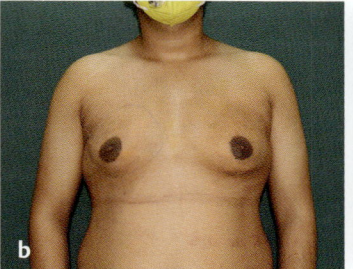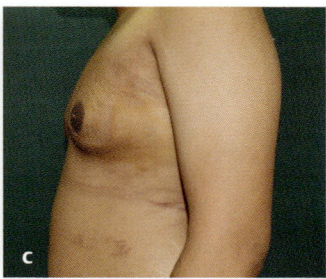

Fig. 23.7 **(a)** Intraoperative photograph of patient in **Fig. 23.6** after liposuction. **(b)** Postoperative photograph of a patient—anterior view; **(c)** lateral view.

- No vertical scar with nipple transposition (Lalonde type).

Q14. What solution is infiltrated and how is it prepared?

The wetting solution is prepared by mixing Ringer's lactate (1 L) with adrenaline (1 mg) (1 mL of 1 in 1000) and 30 mL of 1% lignocaine (300 mg).

Q15. What are the postoperative instructions and follow-up in these patients? (Fig. 23.7a–c)

Following surgery, pressure dressing is done and patients are advised to wear pressure garments for 4 to 6 weeks and sometimes up to 3 months depending on the grading of gynecomastia; oral antibiotics are given for 5 to 7 days.

Q16. What could be the differential diagnosis?

- Lipoma.
- Hematoma.
- Fat necrosis.
- Sebaceous cyst.
- Breast cancer.
- Pseudogynecomastia.

Q17. How to differentiate between gynecomastia and pseudogynecomastia?

It is based on physical examination. Pseudogynecomastia is seen in obese patients with extra fat in the chest area. The patient is asked to lie on his back keeping his hands behind his head and the surgeon places his thumb and forefinger on each side of the breast and slowly brings them together. In cases of true gynecomastia,

a disc or firm tissue that is concentric with the nipple-areolar complex is felt by the surgeon. In patients with pseudogynecomastia there will not be any resistance until the fingers reach the nipple.

Q18. Is there any role of medical treatment?

There is no role of medical treatment; however, it may provide partial regression, or symptomatic relief. Options are androgens, antiestrogens, and aromatase inhibitors.

Q19. Complications after gynecomastia surgery?

- **Hematoma:** It is the most common early complication. It should be evacuated as early as possible.
- **Under-resection:** It is the most common long-term complication of gynecomastia surgery. This is common in cases of liposuction, when a residual mass of tissue is not removed. This can be avoided by using the pull-through technique.
- **Over-resection:** Over-resection in the area of nipple-areola is also common. It can result in a saucer-type deformity which is difficult to correct.

Suggested Readings

1. Malata CM, Wong KY. Gynecomastia surgery. In: Neligan PC, ed. Plastic surgery breast. Vol. 5. 4th ed. Canada: Elsevier; 2018:236–261
2. Amalfi AN, Sommer NZ. Gynecomastia. In: Chung KC, ed. Grabb and Smith's plastic surgery. 8th ed. Lippincott Williams and Wilkins; 2019:2034–2051

Index